Plant Pathogens and Principles of Plant Pathology

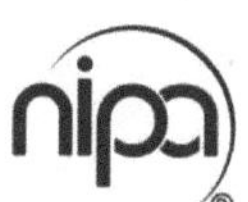

NIPA® GENX ELECTRONIC RESOURCES & SOLUTIONS P. LTD.
New Delhi-110 034

Plant Pathogens and Principles of Plant Pathology

Sanjeev Kumar, *Scientist*
Department of Plant Pathology
Office of the Dean, Faculty of Agriculture
Jawahar Lal Nehru Krishi Vishwavidyalaya-Jabalpur,
MP-482004, India

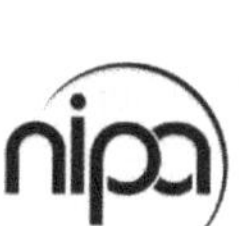

NIPA® GENX ELECTRONIC RESOURCES & SOLUTIONS P. LTD.
New Delhi-110 034

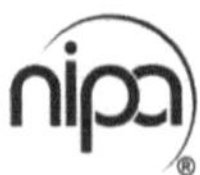

NIPA® GENX ELECTRONIC
RESOURCES & SOLUTIONS P. LTD.

101,103, Vikas Surya Plaza, CU Block
L.S.C. Market, Pitam Pura, New Delhi-110 034
Ph : +91 11 27341616, 27341717, 27341718
E-mail: newindiapublishingagency@gmail.com
web: www.nipabooks.com

For customer assistance, please contact
Phone: + 91-11-27 34 17 17
Fax: + 91-11- 27 34 16 16
E-Mail: feedbacks@nipabooks.com

ISBN: 978-81-19254-94-1

Composed and Designed by NIPA®.

Preface

This would be a long preface if I was to set down in detail the reasons why I attempted to write this book in present form. Suffice it to say that the text is based on course which I have been teaching to undergraduate students. The purpose is to provide the basic and emerging facts whereby the students may be introduced to the scientific foundation of this noble course called "Plant Pathogens and Principles of Plant Pathology". This course is offered at undergraduate levels in all Indian Agricultural Universities. There are several books especially on the subject. However, the course requirement of Indian students is not fulfilled by any single source. The prime objective of writing this book is to fill up the gap and help Indian students. The main features of this volume are as follows;

1. The subject matter has been presented systematically with suitable examples.
2. Efforts have been made to provide recent information.
3. The language is simple and easily understandable.
4. It covers, in its 41 chapters, the major part of syllabi offered by Indian universities especially in Plant Pathology.
5. The glossary of technical terms has been presented at the end for ready reference.

I do not claim originality in the preparation of this book and has taken help from a large number of books, journals, periodicals, bulletins, internet, etc. I humbly thank authors, editors, and publishers of the books, journals, etc. I am also indebted to my wife Dr. (Mrs) Archana Rani for inspiration and help and children Saumya and Adyan for bearing with me during the preparation of this book.

Hope this volume will be useful to the students, teachers and researchers engaged in the field of plant pathology. It will also useful to those commencing post graduate work and preparing for competitive examinations such as ARSE,NET and SET. Suggestions for further improvement of this volume shall be highly appreciated.

June, 2015 Sanjeev Kumar
Jabalpur

Contents

Chapter - 1

Introduction and Importance of Plant Pathology in Agriculture

Plants make up the majority of the earth's living environment as trees, grass, flowers, etc. Plants are the only higher organisms that can convert the energy of sunlight into stored, usable chemical energy in carbohydrates, proteins and fats. Directly or indirectly, plants make up all the food on which humans and all animals depend. Plants however also gets sick, grow and exhibit various types of symptoms and sometimes whole plant die. It is not known whether diseased plant feel pain or discomfort. If a plant is looking different from its community then it is equal to be disease one. Any biotic or abiotic agents which induce the disease in plant is referred as the cause of diseases.The causative agents of disease in plants are pathogenic such as fungi, bacteria, viruses, protozoa and nematodes and environmental conditions such as lack or excess of nutrients, moisture, light, etc to presence of toxic chemicals in air or soil. These biotic constraints can, at times, seriously compromise food security, For example, potato late blight, caused by *Phytophthora infestans*, struck Europe like 'a bolt from the blue' in the 1840s. In Ireland, about a million people died of starvation and more than a million attempted to emigrate. The reasons for this calamity were the arrival in Europe of a virulent strain of the pathogen, the high dependence of much of the Irish population on potato for sustenance, the lack of resistance in the plant to the pathogen, and weather conditions favorable to epidemic development. There have been other disasters caused by plant diseases such as the Great Bengal Famine of 1943 and the southern corn blight epidemic of 1970-71 in the USA, to name but two. In the former, an estimated 2 million people died owing to the high dependence of most of the population on a single crop, rice, which was attacked by the fungus *Cochliobolus miyabeanus*. In the USA, by contrast, although in some genus, *Cochlobolus heterostrophus*, alternative sources of nutrition were plentiful so no one died, although the effect on the agricultural economy was severe.

The first two of these heartbreaking examples demonstrate with brutal clarity that in areas of the world where a large proportion of the population is dependent on a single crop or a few crops, they are at risk should that crop fail owing to one or more devastating diseases. At the present time, the threat is partially great in developing countries, where populations are growing fastest, poverty is endemic , the population depends upon on locally produced staples, and the infrastructure of extension and R&D is often poorly resourced. The losses due to weeds, disease and insects have been estimated to around 40% in the developing and underdeveloped countries. If the post harvest losses (15-20%) are also added , the situation becomes even more alarming.

In India, the need to increased food production to meet the demands of rapidly increasing population in a limited land resource, necessitated the use of intensive farming system, with the inputs like narrow genetic base, high fertilizers, irrigation, non traditional areas, multiple cropping etc. which favors disease development and show little concern to ecology. The intensive agriculture, specially the introduction of high yielding genotypes but susceptible to the race of the pathogen already present in the area/India and changing cropping patterns including cultivation in non traditional areas have resulted in a spurt of diseases in various crop pathosystem, remarkably changing the disease scenario.

In wheat, rusts were the most serious problems until the mi-seventies, but currently with the wide use of rust resistant varieties, a minor disease of the past, namely karnal bunt has assumed serious proportion. The rice tungro and the bacterial blight of rice are the most devastating diseases in the new varieties. Sheath blight becomes serious on rice in the unconventional areas. Maize and millets are now devastated by downy mildews. Blight of cotton became a major problem when the indigenous diploid cottons were replaced by exotic tetraploid cottons. The new exotic cotton varieties are also highly susceptible to a new disease known as parawilt of cotton of unknown etiology. During the past of few years white fly transmitted leaf curl of cotton has become dangerous, and required special efforts to check the spread to different areas. Such examples of changing disease scenario are available for pulses, oil seeds, vegetables, fruits etc, i.e. the crops in which productivity has increased tremendously. Certain diseases of complex or unknown etiology i.e. parawilt of cotton, coconut root wilt, citrus die back, mango malformation, rot of oilpalms, brown bast disease of rubber, etc., need special efforts to develop management practices to minimize losses. The crop yield losses, on field and during post harvest period, caused by pests, diseases and weeds are of paramount importance. The crop losses due to pests, diseases and weeds are approximately assessed to be ranging between 10-30 % of crop productions. If we consider, on a average, crop loss of 20% , and the present gross value of our agriculture produce as Rs. 7 lakh crore, the loss comes to Rs. 1,40,000 crore, which is very collosal. Even if we could save 50 percent by using plant protection, it will add Rs. 70,000 crore additional income to our farmers. At a same time, when all of us are concerned about National

Food Security, can the country afford these losses?

Various type of direct and indirect losses caused by plant diseases include, reduced quality and quantity of crop produce, increased cost of production, threat to animal health and environment, limiting the type of crops/varieties grown, loss of natural resources and less remunerative alternatives adopted. In order to combat the losses caused by the plant diseases, it is obligatory to define the problem and seek remedies. At the biological level, the requirements are for the speedy and accurate identification of the causal organism, accurate estimates of the severity of diseases and its effect on yield, and identification of its virulence mechanisms. Disease may then be minimized by the reduction of the pathogen's inoculums, inhibition of the virulence mechanisms, and promotion of genetic diversity in the crop.

Success in disease management, as in most walks of life, depends on having the right tools and the confidence to apply them. The key tool for disease management is knowledge and having knowledge give confidence. Diagnostic and advisory support systems are facing very big challenges in market relevant and effective knowledge and support available to farmers and market chains and ensuring that upstream researchers are informed of the real priority problems and issues requiring resolution.

Chemical pesticides have reduced crop losses in many situations, but even with a substantial increase in pesticide use, the overall proportion of crop losses and the absolute value of these losses from diseases appear to have increased over time. Despite this perverse relationship, an increase in pesticide use still appears to be profitable. Increased monoculture, reduced crop diversity and rotation, and use of herbicide have all increased vulnerability to diseases as well. Diseases tends to develop resistance to pesticides, requiring higher use to sustain production. Inappropriate and excessive pesticide use have led to increased and unnecessary disease out breaks and additional disease loss because of the inadvertent destruction of natural enemies of diseases, disease resistance and resurgence of secondary diseases. Ultimately, overuse of pesticides can reduce food production. Proponents with varying perspective on chemicals agree that IDM must be science based and economically viable for farmers. The emphasis in on disease problems and preventing them form reaching damaging levels.

Current sensitivities about environmental pollution are a consequence of improper synthetic pesticide use. Host – plant resistance, natural plant products, biopesticides, natural enemies and agronomic practices offer a potentially viable option for integrated disease management (IDM). They are relatively safe for the non target organisms and humans. Biotechnological tools such as marker assisted selection, genetic engineering, and wide hybridization to develop resistant crop cultivars will have a great bearing on future disease management programs. Disease modeling, decision support systems, and remote sensing would contribute to scaling up and dissemination of IDM strategies.

Plant Pathology is challenging and an important science that deals with science of disease development and art of managing diseases. Society, consumers and growers will only be able to continue to benefit from plant pathology if the discipline can evolve appropriate disease management schemes that can respond to the significant changes in agricultural practices in India; the ultimate goal to produce more and safer food in sustainable agricultural systems that conserve natural resources and the environment. Information technology, communication and the integration of conventional and new technologies are essential that must be integrated by the modern practitioners of plant pathology into effective disease management schemes that can be implemented at the farm level.

Some Past and Present Examples of Losses Caused by Plant Diseases

Plant diseases have affected the existence, adequate growth, and productivity of all kinds of plants, and thereby have affected one or more of the basic prerequisites for a healthy, safe life for humans since the time humans began to practice agriculture. A vast number of plant pathogens from viroids of a few hundred nucleotides to higher plants cause diseases in our crops. Their effects range from mild symptoms to catastrophes in which large areas planted to food crops are destroyed. It has resulted in malnutrition, starvation, migration, and death of people and animals on several occasions. Similar effects are observed yearly in developing, agrarian societies, in which families and nations are dependent for their sustenance on their own produce. Catastrophic plant disease exacerbates the current deficit of food supply in which at least 800 million people are inadequately fed. Some examples of plant diseases that have caused severe losses in the past are shown in table-1&2.

Table 1 : Examples of severe losses caused by plant diseases

Sl.no	Disease	Location	Impact/ Remarks
Fungal diseases			
1.	Late blight of potato	Cool and humid climates	Irish famine (1845-46)
2.	Brown spot of rice	India	Bengal famine (1943)
3.	Powdery mildew of grapes	Worldwide	European epidemic (1840s-50s)
4.	Downy mildew of tobacco	U.S, Europe	European epidemic (1950s-60s)
5.	Coffee rust	South East Asia	Destroyed all coffee in Southeast Asia (1870s-1880s)
6.	Downy mildew of grapes	U.S, Europe	European epidemic (1870s-80s)

Contd...

7.	Chest nut blight	U.S	Destroyed almost all American chest nut trees (1904-1940)
8.	Dutch elm disease	U.S, Europe	Destroys all American elm trees (1930 till date)
9.	Cereal rusts	Worldwide	Frequent severe epidemic, huge annual losses.
10.	Sigatoka of banana	Worldwide	Great annual losses
11.	Rubber leaf blight	South America	Destroys rubber tree plantations
Bacterial diseases			
12.	Fire blight of pome fruits	North America, Europe	Kills numerous tree annually
13.	Citrus canker	Asia, Africa, Brazil	Responsible for eradication of millions of trees in Florida in 1910s and again in 1980s and 1990s.
14.	Soft rot of vegetables	Worldwide	Huge losses of vegetables
Viral diseases			
15.	Tristeza	America, Africa	Millions of trees being killed
16.	Tomato yellow leaf curl	Caribbean basin, Mediterranean countries	Severe losses of tomatoes and beans
17.	Sugarcane mosaic	Worldwide	Great losses on sugarcane
18.	Swollen shoot of cacao	Africa	Continuous heavy losses
Phytoplasmal diseases			
19.	Pear decline	Canada, Europe	Millions of pear tree killed
20.	Pear yellows	Russia, Eastern U.S.	10 million peach trees killed
Nematode diseases			
21.	Root knot	Worldwide	Continuous losses on vegetable and most other plants
22.	Sugar beet cyst nematode	Northern Europe and Western U.S	Severe annual losses on sugar beets

Table 2 : Diseases likely to cause severe losses in the future

Sl. no.	Disease	Remarks
Fungal diseases		
1	Late blight of potato and tomato	New compatibility type of fungus spreading worldwide
2	Rust of soybean	Spreading in South east Asia, Russia, Hawaii and Puerto Rico
3	Karnal bunt of wheat	Destructive in Pakistan , India, Nepal, also introduced in Mexico and US
4	White rust of chrysanthemum	Important in Europe, Asia, and recently in California
5	Rust of sugarcane	Destructive in the America and elsewhere
6	Black spot of citrus	Severe in Central and South America
7	Downy mildew of corn and sorghum	South east Asia
8	Scab of sweet orange	Severe in Australia
Bacterial diseases		
9	Bacterial leaf blight	Destructive in Japan and India
10	Moko or Bacterial wilt of banana	Destructive in America; spreading elsewhere
Viral diseases		
11	Bunchy top of banana	Destructive in Australia, Asia, Egypt etc.
12	Rice tungro virus	Destructive in Southeast Asia
13	White tip (*Hoja blanca*) of rice	Destructive in the America
14	African cassava mosaic	Destructive in Africa, Asia and America
15	Bean golden mosaic	Central America, Florida, Caribbean basin
Phytoplasmal diseases		
16	Lethal yellowing of coconut palms	Destructive in Central America
Viroid diseases		
17	Cadang-cadang disease	Killed more than 15 million trees in th Philippines till date
Nematode diseases		
18	Red ring of palms	Severe in Central America and the Caribbean
19	Burrowing nematode	Severe in banana in many areas and citrus in Florida

CHAPTER - 2

Plant Pathology-The Science

DEFINITION

The term Plant Pathology is derived from Greek words-*pathos* (suffering) + *Logos* (study) i.e. the study of the suffering plant. Plant Pathology has two phases broadly-

- **Science**- understanding of the disease i.e. the theoretical consideration of the suffering plants and how do pathogens invade, how do plants defend themselves, what causes symptoms etc.
- **Art**- the application of the science to the field problems i.e. Diagnosis and Control.

Plant pathology or phytopathology is the branch of agricultural, botanical or biological science which deals with the cause, etiology, resulting in losses and management methods of plant diseases.

Plant pathology can also be defined as the study of the nature, cause and prevention of plant diseases. Plant pathology is related to most of the old and new sciences like biology, physics, chemistry, physiology, mathematics, genetics, soil science, biochemistry, biotechnology etc.

Study of plant pathology includes the study of sciences viz, microbiology, bacteriology, virology, mycology, nematology, protozology, phycology, unfavorable environmental factors, nutritional deficiencies and flowering plant parasites.

1. Microbiology : Study of Microorganisms
2. Bacteriology : Study of Bacteria
3. Virology : Study of Viruses
4. Mycology : Study of Fungi
5. Nematology : Study of Nematode
6. Protozology : Study of Protozoa
7. Phycology : Study of Algae.

Major Objectives

1. To study biotic (living), mesobiotic and abiotic (non-living and environmental) causes of diseases or disorders.
2. To study the mechanisms of disease development by pathogens.
3. To study the plant (host)—pathogen interaction in relation to environment.
4. To develop methods of management of plant diseases.

Plant Diseases

Disease is one of those terms that are very difficult to define. It is realized that disease (literally dis-ease) implies lack of 'comfort'and therefore, involves deviation form normal functioning. From time to time several definitions which have been proposed, in fact descriptive but not simultaneously exclusive. Plant diseases are recognized by the symptoms (external or internal) produced by them or by sick appearance of the plant. The term plant disease signifies the condition of the plant due to disease or cause of the disease. Plant disease is mainly defined in terms of the damage caused to the plant or to its organ. The other definitions for the term disease are:

1. Disease is a malfunctioning process that is caused by continuous irritation, which results in some suffering producing symptoms.
2. Disease is an alteration in one or more of the ordered sequential series of physiological processes culminating in a loss of coordination of energy utilization in a plant as a result of the continuous irritation from the presence or absence of some factor or agent.
3. Disease is any morphological or physiological abnormality in a plant or any of its parts caused by continuous irritation and results in economic losses to human beings.
4. Any deviation from normal growth or structure of plants that is sufficiently pronounced and permanent to produce visible symptoms or to impair quality and economic value.
5. A plant is said to be diseased when there is a harmful deviation from normal functioning of physiological process.
6. The disease can also be defined as any disturbance brought about by a living entity or non-living agents or environmental factors which interfere with manufacture, translocation or utilization of food, mineral nutrients and water in such a way that the affected plant changes in

appearance with or without much loss in yield than that of a normal healthy plant of the same variety. In general disease is an interaction among the host, parasite and the environment.

All these definitions indicate that disease;

- Is not a pathogen but it is caused by a pathogen.
- Is not symptom but results in symptoms.
- Is not a condition as the condition results from disease and is not synonymous with it.
- It is not an injury.
- Cannot be infectious , it is actually the pathogen which is infectious.
- Results from continuous irritation.
- And is a malfunctioning process and this result in some suffering and therefore disease is a pathological process.

THE CONCEPT OF DISEASE IN PLANTS

Old Concept

Plant diseases were considered to be a curse and punishment to the people by god for wrongs and sin they had committed (religious belief and superstition). The greak philosopher Theophrastus (300, B.C) was the first to study and write about diseases of trees, cereals and legumes. He wrote a book named "Enquiry into Plants". In this book he mentioned his experience about plant diseases. His experience was not based on experimentation. He being unable to explain diseases bellieved that god controlled the weather that brought diseases. Plant diseases were a manifestation of the worth of God. It is due to religious belief, occulation, superstitions or it is the effect of star moon and bad wind. E.g. Romans actually created a special rust God called Robigo for rust diseases of grain crops. They offered sacrifice of red dogs and sheeps.This was continued for almost 2000 years after Theophrastus. After invention compound microscope in the mid 1600 scientist enable to see many microorganisms associated with diseased plants and they come to believe that the mildews, rust, and other symptoms observed on plants and microorganisms found on diseased plant. Plant parts were the natural product of diseases than the cause and effect of disease.

New Concept

Louis Pasteur (1860 -63) provided irrefusable evidence that microorganisms arises only from pre-existing microorganisms and fermentation is a biological phenomenon not just a chemical one. It is accepted that a plant is healthy, or normal, when, it can carry out its physiological functions to the best of its genetic potential. Whenever the ability of the cells of a plant or plant part to carry out their essential functions like photosynthesis, respiration, transpiration, reproduction etc is interfered with by either a pathogenic microorganism or an adverse environmental factor, the activities of the cells are disrupted, altered, or inhibited, the cells malfunction or die, and the plant become diseased. At first, the association is localized to one or a few cells and is invisible. Soon, though, the reaction becomes more widespread, and affected parts develop changes visible to the naked eye. These visible changes are the symptom of the disease. The visible or otherwise measurable adverse changes in a plant, produced in reaction to infection by a microorganism or to an unfavorable environment factor, are a measure of the amount of disease in the plant. Disease in plants, then, can be defined as the series of visible and invisible responses of plant cells and tissues to a pathogenic microorganism or environmental factor that result in adverse changes in the form, function, or integrity of the plant and may lead to partial impairment or death of the plant.

The type of cells and tissues that become affected determine the type of physiological function that will be disrupted first. For instance, infection of roots may cause roots to rot and make them unable to absorb water and nutrients from the soil; infection of xylem vessels, as happens in all vascular wilts, interferes with translocation of water and minerals to the top of the plant; infection of phloem cells in the veins of leaves and in the bark of stems and shoots, as happens in cankers and in diseases caused by mollicutes, viruses, and protozoa, interferes with the downward translocation of photosynthetic products; infection of the foliage, as happens in blights, leaf spots, mildews, rusts, mosaics etc. interferes with photosynthesis; infection of flowers and fruits interferes reproduction. Even if most infected cells are weakened or die, in some diseases, for instance, in crown gall, infected cells are induced to divide much faster (hyperplasia and hypertrophy) than normal cells and to produce abnormal overgrowth (tumors) or abnormal organs.

The biotic agents commonly referred to as pathogens, usually cause disease in plants by upsetting the metabolism of plant cells through toxins, enzymes, growth regulators, and other substances they secrete, and by absorbing food stuffs from the host cells for their own use. Several pathogens may also cause disease by growing and multiplying in the vascular bundles of plants and, thereby, blocking the upward transportation of water or the downward movement of sugars, respectively, through these tissues. Abiotic factors *viz*, moisture, temperature, mineral nutrients, pollutants, etc., can cause disease in plants when it occur at levels above or below a certain range tolerated by the plants.

Disease Triangle

A plant becomes diseased in most cases when it is attacked by a pathogen (biotic) or affected by an abiotic agent. Therefore, in first case, for a plant disease to occur, at least two components (i.e Plant and Pathogen) must come in contact and must interact. Even through the host and pathogen come in contact and interact, but if the environmental conditions are not congenial or within a favourable range, then disease can not develop. Therefore, the third component, environmental conditions must be favourable for a disease to develop. Each of these three components (host, pathogen and environment) can display considerable variability and as one component changes it affects the degree of disease severity within an individual plant and within a plant population. The environment may affect both the growth and resistance of host plants and also multiplication, virulence and dispersal of pathogen. The interactions of the three component of disease have been visualized as a triangle generally referred to as the "**disease triangle".** Each side of the triangle represents one of the three components. The length of each side is proportional to the sum total of the characteristics of each components that favour disease i.e if the host is resistant, matured and widely spaced, the host side and amount of disease would be small or zero, whereas if the host or plants are susceptible, at susceptible stage of growth or densely planted, the host side would be long and the amount of disease could be great. Similarly, the virulent, abundant and active the pathogen, the longer the pathogen side and greater the amount of disease. Also more favourable the environmental conditions (E .g. Temperature, moisture and wind) help the pathogen or that reduces the host resistance, longer will be the environmental side and greater will be the amount of disease.

When these three components of the disease triangle are quantified, the area of the triangle represents amount of disease in a plant or in a plant population. If any of the three components is zero, there can be no disease.

IMPORTANCE OF PLANT DISEASES

1. Plant diseases may limit the kinds of plants and industries in the area: Plant diseases may limit the kinds of plant that can grow in a large geographical area. For example, the European grape *Vitis vinifera*, which provides all high quality table and wine grapes all over the world, cannot be grown in the south eastern United States because there it is devastated by the Pierce's diseases of grape. Plant diseases may also determine the kinds of agricultural industries and the level of employment in an area by affecting the quantity and kind of produce available for local processing. On the other hand , plant diseases are responsible also for creation of new industries that develop chemicals , machinery and methods to manage plant diseases.

2. Plant diseases reduce the quality and quantity of plant produce: Severe losses my be incurred due to plant diseases by reduction in the quality of plant products. For example, apples infected with apple scab, even as little as 5 percent disease may cut the price in half. Potatoes infected with potato scab, there may be no effect on price in a market with slight scarcity, but there may be considerable price reduction in years of even minor gluts of produce. The quantity of losses caused by plant diseases range from slight to 100 percent. Plant or plant products may be reduced in quantity by disease in the field, as indeed in the case with most plant diseases, or by disease during storage, as is the case of the rots of the stored fruits, vegetables, grains, and fibres.

3. Plant diseases may make plants poisonous to humans and animals: Several grains and at times other seeds and plant products such as hay, purees, etc., are frequently contaminated or infected with one or more fungi that produces highly toxic compounds known as mycotoxins. Humans or Animals consuming such products may develop severe diseases of internal organs, the nervous system, etc., and may die. Some diseases *viz.*, ergot of rye and wheat , make plant products unfit for human or animal consumption by contaminating them with poisonous fruiting structures.

4. Plant diseases may cause financial losses: Financial losses from plant diseases can be arise in the following ways.

- Farmers may have to plant varieties of plants that are resistant to disease but are less productive and commercially less profitable than other varieties.
- They may need to spray the crop to control a disease thus, incurring expenses for chemicals, labour, machinery and storage place.
- Shippers may have to make available refrigerated warehouses and transportation vehicles, thereby increasing expenses.
- Healthy and diseased plant products may require to be separated from one another to avoid spreading the disease, thus escalating handling costs.

5. The cost of controlling plant diseases is also a direct loss to diseases: Some plant diseases can be controlled almost entirely by one or another method, thus resulting in financial losses on to the amount of the cost of the control. Sometimes, however this cost may be almost as high as , or even higher than, the return expected from the crop, as in the case of certain diseases of small grains.

CHAPTER - 3

History of Plant Pathology

History in general reveals chronological account of important events, contribution of persons who significantly influenced the thinking of their era and the interpretations of the observed facts or phenomenon over the period of time. The progress in plant pathology leading to the major land mark in mycology, plant bacteriology, plant virology and plant disease control has been described in chronological order for easy and better understanding of the student in following sub-headings.

Mycology

Year	Contributor (s)	Description
1500	Surapal	Wrote 'Vraksha Ayurveda', the first book in which plant diseases were discussed
1665	Robert Hook	First observed Teliospore of *Pharagmidium disciflorum* under microscope
1676	Anton von Leeuwenhoek	Developed the first microscope
1729	PA Michaeli	Studied fungi and saw their spores on the pieces of water melon. Wrote *'Nova Plantarum Genera'* Known as Father of Mycology
1743	John Needham	Reported plant parasitic nematodes in wheat galls.
1755	M. Tillet	Demonstrated that the bunt of wheat was contagious thought that the spores contained a poisonous entity.
1807	B.Prevost	Proofed the role of a micro organism in the causation of disease.Demonstrated the control of wheat smut by steeping seed in copper sulphate solution
1821	E.M.Fries	Reported that smut and rust fungi as product of diseased plants.Wrote " Systema Mycologium", Known as Linnaeus of Mycology
1827	Cragie	Showed function of pycniospores in rust fungi.
1840	LR Tulasne & C Tulasne	Confirmed the observation of Prevost with regard to the causal organism of wheat bunt.Known as Reconstructor of Mycology

Contd...

1858	JG Kuhn	Published first text book on Plant Pathology namely "The Diseases of Cultivated Crops: Their causes and Their Control"
1861-65	Anton de Bary	First to indicate the nature of obligate and facultative forms. Proved the real cause of late blight of potato is *Phytophthora infestans*.Described the sex and account of development in number of Phycomyetes and Ascomycetes.Described the role of enzymes in tissue disintegration while working on soft rot of carrots caused by *Sclerotinia* spp. Demonstrated heterocious nature of stem rust of wheat
1875	O. Brefeld	Developed pure culture technique
1878	M. S. Woronin	Found out the life cycle of potato wart disease
1881	H.M. Ward	Reported the role of environment in the epidemiology of coffee rust. Father of Tropical Plant Pathology
1882	Robert Hartig	Published a textbook -Diseases of Trees. He is called as "Father of Forest Pathology"
1885	PM Millardet	Discovered the Bordeaux mixture for the control of downy mildew of grapes
1885	Frank	Discovered Mycorrhizal fungi
1887	Mason	Introduced Burgundy mixture
1887	Jensen	Developed hot water technique for wheat smut
1894	Ericson	Reported Physiological specialization in stem rust of wheat
1904	A. F.Blakeslee,	Founded heterothallism in *Rhizopus*
1904	R. H. Biffen	First to show that resistance to pathogens in plants can be inherited as a Mendelian character
1905	RH Biffen	Demonstrated inheritance of rust resistance in wheat in a Medelain fashion
1917	EC Stakman	Distinguished biological forms in cereal rusts
1923	Hansen and Smith	Term Heterokaryosis
1931	PA Saccardo	Wrote "Syllogue Fungorum"
1931	J.C. Luthra	Solar heat treatment for loose smut of wheat
1946	HH Flor	Gave gene for gene hypothesis while working on linseed rust
1952	G Pontecorvo and JA Roper	Discovered parasexuality in *Aspergillus nidulans*
1968	Vander Plank	Concept of horizontal and vertical resistance. Father of Plant Epidemiology
1990	DF Klessig and I Raskin; JP Metraux and J Tyals	Demonstrated that salicylic acid is associated with systemic acquired resistance
2005	RA Dean and Co-workers	The first complete genome sequencing of a plant pathogenic fungus *Magnaporthe grisea*

Plant Bacteriology

Year	Contributor (s)	Description
1683	Anton von Leeuwenhoek	First observed bacteria
1876	Robert Koch	They proved that anthrax disease of cattle was caused byspecific bacterium
1876	Louis Pasteur	Demonstrated role ofbacteria in fermentation and decay
1876	Robert Koch	Described the theory called "Koch's postulates." He established the principles of pure culture technique
1876	Robert Koch and Pasteur	Disproved the theory of spontaneous generation of diseases and propose germ theory in relation to the diseases of man and animal
1876	Woronin	Isolated and described the root nodule bacteria in leguminous plant
1878	TJ Burril	Described first bacterial disease (Fire blight of apples) caused by *Erwinia amylovora*
1879.	Prilleaux	Reported the bacterial decay of wheat kernels
1883	J.H. Wakker	Investigated yellow slime disease of hyacinth caused by bacterium
1885-1887	J.C. Arther	Confirmed Burrill's work
1887	EF Smith	Gave the final proof that bacteria could be the incitants of plant diseases First to notice and study the crown gall disease.Father of Phytobacteriology
1980	DW Dye and Co-workers	Introduced pathovar system in taxonomy
1910	C. O. Jensen.	Related crown gall of plants to cancer of animals
1952	J. Lederberg	Coined the term plasmid
1952	S. A. Waksman	Discovered streptomycin
1952	Zinder and J. Lederberg	Discovered transduction in bacteria
1962.	H. Stolp	Discovered bdellovibrios
1972	P. B. New and A. Kerr	Success in biological control of *A. radiobacter* strain K
1972	I. M. Windsor and L. M. Black.	Observed a new kind of phloem inhabiting bacterium causing clover club leaf disease
1972	Windsor and Black	Observed rickettsia like organisms in the phloem of clover plants infected with the club leaf disease
1974	I. Zanen *et al.*	Demonstrated Ti plasmid in *Agrobacterium tumefaciens*
1977	Chilton *et al.*	Showed that the crown gall bacterium transforms normal plant cells into tumor cells by introducing into them a plasmid, part of which becomes inserted into the plant cell chromosomes DNA

Plant Virology

Year	Contributor (s)	Description
1576	C. Clusius	Recorded Breaking of tulips owing to viral infection
1857.	Swietch	Identified Tobacco mosaic
1886	AE Mayer	First to point out that tobacco mosaic is readily transmissible and infectious.Demonstrated the sap transmission of the TMV
1892	D Ivanowski	Demonsrated that the agents of TMV could pass through filters that retained bacterial cells (bacteria proof filter)
1894	Hashimoto	Showed transmissibility of rice dwarf disease by leaf hopper (*Nephotettix apicalis var. cincticeps*).
1898	MW Beijernick	Concept of contagium vivum fluidum. Father of Plant Virology
1917	d'Herelle	Discovered bacteriophage
1932	Knoll and Ruska	Invented Electron microscope
1935	WM Stanley	Crystallized Tobacco mosaic virus
1936	Bawden and N.W. Pirie	Found that the crystalline nature of the virus contains nucleic acid and protein
1939	Kausche, Pfankuch and Ruska	Saw virus particles for the first time with the electron microscope. Confirmed that TMV was rod shaped
1942 & 1944	Muller Williams and Wycoff	Developed shadow casting technique with heavy metals which was useful for determining the overall size and shape of the virus particles
1949	Markham and Smith	Isolated TYMV and showed that it contained (1) An infectious nucleoprotein (about 25%) and (2) non inferious protein
1952	Morel and Martin	Showed that virus free plants could be obtained from totally infected parents using meristem tip culture
1954	Kassanis	Showed that virus could be eradicated from infected plants by high temperature treatment
1956	Gierer and Schramm	Proved that the nucleic acid fraction of the virus is actually the infectious agent
1966.	Kassanis	Discovered the satellite viruses
1963 &	Black and Markhan;	Showed that wound tamour and rice dwarf
1966	Miura *et.al.*	viruses contain double started RNA
1967	Doi and Co-workers	Discovered Mycoplasma like organism
1967	Ishiie *et.al.*	Showed that the MLO bodies and the symptoms disappeared temporarily when the plants were treated with tetracycline antibodies
1967	Diener and Raymer	Discovered viroid

Contd...

1968	Shephard et.al.	Showed that cauliflower mosaic virus contains double stranded DNA
1974	Davies &Worley	Coined the term spiroplasma
1977	Clark and Adams	Develpoed ELISA assay for detection of plant viruses
1981	TW Randles and co-workers	Discovered virusoids
1982	Prusiner	Discovered prions
1994	Sears and Krikpatrick	MLO that infects plants have been reclassified as Phytoplasmas

Plant Disease Control

Year	Contributor (s)	Description
1000	Homer	Mentioned about the use of sulphur in plant disease control
1807	B Prevost	Recommended copper sulphate for wheat seed treatment against bunt and demonstrated first time the fungitoxic value of copper compounds
1882	PMA Millardet	Discovered Bordeaux mixture for control of downy mildew of grape vine
1887	Mason	Discovered burgundy mixture
1921	Bewley	Developed chestnut compound
1934	Tisdale and Williams	Reported fungitoxicity of dithiocarbamates
1942	Singh	Delveloped Chaubatia paste
1943	SA Waksman and A Schatx	Discovered Streptomycin
1952	Kittleson	Discovered captan, also known as Kittleson's Killer
1966	Von Schmeling and M Kulka	Discovered Systemic fungicides oxanthin

Plant Pathology in India

Year	Contributor (s)	Description
1885	KR Kritikar	First Indian scientist who collected and identified fungi
1886-1971	JF Dastur	First Indian Plant pathologist known for the establishment of genus *Phytophthora* and diseases caused by it in castor and potato
	TS Sadasivan	Developed concept of vivotoxins and worked out the mechanism of wilting in cotton owing to *Fusarium oxysporum f.sp. vasinfectum*
	SN Dasgupta	Carried out extensive study on black tip of mango
	MJ Thrimalachar	Discovered several antifungal , antibiotics *viz* aureofungin, haymycin etc.

Contd...

	YL Nene	Reported Khaira disease of rice caused due to Zn deficiency. Authored book "*Fungicides in Plant Disease Control*"
1889	DD Cunningham	Reported the causal organism of red rust of tea in Assam caused by *Cephaleurous virescens*
1920	EJ Butler	First director of Imperial Mycological Institue in England. Initiated an exhaustive study on Indian fungi and the disease caused by them. Discovered genus Allomyces. Wrote "*Fungi and Diseases in Plants*". Father of Indian Plant Pathology.
1940	K.C.Mehta	Studied epidemiology of cereal rusts in India. Write monograph on "*Further studies on cereal rust in India*". *Father of Indian Rust.*
1948	BB Mundukar	Established Indian Phytopathological Society with its journal "*Indian Phytopathology*"
1953	JC Luthra and A Sattar	Developed solar heat treatment for loose smut of wheat
	Ramanujam and Co-workers	Developed seed plot technique for virus free seed potato production in Indo Gangetic plains
1975	S Nagrajan and H Singh	Formulated Indian Stem Rust Rules for *Puccinia graminis tritici*

CHAPTER - 4

Important Plant Pathogenic Organisms

Plant diseases are classified on the basis of type of pathogenic or non-pathogenic causes of the disease. The classification is based on the plant pathogenic organisms as follows.

PARASITES

They include both biotic and mesobiotic agents. The diseases are incited by parasites under a set of suitable environment. Association of definite pathogen is essential with each disease.

i. Biotic agents: They are also called as animate causes. They are living organisms. Biotic agents include:

1. Prokaryotes

a. True bacteria or bacteria (Facultative parasites) e.g. Citrus canker.

b. Rickettsia-like bacteria (RLB) e.g. Citrus greening, Pierce's disease of grape.

c. Mollicutes or wall-less prokaryotes.

   i. Mycoplasma-like organism (MLO) e.g. Sesame phyllody, egg plant little leaf.

   ii. Spiroplasma e.g. Corn stunt, Citrus stubborn.

2. Eukaryotes

a. Protists (Unicellular, coenocytic or multicellular with little or no differentiation of cells and tissues).

   i. Fungi e.g. wilt of cotton

   ii. Protozoa e.g. heart rot of coconut

   iii. Algae e.g. red rust of mango

b. **Plants** - Parasitic flowering plants or phanerogamic parasites - Broomrape of tobacco etc.

c. **Animals-** Nematodes –Root knot nematode etc.

ii. Mesobiotic agents: They include viruses and viroids. They are infectious agents. They can be crystallized and are considered non-living. But their multiplication in the living plants ensures that they are living. Hence they are called as mesobiotic agents.

a. Viruses e.g. yellow mosaic of blackgram

b. Viroids e.g. spindle tuber of potato

NON-PARASITES OR ABIOTIC AGENTS

They are also called as non-infectious or physiological disorders. When no pathogen is found, cultured from or transmitted from a diseased plant, then the disease is said to be caused by a non-living or environmental factor. These diseases occur because of disturbances in the plant system by the improper environmental conditions in the air or soil or by mechanical influences. They are listed below.

i. Too low or too high temperature

ii. Lack or excess of soil moisture

iii. Lack or excess of light

iv. Lack of oxygen

v. Air pollution (Toxic gases in the atmosphere etc.)

vi. Mineral deficiencies or toxicities

vii. Soil acidity or alkalinity

viii. Toxicity of pesticides

ix. Improper agricultural practices.

Table 3 : Comparison between different plant pathogens

Features	Fungi	Bacteria	Viruses	Viroids	Phytoplasma	Spiroplasma	RLO	Protozoa	Algae	Nematodes
Visibility in microscope	Yes	Yes	No (visible under Electron microscope)	No (visible Electron microscope)	Yes	Yes	Yes	Yes	Yes	Yes
Prokaryote/ Eukaryote	Eukaryote	Prokaryote	Kingdom- Virus	-	Prokaryote	Prokaryote	Prokaryote	Eukaryote	Eukaryote	Eukaryote
Cell Wall	Present	Present	Absent	Absent	Absent	Absent	Present	Present	Present	Present
Cell wall with mucopoly saccharides	No	Yes	Yes	No	No	No	Yes	No	No	No
Nucleic acid	Both DNA & RNA	Both DNA & RNA	Either DNA & RNA	RNA	Both DNA & RNA	Both DNA & RNA	Both DNA & RNA	Both DNA & RNA	Both DNA & RNA	Both DNA & RNA
Protein synthesis by their own enzyme	Yes	Yes	No	No	Yes	Yes		Yes	Yes	Yes
Culture in cell free medium	Yes	Yes	Yes	No	No	No	Xylem inhibitory fastidious vascular bacteria can be cultured	Yes	Yes	Yes
Re-production	Asexual &Sexual	Binary fission	Replication	Replication	Binary fission	Binary fission	Binary fission	Asexual &Sexual	Asexual &Sexual	Asexual &Sexual

Difference between Disease and Disorder

Features	Disease	Disorder
Symptom expression	Appear progressively at definite stage.	Appear suddenly, nearly all at once in their fullest nature and intensity
Proportion of affected plants in an area	May vary in their extent of disease development	Tend to be affected with similar extent or in a similar way
Symptom variability	Symptoms variable in type, pattern and occurrence, although recognizable other wise	Symtom on individual plant or plant parts are regular or uniform in nature and pattern
Sign	Present	Absent
Distribution of affected plants	Usually irregular or uneven distribution	Fairly regular or uniform in field or tightly clustered in affected area with no apparent spread pattern.

Difference between Pathogen and Parasite

Features	Pathogen	Parasite
Definition	Any agent that causes damage or disease	Organism existing in an intimate association with another living organisms and derives its nutrition from that host
Plant Pathogen relationship	Most (not all) pathogens are parasites	All parasites are not pathogens
Exapmle	*Ustilago tritici*	Root nodule bacteria (Rhizobium leguminoserum on the roots of pulses).Mycorhizal fungus parasitic on roots of trees
Sign	Present	Absent
Distribution of affected plants	Usually irregular or uneven distribution.	Fairly regular or uniform in field or tightly clustered in affected area with no apparent spread pattern.

Chapter - 5

The Pathogens- Fungi

GENERAL CHARACTERISTICS OF FUNGI

1. Thallus

The body of the fungus is called as **Thallus**, which is without stem root and leaves. It may be Plasmodial, Pseudoplasmodial , Pseudomycelial or Mycelial. A single thread like filament is called as **hypha.** A hypha is made up of a thin, transparent tabular wall filled or lined with a layer of protoplasm.

A group of hypha constituting the body of fungus is called as **mycelium** may be septate or aseptate. i.e coenocytic.

a) Coenocytic or Nonseptate or Aseptate Mycelium

When mycelium is not divided by cross walls called as **Cornocytic** mycelium.

Depending upon the nature of parasitism with the host plant, mycelium is either ecotophytic or endophytic.

b) Septate Mycelium

When mycelium is divided by cross walls or septa called as **septate** mycelium.

i) Ecotophytic Mycelium

The hyphae grows on external/epidermal surface by means of special sucking organs called as **haustoria.** is called **ecotophytic mycelium** e.g. Powdery mildew fungi.

ii) Endophytic Mycelium

When hyphae grows inside the epidermal layer of plant or host tissues, is called as **endophytic mycelium**. e.g. Downy mildew fungi. Endophytic mycelium is of following types.

a) Intercellular

b) Intracellular

c) Vascular

a) Intercellular Mycelium: Mycelium growing in between the cells.

b) Intracellular Mycelium: Mycelium growing within the host cell. e. g Smut Fungi.

c) Vascular Mycelium: Mycelium growing in vascular tissues of the plant. e. g Wilts

2. Cell Wall

Cell wall is well defined, typically chitinised which contains **chitin or cellulose** or both (Cellulose in oomycetes), living structure of the cell called as organelles (Cytoplasm, nucleolus and protoplasm). Nonliving structure of the cell called as Inorganelles (Chitin , cellulose).

3. Nutrition

Nutrition is **heterotrophic** i.e. Photosynthesis lacking and absorptive (They lack chlorophyll and can't manufacture their own food from CO2 and water). Their mechanism of nourishment is **absorption** which takes place by **osmosis** through the cell walls.

Fungi are divided into three groups according to the manner they obtain their food as:

a. Saprophytes

b. Symbionts

c. Parasites

a. Saprophytes

Those organism which requires dead organic matter to complete its life cycle as saprophytes. e.g. Mucor and Rhizophus.

b. Symbionts or Symbiosis

When two dissimilar organisms lives together in close association for mutual benefits is called as **symbiosis**. When two or more organisms lives together in close association for mutual benefits is called as **mutualism**.e.g. Lichen-Fungus and algae Mycorrhiza- Fungi and roots of higher forest plants.

c. *Parasites*

An organism that lives within or upon another living organism from which it derives nourishment and in which it may cause various degrees of injury is called as **parasite** or An organism which completely depends on its host for food called as **parasite.**

Among the parasite one can distinguish different degree of parasitism as i) Obligate parasites ii) Non obligate parasites, iii) Facultative saprophytes iv) Facultative parasites.

i) Obligate Parasites or Biotrophs

Those organisms which requires living hosts or tissues to complete their life cycle, are called as obligate parasites or An obligate parasite is an organism that can live only on living tissue They can never be grown on dead, artificial food material. Rust, mildews, viruses.

ii) Non Obligate Parasites or Necrotrophs

Those organisms when kills the tissue in advance of penetration and then lives on it as saprophytically. E.g. *Sclerotium rolfsii, Ventruria, Claviceps,*

iii) Facultative Saprophytes

An organism that is ordinarily parasitic but under proper conditions may be saprophytic. e.g. *Smut, Sphacelotheca* sp.

iv) Facultative Parasites

An organism that is ordinarily saprophytic but under proper conditions may be parasitic. e.g. *Pythium, Phytophthora.*

4. Nuclear Status

Fungi multinucleate, mycelium being homokaryotic or heterokaryotic or haploid or diploid or dikarytoic limited duration. Well defined structures i.e. nuclear membrane, nucleolus, and chromatin material etc.

5. Sexuality

Asexual Sexual or and homo or heterothallic.

6. Life Cycle

Simple to Complex.

7. Sporocarps

Microscopic or macroscopic and showing limited differentiation.

8. Distribution

Cosmopolitan.

DEFINITION OF FUNGUS AND SOMATIC STRUCTURES

Definition

Fungus is Latin word meaning **'mushroom'**

Alexopoulus and Mims 1979 defined fungus as eukaryotic or nucleated spore bearing , achlorophyllous organism generally produced by sexual or asexual method and whose filamentous branched somatic structure is typically covered by cell wall and cell wall further consists of either cellulose or chitin or glucon or some other complex organic carbohydrate.

Somatic Structures

1. Haustoria

A modified mycelial branch that grows into a plant cell, makes intimate contact with the protoplast, and absorbs food. They are of different shapes and size ranging from knob like structures to simple, lobed, branched, and coiled and they are able to penetrate only in the cell wall and not in the plasma membrane.

2. Appressoria

These are localized swellings of the tip of germ tube or older hyphae that develop in response to contact with the host. In simple these are special structures for attachment in the early stage of infection. From these a minute infection peg usually grows and enters the epidermal cell of the host.

Types of Fungal Thalli

1. Homothallic Fungi:

(Gr. *homo*= same + *thallos* = shoot, tallus): Fungi in which sexual reproduction takes place in a single thallus or If male and female sex organs or both the gametes are produced on the same Thallus, they are self fertile or self compatible.

e.g. Powdery mildew of mung –*Sapharotheca fulginae.*

2. Hetrothallic Fungi:

(Gr. *Hetero*= different + *thallos* = shoot, tallus). If male and female sex organs or both the gametes are produced on the different Thallus, they are self sterile or self incompatible. e.g. Rust fungi.

Fungus Tissue

1. Plectenchyma; During certain stages of fungal development, the mycelium becomes organized into loosely or compact woven tissues, as against the loose hyphae ordinarily found in the mycelium. The organized fungal tissues are called **Plectenchyma.**

The Plectenchyma is of two types

a. Prosenchyma

b. Pseudoparenchyma.

a. Prosenchyma

The loosely woven tissuc in which the component hyphae with elongated cells lie more or less parallel to one another is called prosenchyma.

b. Pseudoparenchyma

The fungal tissues which ar closely packed, in the form of more or less isodiametric or oval cells resembling the parenchyma cells of higher plants are called pseudoparenchyma.Both prosenchyma and pseudoparenchyma compose various type of vegetative and reproductive structures. Both stromata and sclerotia are somatic structure of fungi.

MODIFICATION OF MYCELIUM OR THALLUS

Rhizomorphs

The mycelium of some fungi forms thick strands, in such strands the hyphae lose their individuality and form complex tissues. The strand are called rhizomorph (root like structures). Its function is believed to be the transportation of water across dry areas. The cables are usually large enough to be readily viewed without a microscope and resemble small roots of a seed plant. They belongs to subdivision Basidiomycotina. e.g. *Arnillaria millea*

Stroma or Stromata

It is a compact mass of the hyphae and appears as pseudoparenchymatous tissue and contain fruiting body of the fungus. e.g. ergot of bajara.

Sclerotium

Asexual, thickwalled, multicelled, overseasoning structurc. Masses of cells that form a hard, rounded structure with a differentiated rind in or a host. It may remain dormant for long periods and germinate under favourable conditions. e.g. *Sclerotium* spp.

Dormant Mycelium

It is the mycelium which hibernates in the host tissue to tide over unfavourable conditions, if remains in a dormant condition for a part of its life cycle and come up into activity when conditions are favourable. e.g. Loose smut of wheat, Downey mildew of grape, , Koleroga of arecanut.

Gemmae

These are the chamydospores produced in lower fungi whose walls are thinner. They occur either singly or in chains a becomes separated after maturing. Gemmae break free from the mycelium and disperse in water. e.g. Mucor sp, Saprolegnia sp.

SPORES IN FUNGI

The fungi reproduce by spores. **Spores** is a minute reproductive or propagative bodies functioning as a seed of fungi. These are produced in three ways.

1. Vegetatively
2. Asexually
3. Sexually

Spores

There are three types of spores:

1) Vegetative

Chlamydospores

2) Asexual

i) Exogenous .e.g. Conidia, Oidia

ii) Endogenous: a. Non motile e.g. Aplanospores, b. Motile, e.g. Zoospores

3) Sexual

i) Zygote

ii) Zygospores

iii) Oospores
iv) Ascospores
v) Basidiospores

I) Vegetative Spores in Fungi

Chlamydospores

A thick-walled asexual resting spore formed by the modification of a fungus hypha. They may be formed terminally or intercalary.e.g. *Fusarium* spp.

II) Asexual Spores in Fungi

Asexual spores form without nuclear fusion or act of breeding. These spores borne of sporophores. They are not usually resistance to unfavourable conditions. They are capable of rapid multiplication. They may be one or many celled borne on specialized hyphae or produced in special structures called as spores fruits.

a. Endogenous (Produced inside)

These spores are formed internally within swollen sac by the division of protoplasm. e.g. Sporangiospores, aplanospore.

i) Sporangiospores

Sporangiospores are produced in a sac or sporangium and are hyaline , unicellular. These spores are liberated by breaking the wall of sporangium. When sporangium gives motile spores, it is known as zoosporangium and the spores as **zoospores.** These spores are **motile** by means of **flagella.**

ii) Aplanospore

A non motile spore produced in the sporangium is knows as **Aplanospore.**

b. Exogenous: (Produced outside)

These spores are borne externally on sporophores. e. g. Conidia, Oidia.

i) Conidia

These spores are produced on sepecialized hyphae i.e. conidiaphore. Conidia differ in their size, shape, septation, colour, and branching within the same species.Conidia may be uni or multicellular, hyaline or coloured. e.g. *Alternaria, Helminthosporium.*

ii) Oidia

These spores are barrel shaped or rectangular in shape and are produced asexually in chains on the stalk called as oidiophore. e.g. Oidia in powdery mildew.

III) Sexual Spores in Fungi

The sexual spores are formed by the fusion between two gametes of opposite sex. Cell carrying the gamete is called gametangium and gamete is unisexual or haploid.

i) Oospores

It is the result of union between female gametes i.e. Oogonium and male gametes i.e. Antheridium. Anthridial nuclei passes to Oogonium through fertilization tube. The Oospores are thick walled and may be smooth or rough, dark in colour. These spores can resist the adverse conditions. e.g. Fungi of sub-division mastigomycotina.

ii) Zygospores

A fungal resting spore produced by the fusion of equal gametes designated as +ve and –ve. The resultant spore is thick walled or spiny. The wall consists of two layer. Outer one is known as exosporium and inner layer as endosporium. These spores resist unfavourable conditions and germinate during favourable season. e.g. Fungi of sub-division zygomycotina.

iii) Zygote

It is form by union of two opposite haploid motile gametes. e.g. Lower fungi of the subdivision mastigomycotina.

iv) Ascospores

Ascospores is a result of union between male gamete. i.e. Antheridium and female gametes. i.e. Ascogonium. Anthridial nuclei passes to Oogonium through trichogyne. Ascospores are produce in a sanction as ascus and are generally eight in number. Ascospores may be single or many celled, hyaline or coloured and having various shapes. e.g. Fungi of sub-division ascomycotina.

v) Basidiospores

A haploid spore formed externally on a basidium on a short stalk or tube known as sterigmata. They are produced exogenously and usually four in number.

In these fungi sex organs are absent, except in rust fungi. e.g. Fungi of sub-division basidiomycotina.

SPORE FRUIT

A spore fruit is an aggregation of spores and spores bearing hyphae, sometimes naked but frequent enclosed in various types of containers or spore cases or receptacles. The spores fruit have a thick wall known as peridium.

Importance of Spore Fruit in Fungi

- The spore fruits are vital in tiding over unfavourable conditions, multiplication and maintenance of inoculum.
- The spore fruit are utilized as taxonomic characters in determining the broad lines of various groups of fungi.

Spore Fruit

There are two types of spores fruit based on whether spore fruit contains the sexual spore or asexual spores.

i) Asexual

a. Sporangium
b. Sorus
c. Coremium
d. Sporodochium
e. Pycnidium
f. Aecium
g. Acervulus
h. Pycnium

ii) Sexual

a. Ascocarps e.g. Cleistothecium, Apothecium, Perithecium
b. Basidiocarps e.g. Puff balls, Todstool

ASEXUAL SPORE FRUITS

1. Sporangium

This type of spore fruit is a characteristic of the fungi belonging to sub division Mastigomycotina and Zygomycotina. The elliptical sporangia are formed by the lower fungi belonging to subdivision Mastigomycotina, which are semi-acquatic in nature, while round sporangia are formed by terrestrial fungi belonging to sub division Zygomycotina

2. Aecium

Aecium is a inverted cup like or bell shaped structure usually formed on lower surface of the leaf, consisting of binuclear hyphal cells producing yellow or orange coloured spores which are usually formed in basipetal manner called **aeciosopores.**

3. Pycnium

A flask shaped structure containing Pycniophores and spermata. e.g. Rust fungi.

4. Acervulus

It is compact mass of hyphae giving rise to short, simple hyaline condiophores, closely packed together forming cushion like mass with or without setae. It is also known as modified open sorus. e.g. *Collectrotrichum* and *Gleosporium.*

5. Pycnidium

Asexual, closed, ostiolate fruiting body with short conidiophores lining inner side which bear spores or conidia called **Pyncidiospores**. The spore fruit usually have an opening is called ostiole. e.g. *Phoma* sp. and *Phomopsis* sp.

6. Sporodochium

A spore fruit having cushion shaped stroma, covered with conidiophores is known as **sporodochium.** The conidia formed inside and ooze out in sticky mass. e.g. Genus *Nectria, Fusarium.*

7. Synnemata

The hyphae, which form conidiophores and erect condiophores, grouped together to form **coremia**. Each Coremium consists of sterile stalk terminating into fertile hyphae bearing conidia. e. g. *Stysannus thyroseides*.

8. Sorus

It is little heap like compact mass of sporophores and spore which usually are covered by epidermis. At maturity, the epidermis breaks and the spores get liberated. e.g. Smut and rust.

SEXUAL SPORE FRUIT

(a) Ascocarps

Ascocarp is the spore fruit produced by the fungi belonging to the sub-division Ascomycotina. Sexual spore produced endogenously are known as **Ascospores** in sac like structure called **ascus**. The spore fruit are of various forms viz. Spherical, flask, cup, saucer and pod shaped etc.

Following are the different types of Ascocarps

1. Apothecium

An open, cuplike, or saucer-shaped sexual fungal fruiting body containing asci. The asci are arranged in palisade layer called hymenium. e.g. *Sclerotinia.*

2. Perithecium

A flask shaped ascocarp with narrow neck like having ostiole through which asci are released. The asci are arranged or lined the inner wall of the Perithecium. The sterile structures present in between the asci known as paraphyses which help asci in nutrition and dispersion. e.g. *Claviceps* and *Glomerella.*

3. Cleistothecium

It is closed, sexual fruiting body of the Ascomycetes containing asci and ascospores adapted as overwintering structure, Ascocarp is round to oval with irregularity arranged or scattered asci having dark brown to black colour and provided with appendages. Cleistothecium breaks open at maturity by wear and tear. e.g. Powdery mildew fungi of order Erysiphales.

4. Ascostroma

The asci formed directly in a locule or cavity within at Stroma. They forms the wall of the ascocarp.

(b) Basidiocarps

These are the fructification of sub-division, Basidiomycotina and consist of mushroom, bracket fungi, and puff balls. They are highly developed and have a compound structure, may be fleshy leathery woody waxy in nature and bear structures known as **gills**. The sexual spores known as **Basidiospores** which are usually **4** in number. The basidia are intermingled with sterile structures called **paraphyses**.

1. Mushrooms

Mushrooms are the fleshy or leathery compound fruictification with variously coloured, commonly found on manure pits, dung heaps and on any rich organic matter. They are borne on stalk and provided with gills and pores to the underside which contains hymenial layer. The mushroom may be edible and non-edible or poisonous. e .g. *Agaricus* sp.

1. Puff balls

It is round or spherical basidiocarp , commonly found on dead organic matter. The Basidiospores are produced in the hymenium which lines the inner surface. On maturity Basidiospores are given off, in the form of puff or smoke.

2. Bracket Fungi

A compound fructification growing on dead tree trunks. These are woody and hard basidiocarp. They are typically bracket, hoof or saddle shaped and highly coloured. They are borne on short stalk. The hymenial layer is found on the honey comb fashioned pores in which basidia and basidiospores are observed.

REPRODUCTION IN FUNGI

Reproduction

Reproduction is the formation of a progeny by either sexual or asexual means. Spore is an unit of reproductions.

Asexual Reproduction

This method of reproduction is characterized by production of identical individuals without the union of the sex organs.

Methods of Asexual Reproduction

1. By fragmentation of soma or cell sap or hyphae
2. Budding
3. Binary fission
4. Production of spores

Sexual Reproduction

Sexual reproduction in fungi involves the union of two compatible nuclei.

Methods of Sexual Reproduction

a. Planogamtic Copulation

b. Gametangial Contact

c. Gametangial Copulation

d. Spermatization

e. Somatogamy

f. Heterokaryasis

g. Dikaryotization.

ASEXUAL REPRODUCTION

1. By fragmentation of soma or cell sap or hyphae
2. Arthrospores or oidia
3. Chlamydospores
4. Budding
5. Binary fission
6. Production of spores

1. By Fragmentation of Soma or Cell Sap or Hyphae

Fragmentation may also occur accidentally by the breaking off of parts of the mycelium through external forces. Such pieces of mycelium under favorable conditions can start a new individual. Laboratory propagation is frequently made from mycelial fragments.

2. By Arthrospores or oidia.

The cells of the hyphae at the distal end round off and separate in basipetal succession. On germination, the arthrospores give rise to new fungus colonies.

3. By Chlamydospores

If the cells become enveloped in a thick wall before they separate from each other or from other hyphal cells adjoining the, they are called **chlamydospores**.

4. Budding

Budding is the asexual production of a small outgrowth from a parent cell. The bud increases in size while still attached to the parent cell. It eventually breaks off and forms a new individual . Sometimes chains of buds form a short mycelium. e.g. Rust and smut fungi, yeast fungi.

5. Binary Fission

Fission can occur through the simple splitting of a cell into two daughter cells by constriction. This is found among the bacteria generally, but some fungal yeasts may do this also.

6. Production of Spores

Spore produced may be conidia or sporangiospores, Basipetal oldest at the top and youngest at the bottom. Acropetal oldest at the bottom and youngest at the top.

SEXUAL REPRODUCTION

Sexual reproduction in fungi involves the union of two compatible nuclei. i.e. haploid.

The process of sexual reproduction consists of three distinct phases.

1. Plasmogamy

It is union of two protoplasts brings the nuclei close together within the same cell.

2. Karyogamy

Actual fusion of two haploid nuclei brought together as a result of plasmogamy, karyogamy immediately follows plasmogamy.

3. Meiosis

The nuclear fusion is followed by meiosis. Meiosis reduces the number of chromosomes to haploid.

The sex organs in fungi are called as gametanigia, Gametangia from differentiated sex cells gametes or may contain one or more gamete nuclei.

METHODS OF SEXUAL REPRODUCTION

a. Planogametic Copulation
b. Gametangial Contact
c. Gametangial Copulation
d. Spermatization
e. Somatogamy
f. Heterokaryosis
g. Dikaryotization.

a. Planogametic Copulation (Gametogamy)

This involves the fusion of two naked gametes one or both of which are motile. Motile gametes are called **planogametes.** Depending on the size and motility of the fusing gametes, there are three types

Isogamy : Union of gametes that are similar in shape and size. e.g. *Synchytricum, Olpidium.*

Anisogamy : Union of gametes that are morphologically similar but differ in size. e.g. Allomyces.

Heterogamy: Union between a motile male gamete with a non motile female gamete is known as heterogamy.

b. Gametangial Contact

In this method, two gametangia of opposite sex come in contact, and one or more gamete nuclei migrate from the male to the female. In no case do the gametangia actually fuse or in any way lose their identity during the sexual act. The male nuclei, in some species, enter the female gametangium through a pore developed by the dissolution of the gametangial walls at the point of contact; in other species, an especially developed fertilization tube serves as a passage for the male nuclei . After the passage of the nuclei has been accomplished the oogonium continues its development in various ways, and the antheridium eventually disintegrates. The zygote formed is called **Oospore**. e.g. Oomycetes, Ascomycetes.

c. Gametangial Copulation

Entire protoplast is transferred into the female gametangia. It involes the fusion of two protoplast in a common cell. Sex gametes are indistinguishable or morphologically identical. Copulation occurs either by complete fusion of two protoplast. It is common in class Trichomycetes and zygomycetes.

d. Spermatization

It involves the formation of small spores or seed like structures or spematia. e.g. Spermatiospores. Spermatia acts as male gamete which is uninucleate or spore like and carried out by wind, insects to the receptive hypha (Female gametangium). A pore developed at the plant of contact and the contents of the spermatia passes into receptive hypha which serves as a female organ. e.g. Pycniospores and Receptive hypha in rusts.

e. Somatogamy

No gametes are involved. Vegetative hypha itself acts as a male and female gamete and bring about sexual reproduction. e. g. Smut Fungi.

f. Dikaryotization

Degenerate type of sexuality. It is accomplished through migration of nuclei from one cell to another cell of vegetative hypha, often through mechanism of clamps. The two nuclei remain in pair and divide as such and only fuse prior to the formation of spores. No special sex cells are produced. Clamp connections are formed during nuclear division. e.g. Class- Basidiomycetes.

g. Heterokaryosis

The phenomenon of the existence of genetically different kinds of nuclei in the same individual is called heterokaryosis (Gr. *heteros*=other + *karyon*=nut,nucleous), and the individuals that exhibit it are heterokaryotic. Heterkaryons may originate in a fungus thallus in four ways:

- By the introduction of genetically different nuclei into a homokaryon, a somatic cell in which all nuclei are similar;
- By the germination of a heterokaryotic spore, which will give rise to heterokaryotic soma.
- By mutation in a multinucleate, homokaryotic structure and the subsequent survival, multiplication, and spread of mutant nuclei among the wild type nuclei, and
- By fusion of some nuclei in a haploid homokaryon, and the subsequent survival, multiplication, and spread of the diploid nuclei among the haploid.

SPECIAL TYPE OF SEXUAL REPRODUCTION

Parasexuality

Some fungi do not go through a true sexual cycle as described. They may derive the benefits of sexual recombination through a process known as parasexuality. In this process, plasmogamy, karyogamy and haploidization take place, but not at specified points in the thallus or the life cycle. The parasexual cycle involves the following steps:

1. Formation of heterokaryotic mycelium
2. Nuclear fusion and multiplication of the diploid nuclei
3. Mitotic crossing over during the divison of the diploid cells
4. Sorting out of the diploid strains
5. Haplodization.

CHAPTER - 6

Taxonomy, Nomenclature and Classification of Fungi

Taxonomy

Taxonomy is the science that deals with the identification nomenclature and classification of organisms.

Nomenclature

It is the system of assigning names to the taxonomic groups or organism according to international rules.

Systematics

It is scientific study of organisms with the ultimate object of characterizing and arranging them in an orderly manner.

Binomial System of Nomenclature

Binomial system of nomenclature was developed by Carlous Von Linnaeus which is now universally used. As per the binomial system the name of organism is composed of two words.. The first word designates the genus and the genus name is always capitalized. The second word designates the species and its name is not capitalized. Binomials when written are underlined and when printed italicized. e.g. *Erwinia amylovora*, in which Erwinia is the genus and amylovora is the species.

Rules of Nomenclature

Following rules should be observed while righting of binomial.

1. The name of the genus should always be capitalized.
2. Species name should not be capitalized.

3. Binomial when written should always be underlined separately; when printed italicized.
4. The name or abbreviated name of the scientist describing the species for first time should be written after binomial. e.g. *Pseudomonas syringae Val Hall.*
5. If the name is revised, the name of the original describer should be written in bracket followed by the name of the revising scientist. e.g. *Xanthomonas compestris pv Oryzae Dye.*
6. To avoid confusion the same binomial should not be used to name two different species.
7. The year in which organism was described should be written after the name of the author or scientist.

Sequence of Taxonomic Categories in Fungi

A sequence of taxonomic categories employed in the classification of microorganism is given below:

Taxa	Standard endings	Description
Super kingdom	Eukaryonta	——
Kingdom	Now Fungi	A group of similar divisions
Sub-kingdom	Mycota	——
Division	mycota (suffix)	A group of similar classes
Sub-division	mycotina (suffix)	——
Class	mycetes(suffix)	A group of similar orders
Sub-class	mycetidae (suffix)	——
Order	ales (suffix)	A group of similar families
Family	aceae	A group or collection of similar genera
Genus	—	A group or collection of similar or closely related species.
Species	—	Collection of strains having similar Characteristics
Strain	—	It is population of organism that descends from a single organism or pure culture isolate.

Whittaker (1969) provided five kingdom system viz., Monera, Protista, Plantae, Animalia and Fungi, and thus Fungi is separated from Protista on the basis of nutrition pattern.

Natural and Artificial Classification

Natural classification: A natural classification attempts to place organisms in an orderly arrangement on the basis of overall resemblances, preferably on genetic basis. This classification reflect degrees of evolutionary relationships and therefore, may be phylogenetic.

Artificial classification: Classification based on one or few convenient characters to serve special purposes, e g. ease of identification, is called artificial classification.

C. Various Classifications of Fungi

Classification of fungi was given by various authors viz. Gwynne-Vaughan and Barnes (1927), Martin (1931, 1941), E.A. Bessey (1950). C.J. Alexopoulos (1962) etc. The classification forwarded by Ainsworth (1966 and 1972) is most widely accepted that has been given below:

KINGDOM : PROTISTA (FUNGI)
SUB-KINGDOM : MYCOTA

1. Division : MYXOMYCOTA (Plasmodium or pseudoplasmodium are present)

Sub-division : Myxomycotina

Class : Acrasiomycetes
Hydromyxomycetes
Myxomycetes
Plasmodiophoromycetes

2. Division: EUMYCOTA (Absence of Plasmodium or Pseudoplasmodium)

1. Sub-div : Mastigomycotina

Class : Chytridiomycetes
Hyphochytridiomycetes
Oomycetes

2. Sub-div : Zygomycotina

Class : Zygomycetes
Trichomycetes

3. Sub-div : Ascomycotina

Class : Hemiascomycetes
Plectomycetes
Pyrenomycetes
Discomycetes

Laboulbaniomycetes

Loculoasomycetes

4. Sub-div : Basidiomycotina

Class : Teliomycetes

Hymenomycetes

Gasteromycetes

5. Sub-div : Deuteromycotina

Class : Blastomycetes

Hyphomycetes

Coelomycetes

CHAPTER - 7

Subdivision: Mastigomycotina

GENERAL CHARACTERS

- The Mastigomycotina includes all eumycota fungi which produce flagellated cells during their life cycle.
- Majority of them are with filamentous hyaline coenocytic mycelium.
- Cell wall contains cellulose.
- They show centric nuclear divison.
- The mode of nutrition is typically absorptive, because a majority of mastigomycotina contains some or other type of haustoria.
- They produce asexual spores called zoospores.
- Oospore is the sexual spores.
- Members of the class oomycetes are mostly aquatic but some are facultative or obligate parasites of vascular plants.

Classification

The Mastigomycotina consists of four classes

- Chytridiomycetes (with posteriorly uniflagellate zoospores)
- Hypochytridiomycetes (with anteriorly uniflagellate zoospores)
- Plasmodiophoromycetes (with anteriorly biflagellate zoospores)
- Oomycetes (biflagellate zoospores)

CLASS: CHYTRIDIOMYCETES

- Characterized by the single posterior whiplash flagellum of their zoospores. It is divided into three orders.

Order: Chytridiales

- True mycelium absent.
- Rhizomycelium present in some species.
- Fungi belonging to this order are only plant pathogenic.

Family: Olpidiaceae

Genus: *Olpidium*

Order: Blastocladiales

- True mycelium present.
- Sexual reproduction by planogametic copulation.
- Thick walled resting spore invariably formed.

Order : Monoblepharidales

- True mycelium present.
- Sexual reproduction by copulation between motile male and non motile female gamete contained in an oogonium (heterogametic copulation).
- No resistant sporangia.

CLASS: PLASMODIOPHOROMYCETES

Order: Plasmodiophoromycetales

Family: Plasmodiophoraceae

- All are obligate parasites of higher plants, algae and fungi.
- It form a wall less, naked **plasmodium** as the somatic phase.
- Plasmodium is a multinucleate mass of protoplasm, which can move in amoeboid fashion.
- It forms zoospores which bear two unequal flagella of whiplash type at their anterior end.

Genus: *Plasmodiophora*

Example: Club root disease of cabbage-*Plasmodiophora brassicae*

CLASS: OOMYCETES

- The cell wall is made of cellulose.

- Zoospores biflagellate (posterior flagellum whiplash-type; anterior tinsel-type).
- In sexual reproduction the union of antheridia and oogonia produces oospores.

Order: Peronosporales

- Hyphae are well developed and aseptate.
- Cell wall is composed of glucan-cellulose complex and hydroxyproline.
- Parasites produce haustoria, which may be knob-like, elongated or branched and are found within the host cells.
- Asexual reproduction is by well-defined sporangia.
- Sexual reproduction is by means of well differentiated sex organs, antheridia (male) and oogonia (female).
- Oospores germinate directly or by producing a sporangium.

Family: Pythiaceae

- Sporangiophores similar to the vegetative hyphae or if different then of indeterminate growth.

Genus: *Pythium* and *Phytophthora*

The Difference between *Pythium* and *Phytophthora* are given below

Sl. No	Pythium	Phytophthora
1.	Hyphal wall contains greater amount of protein.	Hyphal wall contains little amount of protein.
2.	Haustoria are absent.	Haustoria are always present.
3.	Sporangiophores are indistinguishable from the somatic hyphae of the mycelium.	Sporangia developed on specialized aerial hyphae, called sporangiophores.
4.	Sporangia are either terminal or intercalary.	Sporangia are always terminal.
5.	Zoospores are not differentiated inside the sporangium; undifferentiated sporangial contents are extruded into a vesicle in which the zoospores are differentiated.	Zoospores are fully differentiated within the sporangium itself: vesicle is formed only rarely.
6.	Appresoria are not formed.	Appresoria may be formed.
7.	Sporangia are hyphal, spherical and rarely ovoid.	Sporangia are limoniform, obpyriform or ovoid.

Important plant diseases caused by *Pythium* and *Phytophthora* spp. are

Fungus	Disease
Pythium	
Pythium debaryanum	Damping of tobacco and chillies
Pythium aphanidermatum	Soft rot of papaya, Damping off of potato
Pythium graminicolum	Rhizome and soft rot of turmeric
Pythium myriotylum	Foot rot of ginger
Phytophthora	
Phytophthora infestans	Late blight of potato
P. colocasiae	Colocasia blight
P. parasitica var. sesami	Leaf blight of Sesamum

Family:Albuginaceae

- Sporangiophores strikingly different from vegetative hyphae, slender or thick, variously club-shaped, arranged in a layer, and bear sporangia in chain at the tip.
- These are obligate parasites.

Genus: *Albugo.*

Important plant diseases caused by *Albugo* spp. are

Fungus	Disease
Albugo candida	White blister on members of Cruciferae
Albugo bliti	White blister on members of Amaranthaceae
A. tragapogonis	White blister on members of Compositae
A. occidentalis	Infects Spinach

Family: Peronosporaceae

- Sporangiophores strikingly different from vegetative hyphae, Sporangia, singly or in clusters borne at the tip of characteristically branched sporangiophores of determinate growth.
- These are obligate parasites.

Classification of Peronosporaceae

Sclerospora	Pernospora	Plasmopara	Pseudoperonospora	Bremia
Sporangiophore is a long stout hypha, with many upright branches near the end, beraing sporangia at its tips	Sporangiophores are dichotomously branched at acute angles and sporangia are borne on pointed tips.	Sporangiophores are dichotomously branched and sporangia are formed on short sterigmata and irregularly spaced.	Sporangiophores are dichotomously branched and sporangia germinate by means of zoospores.	Sporangiophores are dichotomously branched and tips of branches into cup shapedapophyses which form sterigamata each bearing sporangia.
E.g. Downey mildew of bajara.- *S.graminicola*	E.g. Downey mildew of onion- *P.destructor*	E.g. Downey mildew of grape *P.viticola*	E.g. Downey mildew of cucurbits - *P.cubensis*	E.g. Downey mildew of Lettuce- *B.lactucae*.

Order: Saproleginiales

- Zoospores are formed in zoosporangia.
- Oogonia never have a periplasm.
- A peculiar character of this group is the production of two types of zoospores in succession. This is called dimorphism or less accurately diplanetism.
- The two types of zoospores are termed primary and secondary zoospores.

Family: Saproleginaceae

Genus: *Saprolegina* and *Achlya*

The differences between *Saprolegina* and *Achlya* are given below:

Characters	Saprolegina	Achlya
Dimorphism	Present	Absent
Sporangial proliferation	Present	Absent
Zoospore liberation	Slow	In one stroke, the zoospores encysted at the tip of the sporangia to form a hollow ball of encysted, primary zoospores

CHAPTER - 8

Subdivision - Zygomycotina

GENERAL CHARACTERS

- The majority of the members are saprobic. A few Zygomycetes are weak parasites, attacking plants and animals.
- Most Zygomycetes produce a well developed and branched mycelium, consisting of coenocytic hyphae.
- Cell wall is mainly composed of chitin.
- Motile cells or zoospores are absent.
- Asexual reproduction takes place by non motile sporangiospores called aplanospores.
- Sexual reproduction takes place by gametangial fusion.
- Gametangial fusion results in the production of a thick walled resting spore, called zygospore.

CLASS-ZYGOMYCETES

Hasseltine and Ellis (1973) and a majority of the other workers divide Zygomycetes into three orders.

(i) **Mucorales** : Chiefly saprophytic; asexual reproduction by spores or occasionally by conidia.

(ii) **Entomophthorales**: Chiefly parasitic on insects, asexual reproduction by modified sporangia acting like conidia or by true conidia. Modified sporangia are discharged with force.

(iii) **Zoopagales**: Chiefly parasitic on insects, asexual reproduction by modified sporangia acting like conidia or by true conidia. Conidia passively discharged.

Only Mucorales are discussed here.

Order: Mucorales

Family: Mucoraceae

Genus: *Mucor* and *Rhizopus*

The major difference between Mucor and Rhizopus are given below

Sl.No	Rhizopus	Mucor
1.	Rhizoids or holdfasts are present.	Absent or less specialized.
2.	Stolons are present.	Stolons are absent.
3.	Food material is absorbed mainly by rhizoids.	Food is mainly absorbed by the entire mycelia surface.
4.	Sporangiophores develop in well organized groups mainly against the rhizoidal hyphae.	Sporangiophores arise singly, and not in groups.
5.	Spores remain adhered to columella and are not easily disseminated.	Spores easily blown away by wind.
6.	Most common Indian species is *R. stolonifer* (Sweet potato rot).	Some common species are *M. indicus, M.hiemalis, M.mucedo.*

CHAPTER - 9

Subdivision: Ascomycotina

GENERAL CHARACTERS

- Ascomycotina includes only such fungi in which the zygospores are absent and the perfect state spores are the ascospores.
- The Ascomycetes and Basidiomycetes are sometimes combindly called 'higher fungi'.
- Cell wall is made up of chitin.
- Mycelium is well developed branched and septate.
- Asexual spores are non-motile conidia.
- Sexual spores are ascospores.
- Ascospores are usually 8 in an ascus.
- They are produced endogenously inside the ascus.
- The asci are usually grouped to form a definite type of multicellular fruiting body called ascocarp.
- The ascocarps are either cup or saucer shaped (apothecium), flask shaped (perithecium), or closed, spherical and indehiscent (cleistothecium).
- The characteristic ascospores are present in sac- like body, called ascus and therefore these fungi are also commonly called 'sac fungi'
- Yeast is single celled organism.

Key to the Classes of Ascomycotina

- Ascocarps and ascogenous hyphae absent, thallus yeast-like - **Hemiascomycetes**
- Ascocarps and ascogenous hyphae present, thallus mycelial: asci

bitunicate, ascocarp an ascostroma - **Loculoascomycetes**

- Asci typically unitunicate, if bitunicate, ascocarp as apothecium: ascocarp a cleistothecium, asci evanescent and scattered - **Plectomycetes**
- Asci regularly arranged as basal or peripheral layer in the ascocarp Insect parasites - **Laboulbeniomycetes**
- Ascocarp perithecium, Not insect parasites, - **Pyrenomycetes**
- Ascocarp apothecium – **Discomycetes**

CLASS: HEMIASCOMYCETES

- Characterized by the lack of ascocarp.
- Vegetative phase comprising of unicellular thallus or poorly developed mycelium. It is divided into three orders:
- **Endomycetales***:* Asci developing parthenogenetically from a single cell or directly from a zygote formed by population of 2 cells.
- **Taphrinales:** Asci arise from binucleate ascogenous cells formed by breaking of cells from hyphae.
- **Protomycetales:** Asci developing in a compound spore sac (syn ascus), produced singly from thick walled chlamydospores.

Order : Endomycetales
Family : Saccharomycetaceae
Genus : *Sacchromyces, Schizosaccharomyces,*

Fungus	
Saccharomycetes cerevisiae	Brewer's and Baker's yeast

Order : Taphrinales
Family : Taphrinaceae
Genus : *Taphrina*

Fungus	Disease
Taphrina deformans	Leaf curl or leaf blister of peach
T. maculans	Leaf spot of turmeric and ginger

Order : Protomycetales
Family : Protomycetaceae
Genus : *Protomyces*

Fungus	Disease
Protomyces macrosporus	Stem gall of coriander

CLASS: LOCULOASCOMYCETES

It comprises the following 5 orders

Myriangiales, Dothideales, Pleosporales (Pseudosphaeriales), Hemisphaeriales (Microthyriales) and Hysteriales

Order : Myriangiales

Family : Myriangiaceae

Genera : *Elsinoe, Myriangium*

Order : Dothideales

Family : Capnodiaceae

Genera : *Capnodium, Limacinia*

Family : Dothideaceae

Genera : *Mycosphaerella, Guignardia*

Order : Pleosporales

Family : Venturiaceae

Genera : *Venturia*

Fungus	Disease
Venturia inaequalis	apple scab

CLASS: PYRENOMYCETES

- Characterized by unitunicate asci which arranged in a definite hymenium, usually inside a perithecium.
- The perithecia may be globose or flask shaped. In exceptional cases (Erysiphales- powdery mildews), the ascocarp may be a cleistothecium.
- Fungi having cleistothecia with a hymenium belongs to Pyrenomycetes.

Order : Erysiphales

Family : Erysiphaceae

It has the following genera.

I. Ascocarps Present

A. Mycelium superficial

1. Ascocarp containing one ascus only
   a. Perithecial appendages simple, myceloid -*Sphaerotheca*
   b. Perithecial appendages dichotomously branched -*Podosphaera*
2. Ascocarp containing many asci
   a. Perithecial appendages simples, myceloid -*Erysiphe*
   b. Perithecial appendages coiled at the top –*Uncinula*
   c. Perithecial appendages dichotomously branched -*Microsphaera*

B. Mycelium partially endophytic

1. Perithecial appendages simple, imperfect state -Oidiopsis, *Leveillula*
2. Perithecial appendages coiled at the tip, imperfect state -Oidiopsis – *Pleochaeta*
3. Perithecial appendages with basal swellings, imperfect state – *Ovulariopsis*

II. Ascocarps Absent

A. Mycelium superficial

1. Basal cell of the conidiophores swollen.
2. Basal cell of the onidiophores not swollen.
   a. Conidia borne in chains –*Euoidium*
   b. Conidia borne singly –*Pseudoidium*

B. Mycelium partly endophytic

1. Conidia ovoid, obclavate -*Oidiopsis*
2. Conidia pyriform -*Ovulariopsis*

Order : Clavicipitales
Family : Clavicipitaceae
Genus : *Claviceps*

Fungus	Disease
Claviceps microcephala (C. fusiformis)	Ergot of pearl millet
C. oryzae	False smut of rice
Claviceps purpurea	Ergot of rye
C. sorghi (Sphacelia sorghi)	Ergot of sorghum

Powdery Mildews

- The fungi produces closed ascocarp called cleistothecium.
- The genera are differentiated based on the number of asci in the cleistothecium and type of appendages on it.
- Obligate parasites of higher plants mostly dicotyledons

They are classified as follows.

I. One ascus in a cleistothecium

i. Myceloid appendages - e.g., *Sphaerotheca*

ii. Dichotomously branched appendages - e.g., *Podosphaera*

II. Many asci in a cleistothecium

i. Myceloid appendages - e.g., *Erysiphe Leveillula.*

ii. Appendage coiled at the tip (circinoid type) - e.g., *Uncinula.*

iii. Dichotomously branched appendages - e.g., *Microsphaera*

iv. Appendage with bulbous base and spear like tip - e.g., *Phyllactinia*

Fungus	Disease
Powdery mildew of grapes	*Uncinula necator*
Powdery mildew of rose	*Sphaerotheca pannosa*
Powdery mildew of wheat	*Erysiphe graminis*
Powdery mildew of shisham	*Phyllactinia corylea*
Powdery mildew of wheat	*Erysiphe polygoni*
Powdery mildew of apple	*Podosphaera leucotricha*

Order : Meliolales

Family : Meliolaceae

Genus : *Meliola*

CLASS- PLECTOMYCETES

- The asci are produced at different levels (not in a definite hymenium) inside the ascocarp, which is mostly a cleistothecium.

- The asci are unitunicate and evanescent (i.e. dehisce at maturity so that the ascospores lie free inside the cleistothecium).

Order : Eurotiales

Family : Eurotiaceae

Genus : *Aspergillus* and *Penicillium*

The Difference between *Aspergillus* and *Penicillium are given below*

Sl.No	Aspergillus	Penicillium
1.	The conidiophores are unseptate and unbranched	The conidiophores are septate and branched
2.	A conidiophores develops from a specialized thick walled cell, called foot cell	Foot cells are absent. Conidiophore develops from any vegetative cell of the mycelium.
3.	Each conidiophores enlarges into a swollen vesicle at its tip	Vesicle are not formed
4.	Metulae are not present	Metulae are present
5.	Mature conidia are yellow, green, brown or black in colour.	Usually the mature conidia are green in colour.

CLASS-DISCOMYCETES

- These are the Ascomycetes with apothecium type of fruiting bodies, which are cup shaped, saucer shaped or disc shaped.
- The shape of the ascocarp provides them the common name 'Cup fungi'.

Discomycetes are classified into seven orders. Only Pezizales and Tuberales are discussed here.

Order : Pezizales

Family : Pezizaceae (uninucleate ascospores present)

Genus : *Peziza*

Order : Tuberales

Family : Tuberaceae

Genus : *Tuber*

Chapter - 10

Subdivision - Basidiomycotina

GENERAL CHARACTERS

- The members are terrestrial, and saprophytic or parasitic.
- The mycelium is well developed, branched and septate. The mycelium is of primary, secondary and tertiary type.
- Dolipore septum is present except rusts and smuts.
- Clamp connections present.
- Cell wall consists of chitin and glucans.
- Basidiomycetes reproduce asexually by conidia, arthrospores, oidia, fragmentation or budding.
- No specialized sex organs develop in Basidiomycetes.
- Plasmogamy takes place by somatogamy or spermatization.
- Sexual spores are basidiospores.
- They are exogenously produced on basidium.
- Usually four basidiospores are develop on basidium.
- The Basidiomycotina includes rusts, smuts, mushrooms, jelly fungi, puffballs, shelf fungi, toadstools, bird's nest fungi, bracket fungi and earth stars.

Key to the Classes of Basidiomycotina

- Basidiocarp lacking and replaced by teliospores grouped in sori or scattered within the host tissues - **Teliomycetes**
- Basidiocarp usually well-developed, Basidia typically organized as a hymenium; Saprobes or rarely parasites. Hymenium present and exposed before the spores mature. Basidiospores are violently

discharged-**Hymenomycetes**

- Basidiocarp remains closed at least until the basidiospores have been released from the basidia. Basidiospores not released with force; Basidium not involved in the discharge of spores.- **Gasteromycetes**

CLASS : TELIOMYCETES

- This class includes rusts and smuts.
- The class is characterized by thick walled, dikaryotic resting spores commonly called as teliospores in rusts and chlamydospores in smuts, Karyogamy takes place in this part and therefore, is actually a probasidium.
- The resting spores on germination produce promycelium (metabasidium) into which diploid nucleus moves and after meiosis four haploid nuclei are produced.
- These nuclei later, result in the formation of haploid basidiospores
- Mycelial hyphae septate and the septa are of simple type.
- Asexual reproduction is uncommon, through dikaryotic spores of conidial nature produced in rusts. In smut fungi, haploid sporidia may bud off into daughter cells.
- Basidiocarps absent.

This class is divided into 2 orders:

1. **Uredinales**
2. **Ustilaginales**

Order Uredinales (The rust fungi)

- These are obligate parasites and cause great losses to many cultivated crops.
- The mycelium is septate without clamp connections.
- It grows intercellularly, frequently producing haustoria.
- The rusts in which life cycle is short and completed by only two types of spores (teleutospores and basidiospores) are called **microcyclic** rust.
- The rust which has all the five spore stages (teleutospore, basidiospore, spermatia, pycniospore, aeciospore and uredospore) in its life cycle

called **macrocyclic** rust.

- A macrocyclic rust in which uredospores are not formed has been named as **demicyclic** rust.
- The rust fungi that complete their life cycle in one host are termed as **autoecious** and those requiring two hosts for the completion of their life cycle are called as **heteroecious**.
- The rust fungi produce upto five types of spores in their life cycle, as given below:

Stage 0 : Spermagonia with spermatia and receptive hyphae
Stage I : Aecia with aeciospores
Stage II : Uredia with uredospores
Stage III : Telia with teleutospores
Stage IV : Basidia with basidiospores

(a) Pycniospores Stage (0)

- These are the spores produced in a flask-shaped structure called as pycnium, containing a palisade of sporogenous cells which produce spores in nectar exuded from the ostiole.
- Periphyses and flexuous hyphae (receptive hyphae) are commonly present in pycnia.
- Pycnia are formed in the host after it is infected by the basidiospores.
- Pycniospores are single celled and behave as spermatia.

(b) Aeciospores Stage (I)

- These are single celled dikaryotic spores produced in chains in cup-like structures known as aecia.
- The spores are yellow to orange in colour with a hyaline characteristically verrucose wall.

(c) Uredospores Stage (II)

- These are single celled binucleate, pedicellate deciduous spores borne in naked or paraphysate sori breaking through the host epidermis, commonly called as uredia or uredinia.
- Uredospores are brown, echinulate having almost conspicuous germ pores.

- They behave as conidia and repeat several cycles in a season and are also called as summer spores.

(d) Teliospores Stage (III)

- These are binucleate, pedicellate or sessile, erumpent or embedded in host tissue.
- They may be single celled, bicelled or more than 2-celled, with dark brown walls, having one or more germ pores.
- They produce basidium and basidiospores upon germination.

(e) Basidiospores Stage (IV)

- They are haploid, unicellular spores borne on sterigma.
- These arise from cylindrical to club-shaped 2 to 4 celled basidia.
- Depending on the reproductive stages present in the life cycle of rusts, rusts can be termed as 'macrocyclic'(all 5 stages present), 'demicyclic' (uredial stage absent) or 'microcyclic' (teliospore only as the binucleate spore).
- Rusts are either homothallic or heterothallic.
- In the former case pycnia, are not necessary and frequently absent.
- Dikaryotic phase starts from two cell nuclei at some point in the life cycle.
- In the case of heterothallic macrocyclic rusts, basidium bears four basidiospores; two of +type or two of -type.
- These basidiospores produce pycnia of + or-type respectively.
- The pycniospores behave as spermatia and fuse with the receptive hyphae of the opposite sex.
- The dikaryotic phase thus resulted, leads to the development of aecia.

Classification

There are four families in Uredinales

A. Teliospores pedicellate, germinating to form a promycelium, which become septate; spores uni -or multicellular, free **- Pucciniaceae**

B. Teliospores sessile

1. Teliospores in single, sessile, germinating to produce a septate promycelium; **- Melampsoraceae**

2. Teliospores in waxy crusts of one or two layers, becoming septate during germination without forming an external promycelium - **Coleosporiaceae**
3. Teliospores in chains - **Cronartianceae**

Family: Pucciniaceae

- The teliospores are pedicellate (Stalked).
- Teliospores are never present in the form of layers of crusts. They may be simple or compound .
- The uredinia may or may not have paraphyses.
- The aecia may be cup-like or naked.
- The peridium may be curved back.
- Spermagonia may be subcuticular and flattened or subepidermal and spherical with an ostiole.
- Both heteroecious and autoecious species are present.
- Other genera in Pucciniaceae are *Gymnosporangium, Phragmidium, Hemileia* and *Ravenelia.*

Classification

Important genera in Pucciniaceae are

1. Teliospores walls colourless; uredospores reniform, basidia slender, symmetrical ***-Hemileia***
2. Teliospore walls coloured, thickened, ornamented or with visible pores. Telia subepidermal, each pedicel bearing single teliospore. Pycnia subepidermal, globose; teliospore wall thicker above than sides or coloured or smooth ***-Uromyces***
3. Telia gelatinous, telial pedicel aseptate; teliospore cells arranged serially, with pedicel attached to the lower one only. On Cupressaceae - ***Gymnosporangium***
4. Teliospores not in fascicles. Pycnia globose, subepidermal; teliospores truly pedicellate, sometimes >2 celled - ***Puccinia***
5. Teliospore cells arranged as in phragmospores; teliospore wall coloured with 2 or more germ pores in each cell; pedicel usually long, teliospore without conspicuous outer hygroscopic layer - ***Phragmidium***
6. Teliospore cells arranged in a radially discoid head; teliospore pedicels

several per head, fused together, telial head with hygroscopic cysts – ***Ravenelia***

Genus - Puccinia

- The genus Puccinia is an obligate parasite and is extremely host-specific.
- The teliospores are brown and are with mostly 2 cells.
- Telia are at first embedded in the host tissue but sooner or later the epidermis is ruptured and the spores become free. Spermagonia are subepidermal and spherical with ostiole.Aecia are cupulate with recurved peridium on maturity. Urediniospores (uredospores) are single and stalked, with long pedicel.
- They are often present in the same sori in which later the teliospores (teleutospores) are formed.
- They mostly parasitize and cause rust diseases in Gramineae and Cyperaceae.
- Uredo- and teliospores are produced on wheat while spermatia and aeciospores are produced on barberry.
- The important plant pathogenic species are as follows:

Fungus	**Disease**
P. recondita	Brown or leaf rust of wheat
P. graminis tritici	Stem or black rust of wheat
P. striiformis	Yellow or stripe rust of wheat
P. graminis hordei	Barley rust
P. graminis avenae	Oat rust
P. malvacearum	Holly hock rust
P. arachidis	Groundnut rust
P.asparagi	Rust of asparagus
P. helianthi	Sunflower rust
P. hordei	Barley rust
P. arachidis	Groundnut rust
P.asparagi	Rust of asparagus

Life Cycle of *Puccinia*

There are three types of rusts based on the life cycle. They are,

1. Macrocyclic rust
   a. Autoecious rust
   b. Heteroecious rust
2. Demicyclic rust
3. Microcyclic rust.

1. Macrocyclic rust: Five spore stages are produced in their life cycle.

a. Autoecious rust: Five spore stages are formed on a single host.

Examples:

- Linseed rust - *Melampsora lini*
- Sunflower rust - *Puccinia helianthi*
- Pea rust - *Uromyces fabae*
- Castor rust –*M. ricini.*

b. Heteroecious rust: Two different hosts (viz., primary host and alternate hosts) are required for completion of its life cycle.

- Primary host is the plant where the teliospores are produced.
- Alternate host is a plant which is required to complete life cycle without which the pathogen cannot survive.
- Uredia and uredospores and telia and teliospores are formed on the primary host.
- Pycnia and pycniospores and aecia and aeciospores are formed on the alternate host.
- Example: Wheat stem rust – *Puccinia graminis* var. *tritici.* For this rust wheat is the primary host and the barberry is the alternate host.

2. Demicyclic rust: Uredial stage absent and spermagonia may be present or absent.

Example- Cedar apple rust - *Gymnosporangium juniperi-virginianae*

3. Microcyclic rust: Teliospore is the only binucleate spore produced in this rust.

Example: Holly-hock *rust-Puccinia malvacearum.*

Comparison between Black, Brown and Yellow rust

Sl. No	**Black rust** (*Puccinia graminis tritici*)	**Brown rust** (*Puccinia recondita*)	**Yellow rust** (*Puccinia striiformis*)
1.	Stems are most seriously attacked, followed by leaf sheaths, leaves and 'ears', in decreasing order.	Attack leaves almost exclusively, very rarely leaf sheaths or stem	Leaves are most severly attacked followed by leaf sheath, stems and ears.
2.	First noticed in plains in March-April	First noticed in January	From January and causes more damage than black rust
3.	Alternate hosts are species of *Barberry* and *Mahonia*	Alternate hosts are species of *Thalictrum* and *Isopyrum*	Alternate host is not known
4.	Uridinia are large, elongated and coalescing	Uridinia are small, oval, round, and never in long rows.	Uridinia are very small, oval and arranged in rows of stripes.
5.	Uredospores oval with four equatorial germ pores	Uredospores round and having 7-8 scattered germ pores	Uredospores round with 6-10 scattered germ pores
6.	Telia are black and found on all green parts with very low frequency of leaf blades	Telia are very rare. If present , they are distributed mainly on undersurface of leaves.	Telia are dull black, and arranged in rows
7.	Teliospores spindle shaped (apex pointed)	Teliospores flattened at the apex, bicelled	Teliospores are dark brown,much flattened at the apex, bicelled
8.	Pycnia and aecia formed on Berberis and Mahonia	Pycnia and aecia formed on Thalictrum and Isopyron but not observed in India	These stages are not reported for yellow rust
9.	The annual recurrence of the disease on the plains is through uredospores blown down from hills late in the wheat season.	The annual recurrence of the disease on the plains is through uredospores blown down from hills late in the wheat season.	In addition to uredospores from hills , the inoculums initiating primary infection is provided by some locally growing 'collateral hosts'

Genus: Uromyces

- It is characterized by the stalked, one celled teliospores on a simple pedicel with a papillum.
- Uredial, aecial and spermagonial characters are similar to *Puccinia*.
- The species may be heteroecious or autoecious.
- The important species causing plant diseases are given below.

Fungus	Disease
Uromyces ciceris-arietini	Gram rust
U. dianthi	Carnation rust
U. fabae	Vicia rust, lentil rust
U. pisi	Pea rust

Family : Melampsoraceae

Genus : *Melampsora*

Fungus	Disease
Melampsora lini	Linseed rust
M. ricini	Castor rust

Order: Ustilaginales

- The fungi included in this order are called smut fungi.
- Mycelium is intercellular and forms haustoria which draw nutrition from the host cells.
- Basidiospores are formed directly on a septate or non septate promycelium prodced by teliospores on germination.
- The teliospores are formed from all the cells of the secondary dikaryotic mycelium by developing a thick resistant wall.
- No sterigmata are formed. The sporidia develop directly on the promycelium.
- The basidiospores are discharge passively.
- Clamp connection and dolipore septum are generally absent.
- Barring one small family- Graphiolaceae, smuts donot form a basidiocarp.

The differences between ustilaginales and uredinales are given in the table below :

Characters	Uredinales (rusts)	Ustilaginales (smuts)
Teliospores	Present, formed by terminal cells of secondary mycelium	Present,formed by intercalary as well as terminal cells of secondary mycelium
Basidiospores	Present in0 definite numbers, usually 4, borne on sterigmata; violently discharged	Not in definite numbers, Sterigmata absent; Basidiospores passively discharged
Basidiocarp	Absent	Present in Graphiolaceae

There are two families in this order.

Family: Ustilaginaceae

- The family includes all the smut fungi in which the promycelium is transversely septate into several, usually four, cells with lateral and terminal sporidia, one or more from each cell. Sometimes there may be only one sporidium on the septate promycelium.
- Occasionally, the basidium (promycelium) develops directly into a mycelium without forming sporidia, as in *Ustilago nuda tritici,* or both conditions may be present (*Sphacelotheca sorghi*).
- Important genera are *Ustilago Sphacelotheca*, *Tolyposporium* and *Melanopsichium*.

Ustilago

- Sori contain 1–celled teliospores, dusty at maturity and are covered by membrane of host origin.
- Germination is by means of septate promycelium, which may become infection hyphae or may produce sporidia laterally near the septa.
- The sporidia germinate easily in water by infection.
- The important species causing plant diseases are given below

Fungus	Disease
Ustilago nuda tritici	Loose smut of wheat
U. zeae	Common smut of corn
U. hordei	Covered smut of barley
U. avenae	Loose smut of oats
U. scitaminea	Whip smut of sugarcane

Family: Tilletiaceae

- The family includes only those smuts in which the promycelium is aseptate with terminal whorl of sporidia.
- The teliospores are single or combined into more or less permanent balls usually including sterile cells.
- Promycelium is simple, usually nonseptate up to the time of formation of sporidia.
- Sporidia are longer than in Ustilaginaceae, produced in clusters at the

apex of the promycelium, fusing or not fusing in pairs, producing similar or dissimilar sporidia or germinating directly into infection threads.

- Important genera are *Tilletia, Neovossia, Urocystis, Entyloma* and *Turbicina.*

CLASS : HYMENOMYCETES

- Well known mushrooms, jelly fungi, bracket fungi, toadstools, fairy clubs, tooth fungi, pore fungi, coral fungi and other similar forms are included under Hymenomycetes.
- This class is characterized by usually well-developed basidiocarp or fruiting bodies.
- The hymenium of the basidiocarps is fully exposed at maturity and consists of large number of basidia arranged in a palisade like manner.
- Basidiocarps are typically gymnocarpic (primordium and mature sporocarp have exposed hymenium) or semiangiocarpic (partially closed till spores are matured).
- Basidiospores are ejected forcibly i.e. these are ballistospores.

Classification

a. Basidia aseptate -Sub-class Holobasidiomycetidae.

b. Basidia septate -Sub-class Phragmobasidiomycetidae

Holobasidiomycetidae

- This class is characterized by an undivided, cylindrical to clavate basidium (i.e. holobasidum), which usually extends into four sterigmata each bearing a basidiospores.
- The basidia are produced in a well developed mycelium.

Phragmobasidiomycetidae

- The metabasidium of these is completely or incompletely divided into 4 cells by transverse or longitudinal septa. The basidiocarp is usually gelatinous, waxy or dry.
- The probasidia may or may not be persistent.
- The basidiospores are often repetitive and sterigmata swollen.

SUB-CLASS : HOLOBASIDIOMYCETIDAE

Order: Exobasidales

- The order is characterized by the 4-spored basidia, which form a layer (hymenium) on the leaf surface and lack the well-define basidiocarps.
- Consisting of the gall-forming plant parasites.

Family : Exobasidiaceae.

Genus : *Exobasidium E. vexans* - blister blight of tea.

Order : Tulasnellales

Family : Ceratobasidiaceae

Genus : *Ceratobasidium* and *Thanatephorus*

Order: Aphyllophorales/ Polyporales

Family : Corticiaceae

Genera : *Chondrostereum, Peniophora, Athelia, Corticium*

Family : Ganodermataceae

Genus : *Ganoderma*

Order: Agaricales

- Commonly called 'gill fungi', which include mushrooms, (edible), toadstools (poisonous) and boletes.
- Mycelium of Agaricales is typically basidiomycetous with primary, secondary and tertiary mycelia.
- The characteristic macroscopic basidiocarp or fruit body is fleshy, generally having a stalk i.e. stipulate, and has a pileus bearing hymenium-covering lamellae on the underside.
- The young basidiocarp may be covered by a universal veil, which becomes broken down by the growth of the stipe and pileus but part may remain as volva at the base of the stipe and as fragments on the upper surface of the mature pileus.
- The developing hymenium may be covered by a partial veil, which later becomes a cortina or an annuals around the mature stipe.
- The hymenium may consist of cystidia of various kinds, setae, or

hyphidia among the basidia the latter producing unicellular, hyaline or coloured ballistospores, typically in fours.

- Asexual reproduction is very rare. Only a few species show the production of thin walled oidia (*Coprinus lagopus*), chlamydospores (*Volvariella volvacea*) or conidiophores as in members of Aphyllophorales.
- Sexual reproduction takes place by hyphal fusion and results in the formation of basidia and basidiospores, present together in the form of fruiting body, called basidiocarp.
- Except a few homothallic species, the majority of the members are heterothallic and show either unifactorial or bifactorial heterothallism.
- The order Agaricales contains 16 families (Smith, 1973). They are Boletaceae, Hygrophoraceae, Tricholomataceae, Entolomataceae, Amanitaceae, Pluteaceae, Lepiotaceae, Agaricaceae Bolbitiaceae, Strophariaceae, Coprinaceae, Cortinariaceae, Paxillaceae, Gomphidiaceae, Russulaceae and Cantharellaceae.

Family : Tricholomataceae

Genus : *Pleurotus,Armillariella, Marasmius,*

Pleurotus

- This genus contains most valuable edible mushroom.
- Stipe is generally eccentric and pileus resupinate in some species. They have white or pigmented range fruiting bodies.
- They grow on wood, on dead or living hosts.

  P. sajor -caju-Oyster mushroom

  P. ostreatus - Oyster mushroom.

Family : Amanitaceae

Genus : *Amanita, Limacella* and *Termitomyces*

Amanita

- The genus is characterized by free gills and the presence of the annulus and volva on the stipe.
- Remnant of the volva may persist as volva scales on the cap.
- More than 5 species are known to be mycorrhizal in habit.
- Some are more attractive and used in decoration. Some are poisonous and produce toxins called phallotoxin and amatoxins.

A. phalloides - Called **'Depth cap fungus'**and it is poisonous.

A. virosa - Called as **'Destroying angel'**; or **Death angel** and it is also poisonous.

Family : Pluteaceae

Genus : *Volvariella, Pluteus, Chamaeota.*

Volvariella

V. volvacea and *V. diplasia*- commonly called the straw, or paddy straw or Chinese mushrooms are edible.

Family : Agaricaceae

Genus : *Agaricus, Cystoagaricus* and *Melanophyllium*

Agaricus

- The characteristic features of the genus are the presence of deep purplish brown free gills, and an annulus but no volva, and stalk that readily separates from the pileus.
- They are commonly found growing on ground in pastures.
- These mushrooms are edible for their delicacy.

  A. campestris - White button mushroom; edible.

  A. bisporus - Edible and cultivated mushroom.

Edible mushrooms

- Mushroom is a fleshy to tough, edible umberella like basidiocarp (sporophores) of certain basidiomycetes fungi.
- The mushroom consists of stipe, a membranous annular ring called annulus, cap or pileus arid gills or lamellae.
- Each gill on cross section shows closely packed elongated fungal cells called **trauma**.
- A subhymenium with spherical cells is formed on both sides of the trauma.
- A fertile layer with palisade like cells called **hymenium** is found over the sub-hymenial layer.
- It consists of club shaped basidia, sterigmata bearing single-celled basidiospores.
- In the hymenial layer stout sterile structure called cystidia are also found.
- The eating of mushrooms is called **mycophagy.**

Morphology of Mushroom

- *Agaricus campestris* is a field mushroom growing on all organic matter in the fields.
- The mycelium is highly organized and the hyphae are often found to form rhizomorphs.
- Clamp connections are also formed by the hyphae and chlamydospores may be produced to resist the adverse conditions.
- The fruiting body or the basidiocarp commonly called as **mushroom** comes out of the soil and it consists of thick stalk called **stipe** on which an umbrella shaped **pileus**(cap) rest.
- The stipe is cylindrical in shape, fleshy and usually swollen at the base.
- Just above the middle the stipe has a membranous ring known as **annulus**.
- The pileus on the under surface exhibits numerous structures radiating from the stipe. They are called **lamellae** or **gills**, which are slender, pink when young becoming brown later.
- The cross section of a lamella or gills show the central loosely packed elongated fungal cells known as **trama**.
- On both sides of the trama are found **subhymenial** layers the cells of which will be spherical in shape. Over the sub-hymenial layer a layer of palisade-like cells known as **hymenial layer** is formed.
- The hymenial layer consist of club shaped **basidia** which have two to four minute **sterigmata** at their tip.
- The sterigmata bear the haploid single celled, basidiospores. In the hymenial layer there are some stout sterile structures known as **cystidia** (sing. cystidium).
- The **basidiospores** are released forcibly and fall near the base of the stipe and form a pink mass.

Agaricus

- *Agaricus* spp. are called button mushroom or **white button mushroom**.
- It has stout, cylindrical, fleshy umberella-like pileus and possess annulus.

- Good crop of mushroom comes at low temperature of 15 to 25° C.
- Well decomposed wheat / paddy straw compost incorporated with nutrients is used as substrate.
- The substrate mixture is filled in trays.
- The compost is now mixed with mycelial pieces(of the sixe of groundnuts) obtained from pure cultures of the fungus. This is called 'spawning.' Hyphae permeate the compost.
- After 2-3 weeks the compost beds are covered with a thin layer, (2.5-3cm) of soil or peat-vermiculite mixture. This is called "casing".
- Without casing the fruiting bodies are not formed.
- The stimulating factor provided by the casing is not known.
- After amonth, fruiting bodies start making appearance.
- Higher temperature of the bed (15-21^{0}C) favour mycelia growth while a lower temperature (13-15^{0}C) favours fruiting body formation. So the temperature is kept below 15^{0}C after the initiation of fruiting.
- 300-350 kg of mushroom can be harvested from one ton of compost in a period of 85-100 days.
- It has two important commercial cultivated species.

  Agaricus bisporus -Temperate mushroom or white button mushroom.

  A. bitorquis- Hot weather mushrooms.

Pleurotus

- *Pleurotus* spp. are called oyster mushroom as it resembles shell of an oyster.
- The stipe is eccentric.
- It is called Dhingri in India.
- It is a tropical mushroom coming up well between 25-30°C.
- The colour may be white or grey or pink depending upon the species.
- It is grown on paddy straw (substrate) in polybags. In a period of 30-45 days, it yield 1.0 to 1.4 kg per kg of paddy straw.
- Commonly cultivated species in India are *Pleurotus sajor-caju, P. citrinopileatus, P. ostreatus, P. eryingii* etc.

CHAPTER - 11

Subdivision : Deuteromycotina

GENERAL CHARACTERS

- Deuteromycotina includes the fungi in which the 'perfect stage'(zygote, ascus, basidium) is either lacking or has not been discovered so far. Because of the apparent absence of any perfect stage or sexual phase, these fungi are commonly called 'imperfect fungi' or technically **'Fungi imperfecti'**.
- The characteristic feature of Deuteromycotina is the absence of sexual reproduction. The members reproduce only be asexual methods, and that too also chiefly by conidia, which develop on conidiophores.
- The conidia are produced either directly on the conidiophores or in some special types of fruiting bodies such as **synnemata**, **acervuli**, **sporodochia** or **pycnidia.**
- Fungi possess branched, septate and multinucleate mycelium except the unicellular yeast like members of Blastomycetes.
- Sexual reproduction is completely absent.
- Parasexuality is shown by some Deuteromycotina. Under this phenomenon, the process of plasmogamy, karyogamy and haplodization take place, but not at specified time or specified points in the life cycle of the fungus.

Classification

The sub-divison Deuteromycotina is divided into following three classes:

1. **Blastomycetes:** True mycelium absent or not well-developed, soma is made up of yeast (budding) cells with or without pseudomycelium.
2. **Coelomycetes:** Mycelium well-developed, assimilative budding cells absent. Reproduction by conidia borne in **pycnidia** or **acervuli.**
3. **Hyphomycetes:** True mycelium is present; mycelium is either sterile

forms o or bear spores on sporophores, which are never aggregated in pycnidia or acervuli.

CLASS: HYPHOMYCETES

- Majority of the members are either saprophytes or parasites.
- Mycelium well developed and septate.
- Majority of the genera reproduce by conidia (Moniliales), but some members reproduce only by fragmentation e.g. *Rhizoctonia* and *Sclerotium.*
- Neither pycnidia nor acervuli are produced by any member.

The class hyphomycetes is divided into following orders

Order

1. **Agronomycetales or Mycelia sterilia**: Conidia absent except for chlamydospores.
2. **Moniliales** : Conidia present, Conidiophores are not organized as synnemata or sporodochia-Conidiophores are organized as synnemata or sporodochia.
3. **Stilbellales:** Synnemata formed.
4. **Tuberculariales:** Sporodochia formed.

Order: Moniliales

- The conidiogenous cells are produced on the conidiophores, which may be either macronematous. i.e. which are morphologically very different from purely vegetative hyphae or micronematous. i.e morphologically similar to vegetative hyphae but are always mononematous i.e. they are sporodochia.
- The order is divided into four families, Moniliaceae, Dematiaceae and Stilbellaceae

Family 1: Moniliaceae

- The members of this form-family are characterized by the production of free conidiophores or conidiogenous cells from the somatic hyphae and all the structures i.e. hyphae.
- Conidiophores and conidia are hyaline or light coloured.

A key to important plant pathogenic genera is given here:

I. **Conidia unicellular**, globose to cylindrical, conidiophore distinct:

(a) Conidia almost similar to apical cells of conidiophores *Monilia*

(b) Conidia not as above; borne in chains; dry:

(i) Phialides in heads on simple conidiophores -*Aspergillus*

(ii) Phialides bush like; upright -*Penicillium*

(c) Conidia not borne in chains; conidiophores verticillate, phialospores in mucilaginous mass-*Verticillium*

(d) Conidiophore branching irregularly or dichotomously; conidia dry, borne on inflated apical cells -*Botrytis*

II. **Conidia bicelled**, ovoid to cylindrical:

(a) Conidiophores reduced to stromal cells - *Rhyncosporium*

(b) Conidiophore distinct, rarely branched, in clusters; conidia cylindrical, in short chains - *Ramularia*

III. **Conidia 3 or more celled:**

(a) Conidia usually of 2 types, multiseptate macroconidia sickle shaped; unicellular microconidia often present -*Fusarium*

(b) Conidiophores rarely branched, conidia simple, attenuated at the apex - *Cercosporella*

(c) Conidiophores usually simple; conidia on denticles –*Pyricularia* *Aspergillus* and *Penicillium* belong here,

Family 2: Dematiaceae

- This family is characterized by the production of dark-conidia and/or conidiophores.
- Conidiophores are simple and not produced in any type of fruiting body.

Genera: *Alternaria* ,*Bipolaris, Cladosporium, Cercospora, Curvularia, Drechslera, Helminthosporium* and *Pyricularia.*

Alternaria

- It is a polyphagous fungus.
- Conidiophores are dark, septate, sometimes inconspicuous, simple or branched, bearing conidia at the apex.
- Conidia (Porospores) solitary or more often produced in acropetal

succession to form simple or branched chains, **muriform** or **dictyospore** (transverse as well as longitudinal conidia), darkly pigmented, ovate to obclavate, tapering abruptly or gradually towards the apex, smooth or roughened.

- The perfect stage of *Alternaria* belongs to *Pleospora infectoria*

Important plant diseases caused by *Alternaria* spp. are

Fungus	Disease
Alternaria alternata	Black point disease of wheat
A. brassicola	Leaf and pod spot of crucifers
A. solani	Early blight of potato and leaf spot of tomato, chillies and tobacco
A. porri	Purple blotch of onion
A. brassicae	Leaf spot of crucifers
A. triticina	Leaf blight of wheat

Cercospora

- *Cercospora* is characterized by long, hyaline or pigmented conidia borne in acropetal succession from a usually simple, sympodially extending, pigmented conidiophores which are frequently aggregated in fascicles .
- The conidia are long slender, narrow, tapering and contain many transverse septa.

Important plant diseases caused by *Cercospora* spp. are

Fungus	Disease
C. arachidicola	Early leaf spot of groundnut
C. personata	Late leaf spot of groundnut
C. coffeicola	Leaf spot of coffee and spinach
C. nicotianae	Frog -eye spot of tobacco
C. kikuchii	Purple stain of soybean
Cercospora musae	Sigatoka leaf spot of banana

Helminthosporium

- Mycelium immersed stromata usually present.
- Conidiophores often in fascicles, erect, brown to dark brown.
- Conidia develop laterally, often in verticils, through pores beneath the septa of the conidiophore while the tip of the conidiophores continues

to grow but growth ceases with the formation of terminal conidia.

- Conidia sub-hyaline to brown, usually obclavate, pseudoseptate and frequently with a dark brown to black protruding scar at the base.
- Colonies effuse, dark and hairy.
- *Helminthosporium* imperfect state is produced in *Pseudo-cochliobolus* belonging to the Dothideales.

List of *Helminthosporium* transferred to *Drechslera*

Helminthosporium sp.	Drechslera sp.	Ascigerous state
H. oryzae (brown leaf spot of rice)	*D. oryzae*	*C. miyabeanus*
H. maydis (Leaf blight of corn)	*D. maydis*	*Cochliobolus heterosporus*
H. gramineum (Leaf stripe of barely)	*D. graminea*	*Pyrenophora graminea*
H. sativum (Leaf blight of wheat)	*Bipolaris sorokiana*	*C. sativum*

Drechslera

- Drechslera is characterized by the sympodially extending conidiophore, which produces an acropetal succession of multiseptate porospores, which are cylindric in shape and germinate from any or all cells.
- Conidiophores are indeterminate, extending by sympodial growth, brown and produce the conidia singly at the apices.
- Conidia are cylindrical, multiseptate and dark.
- *Cochliobolus, Pyrenophora, Pleospora* and *Trichometasphaeria* are imperfect states of *Drechslera.*

Bipolaris

- It is characterized by germination of conidia from the end cells only.
- Conidiophores brown, producing conidia through an apical pore and forming a new apex by growth of the sub-terminal region.
- Conidia fusoid, straight or curved, germinating by one germ tube from each end cell.
- The perfect state is *Cochliobolus*.

Pyricularia

- Conidiophores are more or less erect, simple or rarely branched, septate, hyaline to lightly pigmented.

- Conidia borne singly and terminally at the apex of conidiophore with successive conidia being produced in acropetal succession.
- Conidia ellipsoid or more often pyriform, broader and truncated at the attachment point, tapering towards the distal end, mostly one septate or two septate, hyaline to lightly pigmented.

Important plant diseases caused by *Pyricularia* spp. are

Fungus	Disease
Pyricularia oryzae	Blast of rice
P. setare	Blast of fox-tail millet
P. grisea	Blast of ragi / finger millet

Curvularia

- Conidiophores are erect, macronematous and mononematous.
- The conidia develop either spirally or in whorls on conidiophores.
- The conidia are usually curved.
- Usually the third cell from the base of the conidium is largest.

Example: *Curvularia Cambopogonis*

Family 3: Stilbellaceae

- Conidia and conidiophores develop in **synnemata**

Genus: *Graphium*

Order: Tuberculariales

- The characteristic features of this order is the production of **sporodochia**.

Family: Tuberculariaceae

Genera. ***Fusarium***

- The **macroconidia** (phialospores) are produced on conidiophores, which may be solitary and simple or aggregated (sporodochia) and with complex branching and the ultimate branched terminating in sporogenous cells.
- **Microconidia** are non-septate or one-septate, ovoid to short cylindric, gathering in short chains or more commonly in spore balls.

- Thick walled **chlamydospores** are also produced either terminally or intercalarily on the somatic hyphae.
- The mycelium, microconidia, macroconidia and sporodochia are bright in colour.
- Perfect state of *Fusarium* is found in Ascomycetes in the family Hypocreaceae in which the genera, *Nectria, Calonectria, Gibberella* and *Micronectriella* are found.

Important plant diseases caused by *Fuarium* spp. are

Fungus	Disease
F. moniliforme	Foot rot of rice
F. oxysporum f.sp. *batatae*	Wilt of sweet potato
F. oxysporum f.sp. *coriandri*	Wilt of coriander
F. oxysporum f.sp. *cubense*	Panama disease of banana
F. oxysporum f.sp. *glycines*	Wilt of soybean
F. oxysporum f.sp. *lagenariae*	Wilt of bottlegourd
F. oxysporum f.sp. *lathyri*	Wilt of Lathyrus
F. oxysporum f.sp. *lentis*	Wilt of lentil
F. oxysporum f.sp. *lini*	Wilt of linseed
F. oxysporum. f.sp. *lycopersici*	Wilt of tomato
F. oxysporum. f. sp. *melongenae*	Wilt of brinjal
F. oxysporum. f.sp. *pisi*	Wilt of pea
F. oxysporum. f. sp. *psidii*	Wilt of guava
F. udum -	Wilt of pigeonpea

CLASS: COELOMYCETES

- The thallus is eucarpic and mycelia septate.
- Conidia are produced either in acervuli or pycnidia.
- The conidia are unicellular, deciduous and hyaline or pigmented.
- Coelomycetes is divided into two orders, Melanconiales and Sphaeropsidales.
    1. **Melanconiales:** Conidia produced in acervuli
    2. **Sphaeropsidales:** Conidia produced in pycnidia

Order: Melanconiales

- The fructifications are acervuli. It contains a single family.

Family: Melanconiaceae

- Characterized by the production of acervuli.
- Conidia may be hyaline to cream, pink, orange or black.
- They cause plant disease known as anthracnose.
- The important genera are *Colletotrichum, Cylindrosporium, Melanconium, Pestalotia, Pestalotiopsis, Gloeosporium*

Colletotrichum

- Acervuli may be subcuticular, epidermal or subepidermal.
- Conidiophores are hyaline to brown, septate, smooth, branched at the base.
- Conidia are hyaline, unicellular, falcate or lunate (sickle shaped) or cylindrical.
- Perfect state of the fungus belongs to *Glomerella.*

Important plant diseases caused by *Colletotrichum* spp. are

Fungus	Disease
C. capsici	Fruit rot and dieback of chillies, anthracnose and boll rot of cotton
C. graminicola	Anthracnose of corn and sorghum
C. circinans	Smudge of onion
C. falcatum	Red rot of sugarcane
C. gloeosporioides	Anthracnose of citrus and banana
C. lindemuthianum	Anthracnose of cowpea
C. musae	Anthracnose of banana
C. coffeanum	Coffee berry disease

Pestalotia

- The genus is characterized by the conidia which are fusiform, straight or slightly curved and five septate.
- There may be 3-9 apical, cellular, simple or dichotomously branched appendages and one basal endogenous cellular, simple or branched appendage.
- The conidiophores are long, branched and septate.
- The fructifications are dark brown.

Important plant diseases caused by *Pestalotia* spp. are

Fungus	Disease
Pestilential palmarum	Grey blight of coconut.
Pestalotia theae	Grey blight of tea and blight of mango, palms and cotton.
Pestalotia mangiferae	Grey blight of mango.

Order: Sphaeropsidales

- The conidia and conidiophores are produced in pycnidia.
- Mycelium may be immersed in the substrate or superficial.
- Conidia are solitary, sympodial catenate etc.
- Sphaeropsidales is divided into four families based on the colour, shape and texture of the pycnidia.
- They are Sphaeropsidaceae ,Nectrioidaceae, Leptostromataceae and Excipulaceae

Family : Sphaeropsidaceae

- This is a large family consisting of both saprobes and a stroma.
- The spores are hyaline spherical or oval and often exude from the ostiole in damp weather in a worm like mass.

Macrophomina

- Mycelium superficial or immersed, hyaline to brown, branched, septate.
- Pycnidia separate, globose, dark brown, immersed, with one cavity, thick walled.
- Ostiole central, circular, papillate.
- Conidiophores absent
- Conidia (Pycnospores) hyaline, aseptate, obtuse at each end straight cylindrical to fusiform,
- Forming mainly sclerotia in cultures, which are black, smooth, hard, formed of dark-brown thickwalled cells.

Genus: ***Macrophomina***

Important plant diseases caused by *Macrophomina* spp. are

Fungus	Disease
Macrophomina phaseolina (syn .*Rhizoctonia bataticola)*	Charcoal rot, ashy stem blight, dry root rot, canker, damping off and leaf lesions on hosts like soybean, groundnut, cotton.

Ascochyta

- Mycelium immersed, branched, septate, hyaline to pale brown.
- Pycnidia are amphigenous, separate, globose, brown, immersed, unilocular and thin-walled.
- Ostiole central, circular, slightly papillate.
- Conidiophores are absent.
- Conidia hyaline, thin-walled, cylindrical, ovoid, oblong to irregular, medianly one-septate, continuous or constricted at the septum.
- Conidia may be guttulate.

Important plant diseases caused by *Ascochyta* spp. are

Fungus	Disease
A. abelmoschi	Leaf, fruit and stem spot of lady's finger.
A. carica	Fruit rot of papaya
A. fabae	Leaf and pod spot of broad beans
A. phaseolorum	Leaf and pod spot of common bean and other legumes.
A. pisi	Leaf and pod spot of pea
A. rabiei	Blight of chickpea
A. sorghi	Leaf spot of sorghum

Septoria

- The pycnidia are immersed in the substratum and are either separate or aggregated .
- They are globose, ostiolate, thin walled and brown.
- Conidia are hyaline, smooth, filiform, continuous or constricted at septa.
- The perfect states in Ascomycotina genera are *Mycosphaerella* and *Leptosphaeria*.

Important plant diseases caused by *Septoria* spp. are

Fungus	Disease
Septoria apii	Celery leaf blight
S. bataticola	Leaf spot of sweet potato
S. glycinea	Brown spot of soybean
S. lycopersici	Leaf spot of tomato
S. nodorum	Speckled leaf blotch of wheat
S. tritici	Leaf spot of wheat

Family: Excipulaceae

Genera : *Excipula, Discula, Dinemosporium, Sporonema*

Order : Agronomycetales or Mycelia sterilia

Genus : *Rhizoctonia* and *Sclerotium.*

Rhizoctonia

- They are facultative necrotrophs i.e. they are capable of prolonged existence as saprophyte in the soil.
- They form sclerotia of irregular size and shape but of uniform texture brown or black, more or less loosely packed.
- The cells of the hyphae are barrel shaped, anastomosing frequently, branching more or less at right angles, and pale brown to brown in colour.
- Perfect states of *Rhizoctonia* are *Ceratobasidium* and *Thanatephorus* (of Basidiomycotina) and *Macrophomina* (Pycnidial state).

Important plant diseases caused by *Rhizoctonia* spp. are

Fungus	Disease
R. bataticola	Dry root rot of pulses, cotton etc. (Pycnidial state: *Macrophomina phaseolina)*
R. solani	Root rot of cotton. (Perfect state: *Thanatephorus cucumeris)*

Sclerotium

It is characterized by hard, brown to black, fairly large sclerotia.

These are produced on sterile, cotton, white mycelium provided with clamp connections.

The perfect states of *Sclerotium* are *Pellicularia* (Hymenomycetes of Basidiomycotina) and *Sclerotinia* (of Ascomycotina)

Important plant diseases caused by *Sclerotium* spp. are

Fungus	**Disease**
Sclerotium cepivorum	White rot of onion
S. rolfsii	Root rot of soybean, black pepper groundnut, cotton, cabbage tomato etc
S. oryzae	Stem rot of rice

Teleomorphic Stage of Some Important Pathogens

Sl.No	**Anamorphic stage**	**Teleomorphic stage**
Cleistothecial ascomycetes		
1.	*Penicillium*	*Talaromyces*
2.	*Oidium*	*Erysiphe*
3.	*Paecilomyces*	*Byssochlamys*
4.	*Aspregillus*	*Eurotium*
Perithecial ascomycetes		
5.	*Colletotrichum*	*Glomerella*
6.	*Fusarium*	*Gibberella*
7.	*Trichoderma*	*Hypocrea*
8.	*Verticillium*	*Hypocrea*
9.	*Graphium*	*Ophiostoma*
10.	*Chalara*	*Ceratocystis*
11.	*Acremonium*	*Epichloe*
Loculoascomycetes		
12.	*Alternaria*	*Lewia*
13.	*Cercospora*	*Mycosphaerella*
14.	*Septoria*	*Mycosphaerella*
15.	*Phyllosticta*	*Guignardia*
16.	*Stemphylium*	*Pleospora*
17.	*Bipolaris*	*Cochliobolus*
18.	*Drechslera*	*Pyrenophora*
19.	*Exserohilum*	*Setosphaera*
20.	*Curvularia*	*Cochliobolus*
21.	*Sphaeropsis*	*Physalospora*

Apothecial ascomycetes		
22.	*Monilia*	*Monilinia*
23.	*Botrytis*	*Botryotinia*
24.	*Melanconium*	*Greeneria*
25.	*Cylindrosporium*	*Mycospharella*
26.	*Entomosporium*	*Diplocarpon*
Basidiomycetes		
27.	*Rhizoctonia*	*Thanatephorus*
28.	*Sclerotium*	*Aethalium*

CHAPTER - 12

Prokaryotes: Classification of Prokaryotes according to Bergey's Manual of Systematic Bacteriology

PROKARYOTES

Prokaryotic organisms are that in which nucleus is primitive type and nuclear material is not enclosed within the nuclear membrane.

Bacteria are placed in the kingdom "Prokaryotae" because of the prokaryotic cellular organization of the members. However, extremely diverse groups of microorganisms differing in morphological, physiological and ecological properties are found within this kingdom. In the beginning, description and information of bacterial systematics or classification was being published in the comprehensive volumes of "Bergey's Manual of Determinative Bacteriology" (1923, first edition). The 9th edition of Bergey's Manual, published in 1984 was the last of such comprehensive manual and from 1984 onwards it was renamed as "Bergey's *Manual of Systematic Bacteriology"*. It is the most widely accepted and used reference document or book for classification and identification of bacteria. In the 9th edition, the kingdom Prokaryota (Monera) is divided into 4 divisons based on nature of the cell wall. These are : ***Gracilicultes***; ***Firmicutes***; ***Tenericutes*** and ***Mendosicutes*** .

Kingdom: Prokaryota

Division 1. Gracilicutes

Important character

1. Usually gram reaction is negative.
2. Cell wall consisting of an outer membrane, a peptidoglycan layer and a unit membrane with fatty acid glycerol ester type lipid.
3. Endospore is not formed.

4. Divided into two classes- Proteobacteria and Oxyphotobacteria on the basis of phylogenetic principles.
5. All gram –ve plant pathogenic bacteria are included in proteobacteria and scattered in three main classes.

Divison 2. Firmicutes

Important character

1. Gram reaction is generally, but not always positive.
2. Cell wall consisting of a thick peptidoglycan and unit membrane but without an outer membrane.
3. Some produce endospores.
4. Divided into two classes of firmibacteria and thallobacteria
5. Bacillus and Clostridium are included into Firmibacteria.
6. Actinomycetes and related bacteria such as *Streptomyces, Clavibacter, Rhodococcus*, *Curobacterium*, and *Nocardia* are included in Thallobacteria.

Divison 3. Tenericutes

Important character

- Prokaryotes that lack a cell wall.
- Highly polymorphic.
- The cells are enclosed by a unit membrane.
- Includes class Mollicutes in which plant pathogenic MLO (Phytoplasma) and Spiroplasma belong.

Divison 4. Mendosicutes

Important character

- The prokaryotes which have a cell envelop without conventional peptidoglycan or cell wall material are included.
- Cell walls are made entirely of heteropolysaccharides and protein macromolecules.
- Gram reaction is positive or negative.
- This divison has a single class- Archaeobacteria

- No plant pathogenic prokaryotes belongs to this divison.

The four divison are further divided into folling classes, orders and families;

Divison I	Gracilicutes	Gram negative bacteria
Class	Scotobacteria	Gram negative, non photosynthetic,bacteria
Class	Anoxyphotobacteria	Gram negative, photosynthetic bacteria that produce oxygen
Class	Oxyphotobacteria	Gram negative, photosynthetic bacteria that produce oxygen

Some families and genera under divisions Gracilicutes

Family	Genus
Neisseriaceae	Neisseria, Acinetobacter
Pseudomonadaceae	Pseudomonas, Xanthomonas
Azotobacteriaceae	Azotobacter
Rhizobcaceae	Rhizobium, Agrobacterium
Enterobacteriaceae	Erwinia, Enterobactor
Vibrionaceae	Vibrio
Bacterioidaceae	Bacterioids
Spirochaetaceae	Spirochaeta
Rickettsiaceae	Rickettsia
Bartonellaceae	Bartonella
Chlamydaceae	Chlamydia

Divison II	Firmicutes	Gram positive bacteria
Class	*Firmibacteria*	Gram positive rods and cocci
Class	*Thallobacteria*	Gram positive branching cells- the actinomycetes

Some families and genera under division Firmicutes

Family	Genus
Microccaceae	Microccaceae
Peptococcaceae	Peptococcus
Bacillaceae	Bacillus, Clostridium
Lactobacillaceae	Lactobacillus
Propionibacteriaceae	Propiniobacterum
Corynebacteriaceae	Corynebacterium
Mycobacteraiceae	Mycobacterium
Nocardiaceae	Nocardia
Actinomycetaceae	Actinomycetes

Contd...

Streptomycetaceae		Streptomyces	
Streptococcaceae		Streptococcus	
Divison III	**Tenericutes**	**Bacteria with soft or no cell walls**	
Class		Mollicutes	The Mycoplasmas
Some families and genera under division Tenericutes			
Family		**Genus**	
Mycoplasmataceae		Mycoplasma, Ureaplasma	
Acholeplasmataceae		Acholeplasma	
Spiroplasmataceaee		Sprioplasma	
Divison IV	**Mendosicutes**	Bacteria that lack peptidoglycan in their cell wall	
Class	*Archaebacteria*	Bacteria with typical compounds in the cell wall and the membranes	

CHAPTER - 13

The Pathogens-Bacteria

DEFINITION

Bacteria belong to prokaryota which encompasses organisms with a primitive type of nucleus lacking a clearly defined membrane .The bacteria are smaller than fungi and measure about 0.5 to 1.0 x 2.0 to 5.0μ.

Structure of Bacteria

1. A bacterial cell consists of a cellwall and a compound membrane enclosing protoplasm.
2. Inside the protoplasm, nucleus, vacuoles, mesosomes, polysaccharides, lipids, mitochondric granules and spores are found.
3. Externally bacterial cells may show capsules, pili, fimbrae and flagella.
4. The bacterial cell contains a characteristics cell wall.
5. The cell wall of bacteria is composed of a **peptidoglycan**. It is composed of **acetyle-glucosamine** and **cetyle-muramic acid**.
6. The rigid peptidoglycan layer is located between the cytoplasmic membrane and an outer multiple tract layer.
7. The latter layer is composed of lipoprotein . It is common in gram negative bacteria.
8. Many bacteria possess other intracellular membrane systems such as mesosomes and chondrioids.
9. The **mesosome** structure is formed by an invagination of the cytoplasmic membrane.
10. Mesosomes serve for compartmentalization and integration of biochemical systems.

11. The cell material contained within the cytoplasmic membrane can be divided into the cytoplasmic are rich in RNA , nuclear area rich in DNA and the fluid portion with dissolved nutrients.
12. Bacteria do not have characteristic **nucleus**. They contain bodies within the cytoplasm that are regarded as a nuclear structure and DNA is confined to this area.
13. Bacteria contain **3 to 70 ribosomes** depending upon the bacteria. Ribosomes are the sites of protein synthesis.
14. Lipids are found in the cytoplasm of bacteria in the form of fat globules.
15. Glycogen accumulates in the cytoplasm at the ends of the cell in the form of granules.
16. Some of the bacteria possess flagella which are useful for motility of the bacteria.
17. The bacteria belonging to Eubacteriales have peritrichous flagellus-flagella at all the sides.
18. Some bacteria transform themselves into small ovals or spheres which are highly resistant to adverse conditions. They are called as **spores**.
19. Bacterial spores have **dipicolinic acid** which is absent in vegetative cells. Dipicolinic acid is found only in bacterial spores.
20. Fibriae are hair like structures that are observed as surface appendages on some bacteria. **Fimbriae** are common in plant pathogenic bacteria.
21. **Pili** are also hair like structures found in some bacteria. They serve as adsorption organs for bacteriophages. **Pili** mediate **conjugation** of bacteria.
22. Most of the plant pathogenic bacteria are rod shaped except *Streptomyces* which are mostly **filmentous**.
23. Majority of plant pathogenic bacteria are **aerobic** except; *Erwinia*
24. Plant pathogenic bacteria required optimum growth temperature ranging between 27-30^{0}C.
25. Most of the plant pathogenic bacteria reproduce by asexual process known as binary **fission** or **fission**.
26. Most of the plant pathogenic bacteria are **gram negative** except *Streptomyces, Clavibactor, Curtobacterium, Nocardia* and *Rhodococcus* which are gram positive in Gram's reaction.

27. In *Streptomyces, Clavibacter* and *Bacillus* a part of cell membrane envaginates into the cytoplasm to form complex membrane infolding called as **mesosomes**.

28. *Bacillus* and *Clostridium* species produce **endosproes** which are dormant structures.

29. Bacterial cell lacking cell wall is called **protoplast**.

30. The naked protoplast may synthesize a portion of cell wall material. Such a protoplast is called **sphaeroplast**.

31. L forms are non rigid bacterial forms. They are soft protoplasmic elements without defined morphology which can be propagated indefinitely on solid medium.

32. L-form of bacteria are usually produced under unfavourable conditions or in laboratory when **penicillin** or other substances that inhibit cell wall production are added to culture medium,

33. The L-form plant pathogenic bacteria reported are *Agrobacterium tumefaciens* and *Erwinia*

34. Protoplast, sphaeroplasts and L-forms are all bacterial forms devoid of the **rigid cell wall**.

35. **Plasmids** are **extra chromosomal DNA** capable of autonomous replication. Some bacteria have plasmids in the cytoplasm. They are not capable of integrated with the chromosome.

36. **Episomes** are similar to plasmids. They are also autonomous and dispensable genetic elements. But unlike plasmids, episomes, can exist even integrated with the chromosome

37. Generally the bacteria contains plasmids do not have episomes and vice versa.

38. **Transposons** are mobile DNA segments that can insert into a few or several sites in a genome .

39. Transponsons are even capable of moving between prokaryotes and eukaryotes.

40. **Siderophores** are produced by many bacateria extracellularly. They are low molecular weight **iron (III) transport agents**. The function of siderophores is to **supply iron** to the cell.The siderophore isolated from *Pseudomonas* sp. is called **pseudobactin.**

41. **Bacteriosins** are non replicationg , bactericidal protein-containing substances which are produced by certain strains of bacteria and are

active against some other strains of the same or closely related species.

42. Bacteriosins are useful in the control of diseases. Bacteriocins produced by avirulent isolates are exploited to control diseases caused by virulent isolates of the same bacterium.

Reproduction of Bacteria

1. Fission

- The most common mode of reproduction in bacteria.
- The bacterial cells divide into two daughter cells.
- It is asexual reproduction.

2. Conjugation

- Genetic material of one cell is transferred to another cell during conjugation.
- The two cells are genetically different.
- The donor cell transfers part of its genome to the recipient cell.
- Conjugation is one type of genetic recombination
- Genetic recombination refers to any process leading to the formation of a new individual which derives some of its gene from one parent and some from another, genetically different, parent.

3. Transforamtion

- DNA from one type of bacterium is incorporated into the genetic makeup of another organism during transformation.
- In this DNA is absorbed through external source. This is a method employed in laboratory to bring about recombination : but it may be occurring in nature as well.

4. Transduction

- Virus that infects bacteria is called bacteriophage.
- Bacteriophage grows within a bacterial cell.
- The infected bacterial cell bursts and the bacteriophage particles are liberated.
- Some of the bacteriophage particles released carry some genetic

material of the host bacterial cell.

- They enter into another bacterial cell and the genetic material brought into the cell by the virus is incorporated into that of the bacteria .
- By this process a new genotype of the bacterium arises and this process is called transduction.

The Genetics of Bacteria

A). The short generation span of bacteria facilitates their evolutionary adaptation to changing environments.

The average bacterial genome is larger than a viral genome, but much smaller than a typical eukaryotic genome.

The major component of the bacterial genome is the *bacterial chromosome*. This structure is:

- Composed of one double-stranded, circular molecule of DNA
- Structurally simpler and has fewer associated proteins than a eukaryotic chromosome
- Found in the *nucleoid* region; since this region is not separated from the rest of the cell (by a membrane), transcription and translation can occur simultaneously.

Many bacteria also contain extrachromosomal DNA in plasmids.

Plasmid = A small double-stranded ring of DNA that carries extrachromosomal genes in some bacteria

Most bacteria can rapidly reproduce by *binary fission*, which is preceded by DNA replication.

- Semi-conservative replication of the bacterial chromosome begins at a single origin of replication.
- The two replication forks move bi directionally until they meet and replication is complete.
- Under optimal conditions, some bacteria can divide in twenty minutes. Because of this rapid reproductive rate, bacteria are useful for genetic studies.

Binary fission is asexual reproduction that produces clones, or daughter cells that are genetically identical to the parent.

- Though mutations are rare events, they can impact genetic diversity in bacteria because of their rapid reproductive rate.

- Though mutation can be a major source of genetic variation in bacteria, it is *not* a major source in more slowly reproducing organisms (e.g., humans). In most higher organisms, genetic recombination from sexual reproduction is responsible for most of the genetic diversity within populations.

B). Genetic Recombination Produces New Bacterial Strains

There are three natural processes of genetic recombination in bacteria: *transformation*, *transduction,* and *conjugation*. These mechanisms of gene transfer occur separately from bacterial reproduction, and in addition to mutation, are another major source of genetic variation in bacterial populations.

1. Transformation = Process of gene transfer during which a bacterial cell assimilates foreign DNA from the surroundings

- Some bacteria can take up naked DNA from the surroundings.
- Assimilated foreign DNA may be integrated into the bacterial chromosome by recombination (crossing over).
- Progeny of the recipient bacterium will carry a new combination of genes.

2. Transduction = Gene transfer from one bacterium to another by a bacteriophage.

Generalized transduction = Transduction that occurs when random pieces of host cell DNA are packaged within a phage capsid during the lytic cycle of a phage

- This process can transfer almost any host gene and little or no phage genes.
- When the phage particle infects a new host cell, the donor cell DNA can recombine with the recipient cell DNA.

Specialized transduction = Transduction that occurs when a prophage excises from the bacterial chromosome and carries with it only certain host genes adjacent to the excision site. Also known as **restricted transduction.**

3. Conjugation = The direct transfer of genes between two cells that are temporarily joined. Conjugation in *E. coli* is one of the best-studied examples:

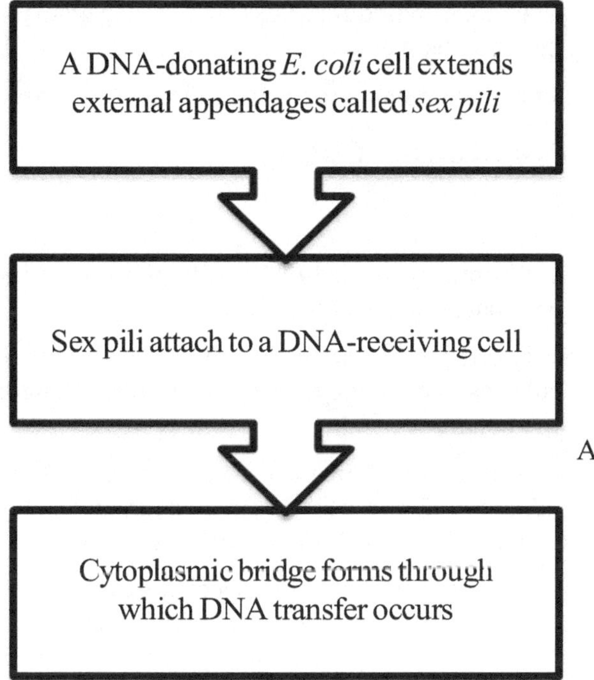

The ability to form sex pili and to transfer DNA is conferred by genes in a plasmid called the *F plasmid.*

GRAM STAINING

- Gram staining is useful to distinguish plant pathogens
- Based on gram stain reaction, the bacteria can be grouped as gram positive and gram negative.
- To do the gram staining the bacterial smear is prepared and subjected to the following solutions in the order listed: crystal violet, iodine solution, alcohol, and saffranin.
- Gram positive bacteria retain the crystal violet and hence appear deep violet in color.
- Gram negative bacteria lose the crystal violet and counter stained by the saffranin, and hence appear red in color.
- Gram negative bacterial cell walls contain minor of lipids. Alcohol treatment extracts the lipid and the crystal violet-iodine complex is also extracted.

- The crystal violet-iodine complex is retained in gram positive bacteria during alcohol treatment.
- Most of the plant pathogenic bacteria is gram negative.

PLANT PATHOGENIC BACTERIA

General Characters

1. Barring Streptomyces, which is filamentous, Almost all plant pathogenic bacteria are **rod shaped**.
2. The rod shaped bacteria are more or less short and cylindrical and in young cultures, they range from 0.6 to 3.5μm in length and from 0.5 to 1.0μm in diameter.
3. Sometimes deviations from the rod shape in the form of a club , a Y or V shaped, and other branched forms occur, and some bacteria may occasionally occur in pairs or in short chains.
4. The cell walls of bacteria of most species are enveloped by a viscous, gummy material, which may be thin (Slime layer) or may be thick, forming a relatively large mass around the cell (Capsule).
5. Most plant pathogenic bacteria are equipped with delicate, thread like flagella.
6. In some bacterial species each bacterium has only the flagellum, others, have a tuff of flagella at one end of the cell (Polar flagella); some have a single flagellum or a tuft of flagella at each end, and till others have peritrichous flagella, that is, distributed over the entire surface of the cell.
7. In the filamentous Streptomyces species, the cells consist of non septate branched threads, which usually have a spiral formation and produce conidia in chains on aerial hyphae.
8. Single bacterium appears hyaline or yellowish white under the compound microscope.
9. Bacteria grow and produce colonies on solid medium.
10. Colonies of different species may vary in size, shape, form of edges, elevation and colour, and are sometimes characteristics of a given species.
11. Bacterial cells have thin, relatively tough, and somewhat rigid cell walls.
12. All the material inside the cell wall constitutes the protoplast.

13. The nuclear material consist of a large circular chromosome composed DNA and appear as spherical, ellipsoidal or dumbbell shaped body within the cytoplasm.
14. Often bacteria also have single or multiple copies of addition smaller circular chromosomes called 'Plasmids' that can move or be moved between bacteria or between bacteria and plants as for example in the crown gall disease.
15. Rod shaped Phytopathogenic bacteria reproduce by the asexual process known as binary fission or fission. Under favourable conditions bacteria may divide every 20 minutes.
16. Almost all plant pathogenic bacteria develop mostly in the host plant as parasites and partly in plant debris or in the soil as saprophytes.

IMPORTANT PLANT PATHOGENIC BACTERIA

Morphology

It is the study of size, shape, structure, and arrangement of cells.

a) Size of Bacteria:

Bacteria are minute, as single drop of water may contains about 50 billions of bacteria are usually measured in micrometer (μm).

1. Size may varies depending upon the species. Size generally ranges from 1 to 10 microns.
2. Most of the bacterial cells 0.5 to 1 μm in width or diameter.
3. Cylindrical or rod (Baclli) 2-3 μm length.
4. Spiral or helical (Spirlli) – 0.75 -1.25 μm.

b) Shape in Bacteria:

The shapes of bacterial cells are

Spherical or Ellipsoidal or Oval – **Cocci**

Cylindrical or rod- **Bacilli**

Spiral or Helical – **Spirilli**

Some species have variety of shapes and thus termed as pleomorphic. e.g. Arthrobacter.

c) Arrangement of Bacterial Cells:

Bacterial cells are arranged in a characteristic manner of the particular species. The typical pattern of cell arrangement in different bacteria is an important characteristics used in identification of bacteria.

d) Cell grouping or Arrangement in Cocci:

i) **Monococcus:** Single spherical bacterial cell.

ii) **Diplococcus:** A coccus divides into two plane and cells remains in pairs.

iii) **Streptococcus:** A coccus is arranged in a long chain e.g. Streptococcus sp.

iv) **Tetrad:** A coccus divides in two plans, second division at a right angle to the first plane of division and forms a square of four cells. e.g. Tetracoccus sp

v) **Sarcina:** A cube of eight coccus cell is formed by three divisions in alternate planes at right angle to each other. A cube of eight cells is known as Sarcina.

vi) **Staphylococci:** A coccus cells divides in three planes in irregular pattern like cluster of cells or bunch of grapes. e.g. **Staphylococcus albus**

vii) **Vibrio:** The short comma shaped cells are called as **Vibrio.** Short tightly coined rods are called **spirillum**. Vey long cell with several cuvves and twiste are called **"Spirochete"**.

e) Cell Grouping or Arrangement in Bacilli:

i) **Monobacilli:** Single rod shaped bacterial cell. e.g. *Monobacillus.*

ii) **Diplobacilli:** Bacilli are arranged in a pair of two cells. e.g. *Bacillus subtilis.*

iii) **Streptobacilli:** Cells are arranged in a chain. e.g. *Lactobacillus bukgaricus.*

iv) **Palisade:** Group of cells lined side by side like matchsticks in a match box called as palisade arrangement.

f) Flagellar Arrangement in Bacteria:

All types of bacteria do not have a flagella they are mostly present in Bacilli and Spirilli and rarely in cocci.

i) **Atrichous:** A cell without flagella.

ii) **Monotrichous:** Single polar flagellum at one end.

iii) **Amphitrichous:** A cell with a single polar flagellum at both the ends. e.g Spirillim.

iv) **Lophotrichous:** A cell having tuft or bunch of flagella at both the ends. e.g. Coli.

v) **Caphalotrichous:** A cell having a pair of flagella at one end.

g) Arrangement in Spirilli:

The Spirilli are predominantly unattached however they differ in frequency of turns and overall length. They are grouped in three types as:

a) Short tightly coiled rod called **spitillium**

b) Short incomplete spirals called as **comma** or **vibrios**.

c) They are long twisted with several curves calls **"Spirochete"**.

CLASSIFICATION OF PLANT PATHOGENIC BACTERIA

The bacteria belongs to the class **Schizomycetes**. Plant pathogenic belongs to 3 different orders.

1. Order: Pseudomonadales

Family : Pseudomonadaceae

Important Characters

- It does not produe non water soluble pigment.
- It produces soluble pigment which is not yellow.
- No acid is produced from lactose.

Genera : *Pseudomonas*

Important Plant Pathogens

Sl.No	Name of Pathogen	Name of disease
1.	*Pseudomonas solanacearum*	Wilts of tomato, banana, brinjal, potato
2.	*Pseudomonas tabaci*	Wild fire of tobacco
3.	*Pseudomonas syringae pv. phaseolicola*	Halo blight of beans

Genera : *Xanthomonas*

Important Characters

- Culture develop an yellow non water soluble pigment
- Produce acid from lactose.

Important Plant Pathogens

Sl.No	Name of Pathogen	Name of disease
1.	*Xanthomons campestris*	Black rot of cabbage
2.	*Xanthomons campestris* pv. *oryzae*	Bacterial blight of rice
3.	*Xanthomons campestris* pv. *citri*	Citrus canker
4.	*Xanthomons campestris* pv. *malvacearum*	Black arm of cotton

2. Order: Eubacteriales

I. Family : Enterobacteriaceae

Important Characters

- The bacterial cells are gram negative and motile with peritrichous flagella.
- They produce acid from sugars.

Genus : *Erwinia*

Important Plant Pathogens

Sl.No	Name of Pathogen	Name of disease
1.	*Erwinia amylovora*	Fire blight of apple
2.	*Erwinia carotovora*	Soft rot of many vegetables

II. Family: Rhizobeaceae

Important Characters

- The cells are rod shaped, gram negative and sparsely flagellated.
- The colonies are white.
- The genus *Agrobacterium* is pathogenic on plants.

Genus : *Agrobacterium*

Important Plant Pathogens

Sl.No	Name of Pathogen	Name of disease
1.	*Agrobacterium tumefaciens*	Crown gall in many fruit trees

III. Family : Corynebacteriaceae

Important Characters

- The bacterial cells are gram positive.
- *Corynebacterium* is the only gram positive plant pathogen while others are gram negative.
- The bacterial cells are pleomorphic rod that show the characteristic arrangement produced by snapping division.
- They are motile rods.

Genus : *Corynebacterium*

Important Plant Pathogens

Sl.No	Name of Pathogen	Name of disease
1.	*Corynebacterium michiganense*	Bacterial wilt of tomato
2.	*Corynebacterium tritici*	Tundu disease of wheat
3.	*Corynebacterium sepedonicum*	Leaf spot and wilt in many crops
4.	*Corynebacterium insidiosum*	Leaf spot of many crops
5.	*Corynebacterium rathayi*	Gummosis in many crops

3.Order: Actinomycetales

Family : Streptomycetaceae

Important Characters

- It produces conidia in aerial hyphae in chains.

- It has characteristic branching mycelium and spores are formed by fragmentation of the plasma straight or rod shaped .

Important Plant Pathogens

Sl.No	Name of Pathogen	Name of disease
1.	*Streptomyces scabies*	Potato scab

MODE OF ENTRY

Bacteria cannot penetrate host tissues as they do not have germ tubes and appresorium. They enter the host through different types of natural opening.

Sl. No.	Pathogen	Enter through	Disease
1.	*Streptomyces scabies*	Lenticels	Scab of potato
2.	*Pseudomonas tabaci*	Stomata	Wild fire of tobacco
3.	*Xanthomonas phaseoli*	Stomata	Bean blight
4.	*Xanthomonas campestris*	Stomata	Black rot of cabbage
5.	*Xanthomonas campestris pv. malvacearum*	Stomata	Angular leaf spot of cotton.
6.	*X.campestris pv. oryzae*	Wounds	Bacterial blight of rice
7.	*Erwinia* spp.	Wounds	Soft rot of vegetables
8.	*Agrobacterium tumefaciens*	Wounds	Crown gall of fruit trees
9.	*Xanthomonas campestris*	Hydathodes	Black rot of cabbage
10.	*Erwinia amylovora*	Floral parts	Fire blight of apple

MODE OF SPREAD

Sl.No.	Transmitted through	Pathogen	Disease
1.	Seed	*Xanthomonas malvacearum* *X.campestris pv. oryzae*	Black arm of cotton Bacterial blight of rice
2.	Soil	*Pseudomonas solanacearum,*	Wilts of tomato, banana,
		X. campestris pv. malvacearum	Wilt of brinjal, potato, cotton
3.	Insect		
I	Honey bees	*Erwinia amylovora*	Fire blight of apple
II	Corn flea beetle	*Xanthomonas stewartii*	Corn wilt
4.	Nemaode		
I	*Anguina tritici*	*Corynubacterium tritici*	Tundu disease of wheat
II	*Meloidogyne var. acrita*	*Pseudomonas solanacearum*	Wilt of tomato
5.	Crop debris	*Xanthomonas malvacearum*	Black arm of cotton

PERPETUATION OF BACTERIA

The Phytopathogenic bacteria do not produce any resting structures. They survive by some of the following ways:

1. Survival on self sown plant, collateral hosts

Bacterial pathogen survives and multiplies on self sown plants of host crop, collateral hosts during the main and the off seasons. The collateral hosts are most often perennial or noxious weeds growing in the host crop fields, or in their vicinity while others may be cultivated economic crop plants. The host range of some bacterial plant pathogens is very wide. e.g. :

- *Pseudomonas solaneceanum* -200 host plants.
- *Agrobacterium tumefaciens*- 150 host plants.

2. Survival on host crop

The pathogens of the bacterial leaf blight and the leaf streak of rice may survive from crop to crop in double or triple – rice culture areas in the tropics. The latent infections as in cankers, galls, bud scales, the cracks in the bark or sheltered place are often further protected by the host mucilage in trees as in the citrus canker or the fire blight.

3. Survival on non host plants

Xanthomonas campestris pv. citri causal agent of citrus canker has been found to survive in the non-host plants. The saprophytic existence of *X. campestris pv. phasebli* on the phyllosphere of *Phaseolus vulgaris* has been found.

4. Survival through crop residues and in soil

Some of the Phytopathogenic bacteria are capable of living saprophytically on plant residues or pearennate in the soil in free state or on any organic matter. e.g *Erwinia* spp. *Pseudomonas solanacearum racee 2, Xanthomoans campestris pv. malvacearum*. Most of the bacterial pathogens of aerial parts can not survive in a natural soil for a long time due to their poor competitive saprophytic ability and antagonism of other microorganisms.

5. Survival through seeds and vegetative propagation parts

Some of the phyopathogenic bacteria survive in seeds of some crops and vegetative plant parts used for propagation e. g *Xanthomonas campestris pv. oyzae* and *Xanthomonas campestris pv. malvacearum* survive through seeds. *Pseudomonas solanacearum* survive in potato tubers.

IMPORTANT PHYTOPATHOGENIC BACTERIA

Sr. No	Genus	Gram Reaction	Characters	Symptoms produced on host	Example
1.	*Pseudomonas*	Gram-ve	1. Rod straight to curved, size 0.5-1 X 1.5-4 μ m, one to many polar flagella. 2. Colonies not yellow, do not produce acid from lactose.	Leaf spot, blights, vascular wilts, soft rots, canker.	1. Brown rot or bacterial wilt of potato 2 Bacterial wilt of brinjal and tomato
2.	*Xanthomonas*	Gram-ve	1. Straight rods, size 0.4-1X 1.2 -3 μ m. One polar flagellum present. 2. Colonies yellow due to Xanthomonadin, produce acid from lactose.	Leaf spot, fruit spots, blight, canker	1. Citrus canker 2. Black arm of cotton 3.Blight of paddy
3.	*Erwinia*	Gram-ve	1. Straight rods, size 0.5-1, 0-3.0 μ m, several peritrichous flagella.	Fire blight, wilt soft rot.	1. Fire blight of apple. 2. Soft rot of vegetables.
4.	*Agrobacterium*	Gram-ve	1. Rod shaped, size 0.8 X 1.5 -3 μ m. 1 to 4 peritrichous flagella. 2. Colonies mostly white do not hydrolyze starch.	Crown Gall	1. Crown Gall of stone fruit.
5.	*Clavibactor (Corynebacterium)*	Gram +ve	Straight to straightly curved rods, 0.5-0.9X 1.5-4.0 μ m. non motile but some species are motile by one or two polar flagella.	Wilt	1. Wilt of potato and Tomato
6.	*Streptomyces*	Gram-ve	Slender branched hyphae without cross walls 0.5-2 μ m diameter.	Scab	1. Potato scab

MANAGEMENT OF BACTERIAL DISEASES

Bacterial plant pathogens directly enter the host tissue either through natural openings or through wounds; therefore, it is tricky to manage them. Some of the general principles of managing the bacterial disease are as follows:

1. Plant Sanitation

These measures are adopted so as to avoid the disease onset and also to prevent spread. e.g.

i) Collection and destruction of diseased fallen leaves, bolls etc. for bacterial blight of cotton.

ii) Removal of dead plant parts from fruit crops and protection of cut surface with suitable bactericides (e. g for citrus canker and fire blight of apple).

iii) Avoiding injuries to the plant parts at the time of cultural operations and during harvest, transport and storage.

2. Exclusion

Exclusion of a disease entry either from a foreign nation or within the country, from a diseased to a healthy tract is an effective measure for avoiding the disease. Quarantine measures are in vogue in several countries. Examle of diseased managed: Citrus canker.

3. Eradication

Eradication is generally carried out for eliminating a well established pathogen and its host plant, collateral hosts, or insect vectors and some times use of cultural measures for starving out or killing the pathogen. Examples of disease managed.

i) Pruning of the infected twigs is followed to reduce the inoculums in orchards for citrus canker.

ii) The destruction of volunteer plants and weed hosts brings down the inoculum level. e.g Brown rot of potato .

iii) The crop residue may be burnt or ploughed deep into the soil with watering to ensure decomposition, which is helpful for the pathogens which cannot live saprophytically in the soil. e. g. Bacterial blight of cotton.

iv). Crop rotation with cereals is advocated for the management of wilt of tobacco.

v) The balanced application of NPK , particularly low and split doses of N, helps to reduce the intensity of the bacterial leaf blight of rice.

vi) The control of vectors is helpful in reducing the citrus canker and soft rot of vegetables.

vii) The avoidance of cultural mismanagement favourable to disease is important viz., flooding or over irrigation in the field (against the soft rot disease) and water logging in the nurseries (against the bacterial leaf blight of rice).

viii) The sterilization of the cutting knife by flame or by 0.1 % KMNO4 solution while cutting the potato tuber for sowing is recommended against the potato wilt.

ix) The seed certification programes to raise pathogen free seeds.

x) Elimination of the externally and internally seed born pathogen by seed treatment. e. g

1. Soaking of rice seeds in 0.025% strp etocyclic solution for leaf blight disease of rice.
2. Delinting of cotton seed with concentrated sulphuric acid for bacterial blight of cotton.
3. Hot water treatment of cotton seed at 56^0 C for 10 minutes for bacterial blight of cotton.

xi) When tobacco is immediately grown after maize there is a considerable reduction in the incidence of *Pseudomonas solanacearum* on the later host.

4. Plant Protection

Plant protection measures are adopted to prevent the commencement and subsequent spread of plant diseases. e. g.

i) Seed treatment of rice and cotton with antibiotics against bacterial blight and leaf streak diseases respectively.

ii) Treatment of seed tubers of potato with streptocycline @ 0.02% for 30 minutes, against brown rot disease.

iii) Foliar sprays with Bordeaux mixture and copper oxychloride against leaf spots and blights.

iv) Foliar sprays of streptomycin sulphate, 100 and 500 ppm against citrus canker and fire blight of apple.

v) Therapy: Pancillin and vancomycin are effective in the disintegration of the crown gall. The application of antibiotics for protection also involves therapy. The bacteriocines have also been demonstrated to be successful against bacterial disease e. g *Agrobacterium radiobacter* against crown gall of peach and tomato seedlings (*Agrobacterium fumetaciens*.)

vi) Immunization: By screening under artificial epiphytic conditions, resistance source for bacterial pathogens can be known. Resistant varieties are evolved by selection, breeding and other methods. e. g BJA-592, P-14, T-12, HC-9, 101-102 B, Reba-B-50, Khandwa-2, DHY-286, B-1007, cultivars of cotton and N-22, IR-22 cultivars of rice resistant to bacterial blight disease of these crops.

CHAPTER - 14

The Pathogens - Viruses

DEFINITION OF VIRUS

Viruses are very small (submicroscopic) infectious particles (virions) composed of a protein coat and a nucleic acid core. They carry genetic information encoded in their nucleic acid, which typically specifies two or more proteins. Translation of the genome (to produce proteins) or transcription and replication (to produce more nucleic acid) takes place within the host cell and uses some of the host's biochemical "machinery". Viruses do not capture or store free energy and are not functionally active outside their host. They are therefore parasites (and usually pathogens) but are not usually regarded as genuine microorganisms.

Mathwas (1981) considers a virus as a set of one or more template molecules normally encased in a protective coat or coats of protein or lipoprotein, which is able to organize its own replication only within suitable host cells where its production is:

i) Dependent on hosts protein synthesizing machinery (ribosomes).

ii) Organised from pools of required material rather than binary fission and

iii) Located at sites which are not separated from the host cell contents by a lipoprotein bilayer membrane.

Bos (1983) defines virus as an infectious agent often causing disease, invisible with the light microscope (Sub-microscopic), small enough to pass through a bacterial filter, lacking a metabolism of its own and depending on a living host cell for multiplication. Viruses are small packages of host alien genetic information of one type. (RNA or DNA), either in one strand or in a few segment. Encapsulated together or separately and enclosed in a coat of one or more types of protein, some time with an extra coat (envelope) and some other constituents.

CHARACTERISTIC OF VIRUS

1. Viruses contain a single type of nucleic acid, either RNA or DNA, never both.
2. The nucleic acid carries the genome of the virus which differs from one virus to another.
3. The genome in the nucleic acid strand directs the synthesis of specific proteins for the protein coat which must be present in all viruses throughout their active phase except at the time of replication when, protein coat and nucleic acid are separated
4. Viruses rely on living host cells for most of the enzymes necessary for their replication.
5. Viruses are in cable of growing for the synthesis of **Lipman system** is absent in Viruses.

NATURE OF VIRUS

Each plant virus consists of two components the **nucleic acid** and the **protein coat** or capsid. The mature particle of a plant virus is generally called **virion** and the whole infective particle is called as **Nuclcocapsid.**

Nucleic Acid of Viruses

1. Nucleic acid portion of the virus particle is called as **Genome**.
2. Genomes are organized as single nucleic acid molecules that are **linear** or **circular**
3. They may have as few as four genes or as many as several hundred.
4. They may be double-stranded DNA, single-stranded DNA, double-stranded RNA, or single-stranded RNA
5. Genome is actual infective component.
6. Majority of plant viruses contain **RNA** .
7. Some viruses (Cauliflower mosaic virus, , maize streak virus, mung bean yellow mosaic virus) contain DNA.
8. Most plant viruses contain single strand of RNA.
9. In double stranded viruses (as RNA or ds DNA) the two strands are coiled around each other helically.

The Virus Protein

1. Protein coat that encloses the viral genome is called **capsid.**
2. Its structure may be rod-shaped, polyhedral, or complex.
3. Composed of many **capsomeres,** protein subunits made from only one or a few types of protein.
4. It helps viruses infect their host.
5. It protects nucleic acid (RNA or DNA) of virus.
6. It is made-up of different amino acid sequences in different viruses.
7. Protein shell or coat protects viral nucleic acid from environment.

DIFFERENT TYPES OF VIRUSES

The following are the examples for different types of viruses

Sl.No	Types		Examples
1.	**RNA viruses**		
	a. Single stranded	With one segment	Tobacco mosaic virus, Lettuce necrotic yellow virus
		With two segments	Cowpea mosaic virus, Tobacco ring spot virus
		With three segments	Cucumber mosaic virus
		With more number of segments	Potato virus x Tomato spotted wilt virus
	b. Double stranded		Wound tumour virus Fiji disease virus Reo virus
2.	**DNA viruses**		
	Double stranded		Cauliflower mosaic virus
	Single stranded		Maize streak virus, 2”X174

3. Satellite Viruses

These are viruses associated with certain typical viruses but depend on the latter for multiplication and plant infection and reduce the ability of the typical viruses act like parasite of the associated typical virus.

4. Helper Viruses

The viruses which help multiplication of satellite RNA are called helper viruses.

5. Virusoids

These are viriod like, small, single stranded , circular RNAs that are present inside some RNA viruses. Virusoids are the part of genetic material of these viruses and therefore , form an obligatory association with these viruses so that neither the virus not the virusoid can multiply and infect a plant in the absence of its partner.

6. Temperate Viruses

Viruses that can integrate their genome into a host chromosome and remain latent until they initiate a lytic cycle.

7. Provirus

Viral DNA that inserts into a host cell chromosome.

8. Retrovirus (Retro = backward)

RNA virus that uses reverse transcriptase to transcribe DNA from the viral RNA genome.

9. Viroid

These are small (250-400 nucleotide), naked, single stranded, circular RNAs capable of causing disease in plants by themselves.

MORPHOLOGY OF VIRUSES

Plant viruses are usually described as

1. Elongated (Rigid rod or Flexious thread)

Sl.No	Morphology	Example	Size(nm)
1.	Rigid rod	*Barley stripe mosaic virus*	20X 10
		Tobacco mosaic virus	15 X 300
2.	Flexuous thread	*Potato virus X*	10-13 X480
		Citrus tristeza virus	10-14 X 2000

2. Spherical (Isometric or Polyhedral)

All spherical viruses are actually polyhedral ranging in diameter about 17 nm to 60 nm. Examples;

Sl.No	Example	Diameter (nm)
1.	Tobacco necrosis satellite virus	17
2.	Wound tumour virus	60
3.	Tomato spotted wilt virus	70-80

3. Rhabdo Viruses

These are short bacillus like rods approximately 3 to 5 times as long as they are wide.

Sl.No	Example	Diameter (nm)
1.	Potato yellow dwarf virus	75X 380 nm.
2.	Wheat striate mosaic virus	65X 270 nm.
3.	Lettuce necrotic yellow virus	52 X 300 nm.

PROPERTIES OF PLANT VIRUS

1. Biological Properties

Each virus produces its own protein, its function is to protect RNA from host enzymes (Ribonuclease), heat, ultra violet light and chemical protein has no infectivity.

a) Viruses can reproduce only within a host cell

Viral reproduction differs strikingly from cellular reproduction, because viruses are **obligate intracellular parasites** which can express their genes and reproduce only within a living cell. Each virus has a specific *host range.*

1. Viruses recognize host cells by a complementary fit between external viral proteins and specific cell surface *receptor sites.*
2. Some viruses have broad host ranges which may include several species .
3. Some viruses have host ranges so narrow that they can: Infect only one species or Infect only a single tissue type of one species .
4. There are many patterns of viral life cycles, but they all generally involve:
   - Infecting the host cell with viral genome
   - Co-opting host cell's resources to:
   - Replicate the viral genome

- Manufacture capsid protein
- Assembling newly produced viral nucleic acid and capsomeres into the next generation of viruses

b) Infectiousness of Virus

1. Viruses are infectious and highly contagious, infectivity depends on virus synthesis.
2. After the entry of pathogen in host through natural opening or wounds or pollen grains, virus comes in contact with host.
3. Since viruses do not produce enzymes. They lack the Lipman Enzymatic system for the conversion of high energy into potential energy required for biological activity.
4. So they have to depend on hosts. This is a major difference between the host parasite relationship in viral diseases and those of other pathogen.
5. The naked RNA induces host cell to form enzyme RNA polymerase. These enzyme in presence of viral RNA and nucleotides produce additional RNA. The new viral RNA induces host cell to produce specific protein molecule required for its coat.

c) Replication of Virus

There are three possible patterns of viral genome replication:

1. DNA'! DNA. If viral DNA is double-stranded, DNA replication resembles that of cellular DNA, and the virus uses DNA polymerase produced by the host.
2. RNA'! RNA. Since host cells lack the enzyme to copy RNA, most RNA viruses contain a gene that codes for *RNA replicase*, an enzyme that uses viral. RNA as a template to produce complementary RNA.
3. RNA '!DNA '!RNA. Some RNA viruses encode *reverse transcriptase*, an enzyme that transcribes DNA from an RNA template.

Regardless of how viral genomes replicate, all viruses divert host cell resources for viral production.

- Viral genes use the host cell's enzymes, ribosomes, tRNAs, amino acids, ATP, and other resources to make copies of the viral genome and produce viral capsid proteins.

- These viral components—nucleic acid and capsids—are assembled into hundreds or thousands of virions, which leave to parasitize new hosts.
- Viral nucleic acid and capsid proteins assemble spontaneously into new virus particles, a process called *self-assembly*.
- Since most viral components are held together by weak bonds (e.g., hydrogen bonds and Van der Waals forces), enzymes are not usually necessary for assembly.
- For example, TMV can be disassembled in the laboratory. When mixed together, the RNA and capsids spontaneously reassemble to form complete TMV virions.

2. Physiological Properties of Virus

i) Dilution End Point (DEP)

Dilution –end point of plant virus is reported between dilutions- the highest dilution of leaf sap that is still not infectious and the next one. This means to say that the greatest dilution at which leaf sap from TMV infected tobacco , for example, is no longer able to produce local lesions on *Nicotiana glutinosa* or it is not able to produce any systemic infection at that dilution on tobacco. Tobacco mosaic virus is reported to remain infectious even in a dilution of 1:1000000, Cucumber mosaic virus retains, virulence at 1: 1000, Potato rugose mosaic virus causes poor infection when diluted to 1:10 or 1: 100.

ii) Thermal End Point (TEP)

TEP is the lowest temperature, applied for a given period (usually 10 minutes) at which virus loses its infectivity. This is to say that it is to determine the lowest temperature which inactivates TMV containing leaf sap. Tomato mosaic virus is destroyed by treating virus containing juice at 85 to 90 degree centigrade for 10 minutes, Lower temp, seems to have no effect on the viability of plant viruses.

iii) Longevity in vitro (LIV)

LIV is the time, the virus remains infectious in crude sap at room temperature as the temperature varies. It also depends on concentration of virus in sap and properties of sap. Although LIV has limited value for identification yet sometimes it is essential to know the rate of change of infectivity. It is important to determine the maximum time leaf sap containing *Cowpea mosaic virus* (as an example) remains infectious at room temperature. This knowledge is useful in purification studies of the virus. TMV in dried leaves or in Juice dried on filter paper remains infective for many years.

3. Chemical Properties

i) Host Range

Host range is useful in distinguishing the viruses from one another. The viruses are inoculated into indicator plant which develops typical symptoms, local lesions, ring spot systemic symptoms etc. Example: TMV and EMV incite symptoms on tobacco but EMV affects cucumber systematically where as TMV does not.

ii) Mutability and Strains

The presence of genetic material in the form of RNA in plant viruses ensure that new strains of the viruses may develop probably by mutation of RNA. In Tobacco mosaic virus alone, there are more than 50 strains.

iii) Serological Reactions

Serology is the study of reaction between antigen produced by microorganisms or viruses and antibodies in the serum of immunized animals. If a virus containing juice is injected into body of a rabbit, the rabbits form antibodies, which will react with viral proteins to give precipitation. The reactions are specific. i. e the antibodies obtained by inoculation of strain A, of a virus will precipitate , the juice containing the same specific type of virus.

DISTRIBUTION AND MOVEMENT OF VIRUSES IN PLANT

1. After introduction into cell, virus moves towards site of synthesis. This movement is passive through protoplasmic stream.
2. The movement of synthesized virus particles between cells occurs through **plasmodesmata** connecting adjacent cells.
3. The rate of spread is greater in young than old tissues. The movement faster at higher than lower temperature due to fast streaming of protoplasm. Some viruses transported through phloem, few through xylem vessels.

CLASSIFICATION OF PLANT VIRUSES

International committee on taxonomy of viruses has classified viruses into different groups. The classification is based on particle morphology and size, naked or enveloped nucleocapsids, number of virion types, number of genome fragements, type of nucleic acid and strandness of nucleic acid.The group name is mostly based on the type virus included in the group.

Group	**Name**	**Pieces of RNA/DNA**	**Shape**
ssRNA			
Bromovirus	*Brome mosaic virus Dahlia mosaic virus*	ssRNA	Elongated
Carlavirus	*Carnation latent virus*	ss RNA	Elongated
Closterovirus	*Beet yellow virus*	ssRNA	Elongted
Comovirus	*Cow pea mosaic virus*	ssRNA	Isometric
Cucumovirus	*Cucumber mosaic virus*	ssRNA	Isometric
Dianthovirus	*Carnation ring spot virus*	ssRNA	Isometric
Geminivirus	*Maize streak virus*	ssRNA	Isometric
Hordei virus	*Barley stripe mosaic virus*	ssRNA	Elongated
Ilarvirus	*Tobacco streak virus*	ssRNA	Isometric
Luteovirus	*Barley yellow dwarf virus*	ssRNA	Isometric
Nepo virus	*Tobacco ring spot virus*	ssRNA	Isometric
Potyvirus	*Pototo virus x*	ssRNA	Elongated
Rhabdovirus	*Lettuce necrotic mosaic virus*	ss RNA	Baciliformed
Sobemovirus	*Southern bean mosaic virus*	ssRNA	Isometric
Tobamo virus	*Tobacco mosaic virus*	ssRNA	Elongated
Tobravirus	*Tobaco rattle virus*	ssRNA	Elongated
Tymovirus	*Turnip yellow mosaic virus*	ssRNA	Isometric, Elongated
Tombus virus	*Tomato bushy stunt virus*	ssRNA	Isometric,
dsRNA			
Fiji virus	*Fiji disease virus*	dsRNA	Isometric
Phytoreovirus	*Wound tumor virus*	dsRNA	Isometric
Orizavirus	*Rice ragged stunt virus*	dsRNA	Isometric
Alphacryptovirus	*White clover cryptic virus 1*	dsRNA	Isometric
Betacryptovirus	*White clover cryptic virus 1*	dsRNA	Isometric
Varicosavirus	*Lettuce big vein associated virus*	dsRNA	Rod shaped
Endornavirus	*Vicia faba endornavirus*	dsRNA	Unknown
ss DNA			
Mastrevirus	*Maize streak virus*	ssDNA	Isometric
Curtovirus	*Beet curly top virus*	ssDNA	Isometric

Topocuvirus	*Tomato pseudo curly top virus*	ssDNA	Isometric
Begomovirus	*Bean golden mosaic virus, Mung bean yellow mosaic virus, Tobacco and Tomato leaf curl virus, Soybean leaf curl virus*	ssDNA	Isometric
Nanovirus	*Subterranean clover stunt virus*	ssDNA	Isometric
Babuvirus	*Banana bunchy top virus*	ssDNA	Isometric
ds DNA			
Caulimovirus	*Cauliflower mosaic virus, Dahelia mosaic virus*	ds DNA	Isometric
Soymovirus	*Soybean chlorotic mottle virus*	ds DNA	Isometric
Cavemovirus	*Cassava vein mosaic virus*	ds DNA	Isometric
Petu virus	*Petunia vein clearing virus*	ds DNA	Isometric
Cheravirus	*Cherry rasp leaf virus*	ds DNA	Isometric
Badnavirus	*Commelina yellow mottle virus*	ds DNA	Baciliformed
Tungrovirus	*Rice tungro bacilliform virus*	ds DNA	Baciliformed

SYMPTOMS OF PLANT VIRUSES

Symptoms are the expression of the diseased condition of the plant. All most all virus disease seem to cause some degree of reduction in yield and the length of life of virus infected plants is usually shortened. The most obvious symptoms of virus infected plants are usually those appearing on the leaves but some viruses may cause striking symptoms on the stem, fruits and roots.

Symptoms

I) External (Macroscopic)

A) Local

These are the symptoms produced at the site of artificial inoculation on leaves with virus.

i) **Chlorotic local lessions**: Infected cell loose chlorophylls and other pigments. For example, TMV on Cowpea host.

ii) **Necrotic local lessions**: Infected cell die. For example, TMV on *Nicotina glutinosa* host.

iii) **Ring spot local lesions**: Consist of central group of died cells near inoculated area (Necrotic ring) For example, Potato Virus: on *Chenopodium amaranticolar* host.

B) Systemic

In almost all viruses of plant occurring in field, the virus is present throughout the plant.

a) Colour Breaking (Variegation)

i) Mosaic

Mosaic are characterized by non uniform foliage coloration, with a more or less distinct intermingling of normal and light green or yellowish patches. Mosaic type symptoms may be described as follows.

a. Streak or stripe: Red stripe of jowar.

b. Vein clearing: BCMV

c. Vein banding: Beat curly top.

d. Inter veinal mosaic light discolouration restricted in between veins.

ii) Mottling

If the discoloured patch of a variegated leaves are rounded the variegation is usually designated as mottling.

iii) Line Pattern

a. Oak leaf pattern (OLP) (Apple oak leaf)

b. Systemic Rings (AMV on tobacco)

b. Malformation

1. Change in leaf form, any deviation from normal.
2. This includes uneven growth of leaf lamina leaves becomes curled, britle (Crinkling) and show, prominances and depressions (puckering) upward and downward curling, vein distortion, leaf enation, galls and tumours.

c. Others

a. Reddening of leaves cotton red leaf due to abnormal accumulation of anthocynanin.

b. Blackening of veins Potato virus 'Y' in potato (Due to more synthesis of melanis).

c. Bronzening: Example. TSWV, in Tomato

d. Etching: Tobacco etch virus.

II) Internal (Microscopic)

These include inclusion bodies. Inclusions are microscopic bodies produced by some of the viruses. These are produced in cytoplasm or nucleic acid.

a) Cytoplasm

1. **Amorphous** or amoeboid also called as X-bodies produced by spherical or oval viruses Example. CMV.
2. **Crystalline:** These type of inclusions are produced by rod shaped viruses. Example. Red clover vein mosaic, Cactus virus, and Petunia ring spot.

b) Nucleus

Example. Tobacco etch virus, rectangular plates. BCMV- Strain pisum Virus -2. Isometric crystals.

Proliferation (Toratonic Symptoms)

1. Asymmetry of leaf lamina. Example, Grape fan leaf.
2. Blistering: Dark green area may be raised to give blistering effect. Margin of leaves twisted Example. BCMV.
3. Tumours: Clover wound tumour virus.
4. Swelling of stem: Cocoa swollen shoot virus.
5. Flattening of branches and distribution of stem: Apple flat limb.
6. Enations: These are the out growth in different shape and form either on veins or leaf lamina.
7. Vein enation: Citrus enation virus, Pea enation mosaic.
8. Leaf enation: Cotton leaf curl: Tobacco leaf curl;
9. Galls: Woody galls of citrus.
10. Pitting:

    A) Stem pitting – Apple stem pitting, Citrus tristeza virus on kagzi lime.

    B) Fruit pitting: Pear stony pit- Apple groove virus on apple.

11. Stunt: Tomato bushy stunt.
12. Dwarfing: Barley yellow dwarf.
13. Leaf Roll: Potato leaf roll.
14. Yellows: Beet Yellows.
15. Pox: Plum pox virus.

LATENT VIRUSES AND MASKED SYMPTOMS

1. Latent Viruses

Many viruses may infect certain hosts without ever causing development of visible symptoms on them. Such viruses are usually called as "**Latent viruses**" and hosts are called as "**Symptomless carriers**".

2. Masked Symptoms

Virus induced plant symptoms that are absent under certain environmental conditions, but appear when the host is exposed to certain conditions of light and temperature.

TRANSMISSION OF PLANT VIRUSES

The plant virus rarely, if ever, come out of plant spontaneously. For this reason, Plant viruses are not disseminated as such by wind or water. Viruses are transmitted from plant to plant in a number of ways such as vegetative, propagation, mechanically through sap and by seed, pollen, insect, mites, nematodes, dodder and fungi.

1. Mechanical Transmissions

Such transmissions may takes place between closely spaced plants after a strong wind by contact , when plants are wounded during cultural operations, virus infected sap adhering to the tools, worker hands or cloth accidently transmitted to the subsequently wounded plants.Example, Potato virus: (PV-X, TMV on Tobacco and Tomato)

2. Transmission by Vegetative Propagation

Plants are propagated vegetatively by budding or grafting or by cutting or by the use of tubers, corms, bulbs or rhizome. Any virus present in the mother plant from which these organs are taken will almost always be transmitted to the progeny. Transmission of viruses may also occur through natural root grafts of adjacent plant.

3. Transmission by Seed and pollen

Plant virus transmission from generation to generation occurs in about 20% of plant viruses. When viruses are transmitted by seeds, the seed is infected in the generative cells and the virus is maintained in the germ cells and sometimes, but less often, in the seed coat. When the growth and development of plants is delayed because of situations like unfavourable weather, there is an increase in the amount of virus infections in seeds. There does not seem to be a correlation between the location of the seed on the plant and its chances of being infected. Little is known about the mechanisms involved in the transmission of plant viruses via seeds, although it is known that it is environmentally influenced and that seed transmission occurs because of a direct invasion of the embryo via the ovule or by an indirect route with an attack on the embryo mediated by infected gametes. These processes can occur concurrently or separately depending on the host plant. It is unknown how the virus is able to directly invade and cross the embryo and boundary between the parental and progeny generations in the ovule. Many plants species can be infected through seeds including but not limited to the families Leguminosae, Solanaceae, Compositae, Rosaceae, Cucurbitaceae, Gramineae. Bean common mosaic virus is transmitted through seeds.

4. Dodder Transmission

Several plant virus can be transmitted from one plant to another plant through the bridge formed between the two plants by twining the stem of parasitic plant, dodder (Cuscuta species), green strain of cucumber mosaic virus on *N. glutinosa*, lucern (alfa-alfa) , mosaic virus to tobacco potato stem mottle virus to tobacco. Bennett (1940) showed dodder transmission, sugar beet curly top virus (BCTV), cucumber mosaic virus.

5. Natural Modes of Transmission

This includes air borne transmission through insects and mites and soil borne transmission through nematodes and fungus.

A) Air Borne through Insects

The most common and important means of virus transmission in the field.

Members of the order Homoptera- Aphids, Jassids, Leaf hopper, White flies, Mealy bug , Scale insects.

Thysanoptera – Thrips, Coleopteran – Beetles.

Insects with sucking mouth parts carry plant viruses on their stylet- stylet borne or non persistances.

B) Circulative

1. Circulative Viruses (Persistent)

A circulative virus is one that passes into a vector through the mouth parts, circulates internally and enlarges through the salivary glands.

2. Propagative Viruses

Propagative viruses are those viruses which multiply in their insect vectors and transmit them for a long time but very often for as long as they live.

C) Insect Vectors

Virus transmitting insect is called vector. Viruses are mostly really on insect for transmission (400 species of insect vector transmitting more than 200 viruses). The viruses are transmitted by diffeent types of insects and most efficient vectors are of sucking and bitting type of insects.

a. White Flies: Yellow vein mosaic of okra, Tobacco leaf curl, Pumpkin yellow mosaic , Mung yellow mosaic, Sweet potato mosaic,Cotton leaf curl, Cassava mosaic.

b. Aphids: These are the most important insect vector of plant viruses and transmit great majority (about 170) of the all stylet borne viruses. Example. Soybean mosaic, Pea enation mosaic, Lettuce necrotic, Potato leaf roll, Red clover mosaic, MCMV, AMV, BYMV.

c. Leaf Hoppers: All leaf hoppers transmitted viruses are circulatory, several are known to multiply in the vector (propagative), cause disturbance in phloem region. Example, Rice tungro viruses, Rice dwarf viruses, Potato yellow dwarf ,Maize mosaic, Beet curly top, Maize rough dwarf.

d. Thrips: Tomato spotted wilt virus.

e. Beetles: Cowpea mosaic virus, Bean pod mottle, Squash mosaic, Cowpea chlorotic mottle virus, Raddish mosaic.

f. Mites: Transmit viruses like Pigeonpea sterility mosaic, Peach mosaic, Fig mosaic, Wheat, streak mosaic.

D. Nematodes

Hewitt and colleagues (1958) first showed that Fan leaf virus of grapevines is transmitted by dagger nematode, *Xiphinema index*. Later, a few other plant viruses were reported to be transmitted by nematodes and now about 24 plant viruses are known to be transmitted by neamtodes. Most nematodes parasitic on green plants belong to order **Tylenchyda**, but none of this group has yet been found to be a vector virus. All species of nematodes known to transmit viruses are members of the order **Dorylaimida** and belong to the five genera: *Xiphineama, Longidorus, Paralongidorus, Trichodorus* and *Paratrichodorus*. Approximately 20 plant viruses have been shown to be transmitted by one or more species of 4 genera of soil inhabiting ectoparasitic Nematodes. Examples of viruses that can be transmitted by nematodes are given below.

Sr.No	Group	Nematode Virus Vectors	Example
1.	NEPO: Nematode transmitted polyhedral soil viruses	*Xiphinema index*	Grape vine fan leaf
		Xiphinema coxy	Cherry leaf roll
		Xiphinema americaum	Ring spot of tobacco, Tomato, Soybean bud blight, Brinjal mosaic.
2.	NETU: Nematode transmitted tubular soil viruses	*Longidorus*	Rasberry ring spot, tomato black ring.
		Trichodorus and para trichodorus	Rod shaped viruses, Tobacco rattle pea early browing.

E. Fungus

Soil inhabiting species of chytrid true fungi belonging to two genera *Olpidium* and *Synchitrium* and 2 species of protozoa (fungal like) belonging to two genera *Polymyxa* and *Spongospora* have been proved to be vectors of certain category of plant viruses. Examples of viruses that can be transmitted by fungi are given below.

Sr.No	Fungus Virus Vectors	Example
1.	*Olpidium brassicae*	Lettuce big vein, Tobacco necrosis , Cucumeber, necrosis, Tobacco stunt virus
2.	*Synchytrium endobioticum*	PU-X virus
3.	*Polymyxa graminis*	Wheat mosaic virus, Beat necrotic yellow vein virus.
4.	*Spongospora subteranea*	Potato mop top virus

HORIZONTAL AND VERTICAL TRANSMISSION OF VIRUS

Plant viruses spread from plant to plant by two major routes: horizontal transmission and vertical transmission.

Horizontal transmission = Route of viral transmission in which an organism receives the virus from an external source.

- Plants are more susceptible to viral infection if their protective epidermal layer is damaged.
- Insects may be *vectors* that transmit viruses from plant to plant and can inject the virus directly into the cytoplasm.
- By using contaminated tools, gardeners and farmers may transmit plant viruses.

Vertical transmission = Route of viral transmission in which an organism inherits a viral infection from its parent.

- Can occur in asexual propagation of infected plants (e.g., by taking cuttings).
- Can occur in sexual reproduction via infected seeds.

RELATIONSHIP BETWEEN INSECT VECTOR AND VIRUS

The virus vector relationship varies widely depending upon the duration of the virus in the vector. In case of persistent viruses, the virus may simply circulate through the body of the vector or propagate also. Hence, this relationship can be classified as

Non-persistant transmission: Vector trasmission of a virus where the vector quickly picks up virus particles on its mouthparts and is infective for a short period of time (hours).

Semi-persistant transmission: Vector trasmission of a virus where virus particles enter the vectors foregut. In this case the vector also picks up the virus quicly but is infective for somewhat longer (days) than with non-persistant transmission.e.g., Beet yellow virus

Circulative transmission: Vector trasmission of a virus where virus particles must circulate through the vectors hemolymph and enter the salivary glands to be tramsitted. In this case the vector aquisition and retention time is longer than with non or semi-persistant transmission.

Propagative transmission: Vector transmission of a virus where virus particles are repliacted in the the vector. In this case the vector retention time is longer than with circulative transmission and, in some cases, the virus can be transovarially transmitted.

Transovarial transmission: Viral transmission from an insect vector to its offspring, meaning offpring of an infected vector are also infective

DETECTION OF PLANT VIRUSES

Due to the inability to observe plant viruses visually by observing them directly through the light microscope, virologists must resort to the following methods of detecting their presence and in diagnosis.

1. Ability to transmit disease via plant sap by rubbing plant, grafting, dodder or insect transmission.
2. Indexing - indicator plants - sensitive to specific virus and will react a certain way if exposed.
3. Visual inspection with electron microscope.
4. By eliminating possibility that symptoms are not due to other sources (e.g., herbicide, nutritional deficiencies).
5. Serological Tests (**ELISA - enzyme-linked immuno sorbent assay**).

ELISA tests are extremely sensitive (small amounts of antisera are needed) results are quantitative, large samples can be run at same time (96 well plates), results can be gathered in a few hours instead of days. ELISAs along with serial dilutions of plant sap and applications of this to the leaves of susceptible hosts (by counting the number of lesions) can be used to quantify the amount of virus present.

Indirect (virus + Ab virus + Enzyme conjugated Ab) and direct (double-antibody sandwich technique) (Ab virus + virus + Enzyme-conjugated Ab).

- Virus or Ab virus added to well and these become attached to walls.
- Antibody or virus added to well and these attach to their counterpart (i.e., antigen to antibody).
- Second antibody with enzyme conjugate attaches to first antibody/ virus complex.
- Substrate is catalyzed by enzyme and this causes a color change.

BACTERIOPHAGES

Bacteriophage is a virus that infects bacteria.Very often the shortened form '*phage*' is used. **Phages** are ultramicroscopic agents that can pass through bacterial proof filter and infects bacteria. Phages are ubiquitous in nature and known to parasitise bacteria from all diverse habitates, such as soil, marine water, plants, intestines of animals.

Structure of T-even phage

A complete virion of T- even phage consists of the following structural units.

1. **Polyhedral head:** The head consists of an outer protein capsid enclosing genetic material or genome. The genome of a phage may contain ssRNA, dsRNA, ssDNA, or dsDNA.The phage genome is between 5 to 500 Kb long with either circular or linear arrangement.

2. **Collar:** The region between head and tail is reffered as collar.
3. **Helical tail:** The helical proteinaceous tail is attached with the head.The tail serves as organ of attachment or adsorption.
4. **Sheath:** In some phages the helical tail is covered by a sheath. The sheath provides a protective .
5. **Base plate:** It provides the support to the tail pins.
6. **Tail fibres:** There are tail fibres surrounding the tail. The tail fibres also helps in attachment process during host infection.
7. **Tail pins:** The tail pins are attached to the base plate connected to the tail and helps in attachment process.

LIFE CYCLE OF BACTERIOPHAGE

The life cycle of bacteriophage is of two types, namely lytic and lysogenic cycle. However in some viruses both the cycle are present.

LYTIC AND LYSOGENIC CYCLES

A. The Lytic Cycle

Lytic cycle = A viral replication cycle that results in the death or lysis of the host cell.

The lytic cycle of phage T4 is illustrated below.

1. Phage attaches to cell surface

T4 recognizes a host cell by a complementary fit between proteins on the virion's tail fibers and specific receptor sites on the outer surface of an *E. coli* cell.

2. Phage contracts sheath and injects DNA.

- ATP stored in the phage tail piece is the energy source for the phage to:
  a. pierce the *E. coli* wall and membrane.
  b. contract its tail sheath.
  c. inject its DNA.
- The genome separates from the capsid leaving a capsid "ghost" outside the cell.

3. Hydrolytic enzymes destroy host cell's DNA

- The *E. coli* host cell begins to transcribe and translate the viral genome.
- One of the first viral proteins produced is an enzyme that degrades host DNA. The phage's own DNA is protected, because it contains modified cytosine not recognized by the enzyme.

4. Phage genome directs the host cell to produce phage components: DNA and capsid proteins.

- Using nucleotides from its own degraded DNA, the host cell makes many copies of the phage genome.
- The host cell also produces three sets of capsid proteins and assembles them into phage tails, tail fibers, and polyhedral heads.
- Phage components spontaneously assemble into virions.

5. Cell lyses and releases phage particles.

- Lysozymes specified by the viral genome digest the bacterial cell wall.
- Osmotic swelling lyses the cell which releases hundreds of phages from their host cell.
- Released virions can infect near by cells.
- Lytic cycle takes only 20 to 30 minutes at 37°C. In that period, a T4 population can increase a hundredfold.

B. The Lysogenic Cycle

Lysogenic cycle = A viral replication cycle that involves the incorporation of the viral genome into the host cell genome

Details of the lysogenic cycle were discovered through studies of phage l life cycle:

1. Phage l binds to the surface of an *E. coli* cell.
2. Phage l injects its DNA into the bacterial host cell.
3. l DNA forms a circle and either begins a lytic or lysogenic cycle.
4. During a lysogenic cycle, l DNA inserts by genetic recombination (crossing over) into a specific site on the bacterial chromosome and becomes a prophage.

Prophage = A phage genome that is incorporated into a specific site on the bacterial chromosome

- Most prophage genes are inactive.
- One active prophage gene codes for the production of *repressor protein* which switches off most other prophage genes.
- Prophage genes are copied along with cellular DNA when the host cell reproduces.
- As the cell divides, both prophage and cellular DNA are passed on to daughter cells.
- A prophage may be carried in the host cell's chromosomes for many generations.

Occasionally, a prophage may leave the bacterial chromosome.

- This may be spontaneous or caused by environmental factors (e.g., radiation).
- The excision process may begin the phage's lytic reproductive cycle.
- Virions produced during the lytic cycle may begin either a lytic or lysogenic cycle in their new host cells.

Lysogenic cell = Host cell carrying a prophage in its chromosome

- It is called lysogenic because it has the potential to lyse.
- Some prophage genes in a lysogenic cell may be expressed and change the cell's phenotype in a process called *lysogenic conversion.*
- Lysogenic conversion occurs in bacteria that cause diphtheria, botulism, and scarlet fever. Pathogenicity results from toxins coded for by prophage genes.

LIFE CYCLE OF PHAGE

The different steps involved in the life cycle of phage include

1. **Attachment**. Glycoprotein spikes protruding from the viral envelope attach to receptor sites on the host's plasma membrane.
2. **Entry**. As the envelope fuses with the plasma membrane, the entire virus (capsid and genome) is transported into the cytoplasm by receptor-mediated endocytosis.
3. **Uncoating**. Cellular enzymes uncoat the genome by removing the protein capsid from viral RNA.
4. **Viral RNA and protein synthesis**. Viral enzymes are required to replicate the RNA genome and to transcribe mRNA.

- Some viral RNA polymerase is packaged in the virion.
- Viral RNA polymerase (transcriptase) replicates the viral genome and transcribes viral mRNA. Note that the viral genome is a strand complementary to mRNA.
- Viral mRNA is translated into viral proteins including:
- Capsid proteins synthesized in the cytoplasm by free ribosomes.
- Viral-envelope glycoproteins synthesized by ribosomes bound to rough ER. Glycoproteins produced in the host's ER are sent to the Golgi apparatus for further processing. Golgi vesicles transport the glycoproteins to the plasma membrane, where they cluster at exit sites for the virus.

5. Assembly and release. New capsids surround viral genomes. Once assembled, the virions envelop with host plasma membrane as they bud off from the cell's surface.

MANAGEMENT OF PLANT VIRUSES

1. **Selection of seed:** Select seed from disease free localities.
2. **Selection of planting materials:** Cutting, bulb, rhizomes, tubers etc should be free from disease.
3. **Soil fumigation:** Nematodes transmitted viruses can be reduced by the soil fumigation to control nematodes.
4. **Eradication:** Eradication of diseased plant to eliminate the inoculum from the field.
5. **Indexing:**Periodical indexing of the mother plants, producing propagative organs is necessary to ascertain these continuous freedom from virus.
6. **Protection against insect vectors:** This can be done by growing trap crops to check the insect vectors. Ex. Cotton reddening, White flies in bhendi.
7. **Weeds:** Removal and destruction of weeds that serve as host. Ex. Broad leaf weeds in banana, orchard reduce bunchy tops.

9. **Use of resistant varieties:** Example. Parbhani Kranti, yellow vein mosaic of the bhendi.
10. **Immunization:** The disease caused by severe strains of virus can be avoided if the plants are inoculated first with a mild strain of some viruses. e.g. Citrus greening.

11. **Temperature treatment:** Sugarcane mosaic can be destroyed or reduce by hot water treatment 52°C for 30 minutes.

12. **Use of insecticides:** Control of insect vector with the use of insecticides.

Insecticide	Insect vector	Dose (ml or g/lit.water)
Malathion 50EC	White fly, Aphids ,Thrips, Hopper, Mites, Mealy bug, Beetles	1-1.5 ml/lit
Dimethoate 30 EC	White fly, Aphids ,Thrips, Hopper, Mites, Mealy bug, Beetles	1.25-1.5 ml/lit
Thiamethoxam 25 WG	White fly, Aphids ,Thrips, Hopper, Mites, Mealy bug, Beetles	0.2-0.25 ml/lit
Oxydemeton methyl 25 EC	White fly, Aphids ,Thrips, Hopper, Mites, Mealy bug, Beetles,	1-1.5 ml/lit
Clothianidin50 WG	White fly, Aphids ,Thrips, Hopper, Mites, Mealy bug, Beetles	0.1-0.5 ml/lit

13. **Quarantine laws:** The best way to control virus disease is to keep it out of an area through a system of quarantine, inspections and certifications.

CHAPTER - 15

The Pathogens-Phytoplasma, Spiroplasma and Fastidious Vascular Bacteria

PHYTOPLASMA OR MYCOPLASMA

Definition

Phytoplasmas are unicellular, ultramicroscopic, wallcss, prokaryotic, self-replicating, highly pleomorphic, filterable organisms or entities.

Mycoplasma lack rigid cell wall, being surrounded only by single triple unit membrane which allows them to be highly plemorphic. They assume vast array of shapes and size. They require sterols (Lipoproteins) for growth. Mycoplasma cannot be grown on artificial media and they reproduce by budding and binary fissions.

Taxonomic Position

Kingdom	Prokaryotic
Division	Firmicutes
Class	Mollicutes
Order	Acholeplasmatales
Family	Acholeplasmataceae
Genus	*Phytoplasma*

Historical Background

1. Plant disease caused by MLO's were known since 1603 in Japan in Mulbery (Mulbery dwarf disease).
2. Mycoplasma –like organism or MLOs were first discovered by Doi *et al.,* in 1967.
3. MLO that infccts plants have been reclassified as Phytoplasmas by Sears and Krikpatrick in 1994.

4. In 2004, the genus name of Phytoplasma was adopted and is currently at *Candidatus status* which is used for bacteria that cannot be cultured.

General Characters

1. They are wall less, surrounded by a unit membrane, and consist of cytoplasm, ribosomes and nuclear material.
2. Pleomorphic or filamentous shape with varying size ranging from 200 to 800 nm and is less than 1 µm in diameter.
3. DNA is present in cytoplasm. Genome is very small (689-1600kb).
4. They are very small and ultramicroscopic.
5. Strictly host dependent and can survive and multiply only in the sap of phloem sieve tubes or insect haemolymph; also in their eggs.
6. Only phloem –feeding insect vectors (Leafhoppers, Plant hoppers and Psllids) that possess piercing/sucking type mouth parts (Hemiptera) can potentially acquire and transmit the phytoplasma in a persistent propagative manner.
7. They cannot be grown on **artificial media** but can grow in alimentary canal, haemolymph, salivery glands, and intercellularly in different body organisms of their insect vectors.
8. Reproduce by **binary fission**.
9. They are sensitive to **tetracycline** but resistant to **penicillin**.
10. MLOs have no flagella, produce no spore and are gram-ve.

Symptoms Produced by Phytoplasma in Plants

1. Phytoplasmas like bodies are now stated to be occur in more than 60 to 70 plant diseases, which are characterized by the growth abnormalities and yellowing of leaves.
2. Characteristic symptom of yellow type disease includes uniform yellowing or reddening of leaves, smaller leaves, shortening of internodes, stunting of plants and proliferation of auxiliary bud.
3. "Witch brooms" includes reduction of leaf size with leaves becoming brittle, excessive proliferation of shoots.
4. "Phyllody" replacement of floral parts of leaves greening or sterility of flowers and reduced yield. Finally more or less rapid dieback,

decline and disorder after several years.

5. MLOs are mostly restricted to phloem tissue becomes; a phloem may provide favourable conditions for growth as phloem elements have a high osmotic pressure and slightly alkaline PH.

Disease Caused by Phytoplasmas

(i) Pear decline

(ii) Grape yellows

(iii) Aster yellows of vegetables

(iv) Apple proliferation

(v) Little leaf of brinjal.

(vi) Coconut lethal yellowing

(vii) Elms yellows

(viii) Pigeonpea witche's broom

(ix) Rice yellow dwarf

(x) Stolbur

(xi) X.disease

(xii) Citrus greening

(xiii) Seasamum phyllody

(xiv) Grassy shoot of sugarcane

Management of Phytoplasmas

1. Most of the control measures against yellow type of disease are avoided at preventing infections.

2. **Heat treatment:** Phytoplasmas are thermolabile and are destroyed or inactivated at or above 40 to 50^0C. It is possible to cure yellow infected plants, grassy shoot of sugarcane by heat treatment.

3. **Use of antibiotics:** Antibiotics are known to suppress the yellow type disease. The most effective antibiotics appear to be chloro tetracycline, chlorotetracycline oxy tetra cycline and tetra cycline with choramphenicol or ledermycin. The application of antibiotics by root dip or paste under tha bark, standing cutting in solution appears to be more effective than foliar spray or soil drenches.

4. **Vector control:** Since most of disease are spread by the vector, control of vector through effective insecticides like Rogar, Malathion, Endosulphan etc.
5. **Killing of alternate hosts:** Weeds may serve as alternate host, hence killing of alternate host.

SPIROPLASMA

Definition

Spiroplasma is a wall less mollicutes bounded by a triple layered unit membrane.

Taxonomic Position

Kingdom	Prokaryotic
Division	Tenericutes
Class	Mollicutes
Order	Endoplasmatales
Family	Spiroplasmataceae
Genus	Spiroplasma

General Characters

1. They lack true cell wall ,bounded by a single triple layered unit membrane .
2. They produce typical **'fried egg'** like colonies on agar medium.
3. They multiplied by **fission**.
4. They produce helical (100-240 nm in dia., 2-4μm inlength) form in liquid culture medium.
5. Can be cultured on nutrient media.
6. Resistant to **penicillin** but inhibited by **tetracycline**.
7. Transmitted only through phloem –feeding insect vectors mostly through **leaf hoppers**.
8. Mostly found in the gut or haemolymph of insects, or in the phloem of infected plants.

Disease Caused by Spiroplasma

(i) Corn stunt

(ii) White bud of maize

(iii) Citrus stubborn

Management of Spiroplasma

1. Use of disease resistant planting stocks.
2. Eradication of infected trees in early stages of infection.
3. **Vector Control:** Since most of disease are spread by the vector, control of vector through effective insecticides like Rogar, Malathion, Endosulphan etc.

FASTIDIOUS VASCULAR BACTERIA (RICKETTESIA LIKE ORGANISMS)

General Characters

1. The fastidious vascular bacteria were formally known as rickettesia like organisms (RLOs).
2. They are usually rod shaped, aflagellate, bounded by a cell membrane and a cell wall measuring 1.0 -4.0x 0.2-0.5μm.
3. They are confined to phloem or xylem of the host plant but never to both.
4. Usually transmitted by **leaf hoppers** exception: Citrus greening bacteria (*Liberobacter asciaticum* is transmitted by citrus psylla (*Diaphorina citri*).
5. Al most all fastidious bacteria known so far are **gram negative**. Exception. Sugarcane ratoon stunting (*Clavibacter xyli pv.xyli*) is gram positive in nature.
6. There are two groups: one in which the fastidious bacteria occur only in phloem (phloem limited) and the other in which they occur in xylem (i.e xylem limited).
7. Xylem limited fastidious bacteria known so far have been successfully grown on nutrient media while phloem limited fastidious bacteria have not been culture so far.
8. They are sensitive to antibiotics such as tetracycline and penicillin and to high temperature.

Disease Caused by Fastidious vascular bacteria

(i) Pierce's disease of grapes

(ii) Almond leaf scorch

(iii) Alfalfa dwarf

(iv) Phony peach

(v) Raton stunting

(vi) Plum leaf scald.

Management

1. **Heat treatment :** Entire plant parts or propagative plant parts, by immersing them in water kept at 45-50^{0}C for 2-3 hours or by keeping the plants or plant propagules in hot air at 45 to 50^{0}C for 2-3 hours.It has been helpful in curing the sugarcane and grapevines from ratoon stunting disease and pierce's disease, respectively.

2. **Use of antibiotics:** Antibiotics are known to suppress fastidious vascular bacteria. The most effective antibiotics appear to be penicillin and tetracyclin.

CHAPTER - 16

The Pathogens-Viroids, Algae, Protozoa and Prions

VIROIDS

Defnition

Viroid is circular, encapsulated, low molecular weight ($1.1\text{-}1.3x10^5$), self replicating, highly infectious ssRNA molecules .

General Characters

1. The viroid exists in *in vivo* as unencapsulated RNA.
2. They never contain any protein coat (capsid).
3. Genome of the viriod naked, single stranded (RNA) with 250-400 nucleotide, either linear or mostly circular. Viroids are smaller in size than viruses i.e 50 nm or 1.1 to $1.3 X 10^3$ molecular weight.
4. Despite its small size, the infectious RNA is replicated autonomously in susceptible cells; that is, no helper virus is required for multiplication.
5. The infectious RNA consists of one molecular species only.
6. Viroids are notable to synthesize protein and replicase enzyme required for replication.
7. Viroids replicate by direct RNA, copying in which all components required for viroid multiplication including RNA polymerase are provided by the host.
8. They cause diseases only in plants.
9. Viroids concentration and translocation is higher in growing parts of the plants (up to 0.2 mm from the apex)
10. Most of the types of symptoms observed with viral diseases also

occurs viroids like epinasty, leaf distortions, vein clearing, localized chlorotic or necrotic spots, mottling of leaves, necrosis of leaves, and death of the whole plants.

Transmission

1. All known viroids are transmissible by mechanical means, either readily or with some difficulty.
2. Farm implements can result in mechanical transmission and spread of viroid infection is best possible by contact which consequently mainly responsible for the spread of the disease in nature.
3. Similarly, mechanical transmission and spread of viroid infection is best possible by using contaminated budding knives and other tools.
4. *Potato spindle tuber viroid*, *Chrysanthemum stunt viroid* and *Chrysanthemum chlorotic mottle viroid* are transmitted through sap quite easily while others such as *Citrus exocortis viroid* is transmitted through sap with some difficulty.
5. Viroids those causing Potato spindle tuber, Coconut cadang- cadang, Tomato bunchy top, and apple scar skin disease appears to be transmitted through the pollen and seed.

Example of diseases caused by viroid

(i) Potato spindle tuber

(ii) Coconut cadang- cadang

(iii) Citrus exocortis

(iv) Chrysanthemum stunt

(v) Tomato bunchy top

(vi) Hot stunt

vii) Avocardo sunblotch

(viii) Peach latent mosaic

Management of viroid diseases

1. Use of viroid free propagating stocks.
2. Removal and destruction of viroid infected plants and following sanitary measures.

3. Washing of hands or sterilizing of tools after handling is very important aspect for viroid disease management.
4. Tools should be disinfected by dipping in a 10-20% sodium hypochlorite solution.
5. Mild strains of viroids are reported to proect the plants from effect of super infection with a severe strain of the same viroid.
6. No chemical are known to inhibit viroid infection.

ALGAE

General Characters

1. Algae are the eukaryotic thallophytes having chlorophyll as their primary photosynthetic pigments. They are aerobic, photosynthetic organisms; contain three types of pigments chlorophyll, cartoenoids and phycocyanin.
2. They are ubiquitous organisms abundantly present in aquatic environment.
3. They have wide range of shapes and size and the common shapes are rhizoidal, filamentous and mucilaginous.
4. The Chlorophycean (green algae) cause disease in plants.
5. Most of the algae are photoautotrophic, may reproduce either sexually or asexually.
6. Algae reproduce asexually by binary fission, fragmentation and formation of spores and sexually by formation of zygotes.
7. They spread through an air borne sporangia and produces 300 spores.
8. They entry in to the host through stomata and other natural openings

Example

Red rust of tea, coffee, mango, citrus, and guava (*Cephaleurous parasitica, C.minimum, C.coffeae)*

Management of Algae

1. Application of nitrogen and potassium significantly reduce the disease. Drainage should be provided.
2. All badly diseased or dead wood should be removed.

3. Pruning is recommended for tea, citrus, and cacao trees for the control of this disease.
4. Close plucking of tea should be discouraged.
5. Irrigation reduces red rust due to an increase in host vigour.
6. Bordeaux mixture, copper oxychloride and cuprous oxide can be sprayed to control the disease.

PROTOZOA

General Characters

1. Protozoa are single celled, non photosynthetic, eukaryotic animal like organisms. They are widely distributed in nature particularly in aquatic, environment or moist habitats.
2. Their size ranges from 2-3 micron.
3. They lack rigid cell wall and do not contain chlorophyll.
4. They make their movements with the help of cilia, flagella or pseudopodia.
5. Most of the protozoa are free living but some are symbiotic or parasitic causing diseases in plants, animals and humans.
6. Free living protozoa are commonly found in fresh water, salt water, sand, soil and decaying organic matter.
7. Protozoa reproduce sexually or asexually.
8. Asexual reproduction is either by binary fission or by budding or by both.
9. Sexual reproduction is by fusion of two gametes.
10. They have characteristic ability to regenerate the lost parts of the body. For example, Genera: Amoeba, Paramecium etc.

Example

1. Phloem necrosis of coffee (*Phytomonas leptovasorum*)
2. Hart rot of coconut and oil palm (Phytomonas)
3. Sudden wilt of oil palm.
4. Empty root of Cassava.

PRIONS

1. Resembling viruses that lacks nucleic acid (DNA or RNA) and have infectious **proteins** molecule which were 100 times smaller than the smallest known virus, for which **Prusiner** coined the term **prions**, which comes from proteinaceous infectious particles that lack nucleic acid.
2. It is the smallest known protein often considered to be the cause of various infectious diseases of the nervous system.
3. Prions are some times called slow viruses because of their slow effect.
4. Prions are transmissible particles and cause **mad cow** disease, **Creutzfeldt- Jakob** disease in humans and **Scrapie** disease in sheep.
5. However, no plant diseases are reported to be caused by prions.

CHAPTER - 17

The Pathogens - Nematodes

INTRODUCTION

1. Nematodes belong to the animal kingdom, and phylum Nematoda.
2. The body of nematodes is elongate (thread like; nema in Greek means thread) without any segment.
3. It is cylindrical, tapering at each end especially towards the tail.
4. Most of the important parasitic genera belong to the order **Tylenchida** and few under **Dorylaimida**.

General Morphology

1. Plant parasitic nematodes mostly measure 300-1000mm with some up to 4 mm long x 15-35mm wide and bilaterally symmetrical.
2. The body of the adult male is cylindrical, filiform, eel-shaped, made up of **cuticle**, **hypodermis** and **somatic muscles**, round in cross section and tapering at each end.
3. The anterior end is smooth, provided with papillae, leading to a buccal cavity and to oesophagus.
4. The body cavity between the gut and the body wall is usually regarded as a **pseudocoelom** containing a pseudocoelomic fluid.
5. Body is smooth, unsegmented without leg or other appendages.
6. The females of some species become swollen at adult stage and have pear-shaped (pyriform) or spheroid bodies.
7. Nematodes can be easily observed under microscope.
8. A valve is located at the junction of oesophagus and the intestine, the latter opening into the rectum and anus at the posterior end of the body.

9. The entire body is covered with a colourless, impermeable (permeable only to water) smooth or transversely striated cuticle with a sub-cuticular and muscular layer.
10. Respiratory and circulatory system absent.

Nervous System

1. The nervous system consists of a **nerve ring** which encircles the gut usually in the region of the oesophageal isthmus.
2. Several nerves extend anteriorly and posteriorly.

Excertory system

1. A excretory duct opens at the exterior via an excretory pore.
2. The gut is an internal tube beginning at the oral opening and ending at the ventrally placed anus in juveniles and females and at the cloaca in male.

Reproductive system

1. Female have avulva in the mid body region with paired reproductive tracts.
2. The reproductive tract consists of an **ovary**, **oviduct**, **uterus**, **vagina** and **vulva**.
3. Male have single or paired testis, **seminal vesicle** and **vasdeferens**.
4. The vasdeferens opens into the cloaca which has a ventrally placed opening.
5. Males usually have a pair of copulatory spicules that lies in an invagination of the cloacal wall.
6. There are sclerotized structures such as a gubernaculums or lateral accessory pieces which guide the spicules.
7. Male and female are found separately (dioecious).
8. Females are oviparous or ovoviviparous and cleavage is determinate.

Life cycle and Reproduction of nematodes

1. The female lay eggs after copulation.
2. The young one from the egg is called **larve**.

3. The nematodes usually moult **four times** to reach the adult stage
4. Appearance and structure of larvae are usually similar to the adults.
5. Larvae start to grow and each larval state is terminated by molt.
6. Nematodes usually moult **four times** to reach the adult stage.
7. Usually, first moult occurs in the egg and the final molt differentiates into adult male and female.
8. Fertile eggs are produced by females after mating with a male, or parthenogenetically in absence of males or can produce sperm herself.
9. A life cycle from egg to egg stage is completed with 3 to 4 weeks or requires slightly longer period in cooler temperature.

Behaviour of nematodes in soil

1. Except free living nematodes, all the plant parasitic nematodes complete a part of the life cycle in soil.
2. Being soil-borne microfauna, the activities of these nematodes are affected by soil temperature, moisture, aeration, soil texture and pH, organic matter, rhizosphere and various cultural operations. Population of nematodes is high in soil layer of 0-15 cm depth and sometimes they can live upto the depth of 150 cm or more.
3. Generally, concentration of nematodes is extremely high in the rhizosphere of susceptible host plants.
4. Movement of nematode in soil is very slow and a nematode can travel a maximum of **one meter** per season.
5. However, they can move faster at certain soil moisture level when pores are lined with thin film of water under water logging conditions.
6. In gall forming nematodes, temperature-moisture interaction determines the emergence of larvae from galls.
7. Most nematodes eggs hatch freely in water in absence of any special stimulus.
8. Nematodes are spread in a local areas by farm equipments, irrigation, flood or drainage water, animal feet and dust storms while spread to a longer distance through farm produce and nursery plants.

Signs and symptoms

Typical root symptoms indicating nematode attack are root knots or galls, root lesions, excessive root branching, injured root tips, and stunted root systems. Symptoms on the above-ground plant parts indicating root infection are a slow decline of the entire plant, wilting even with ample soil moisture, foliage yellowing, and fewer and smaller leaves. These are, in fact, the symptoms that would appear in plants deprived of a properly functioning root system. Bulb and stem nematodes produce stem swellings and shortened internodes. Bud and leaf nematodes distort and kill bud and leaf tissue.

Examples of highly damaging plant parasitic nematodes

Tle plant parasitic nematodes belong to class: **Nematodea**; Subclass : **Secernetia:** Order: **Tylenchida:** Suborder: **Tylenchina** and **Aphlenchina.** A number of genera and species of nematodes are highly damaging to a great range of hosts, including foli-age plants, agronomic and vegetable crops, fruit and nut trees, tuffgrass, and forest trees. Some of the most damaging nematodes are:

1.	Root knot	*Meloidogyne* spp
2.	Cyst	*Heterodera* and *Globodera* spp
3.	Root lesion	*Pratylenchus* spp.
4.	Spiral	*Helicotylenchus* spp.
5.	Burrowing	*Radopholus similis*
6.	Bulb and stem	*Ditylenchus dipsaci*
7.	Reniform	*Rotylenchulus reniformis*
8.	Dagger	*Xiphinema* spp.
9.	Bud and leaf	*Aphelenchoides* spp.

Nematodes as vector of plant pathogens

1. Some species of nematodes viz., dagger nematode (*Xiphinema* sp.), needle nematode (*Longidorus* spp. and *Paralongidorus* spp.) and stubby-root nematodes (*Trichodorus* spp. and *Paratrichodorus* spp.) can carry plant viruses.

2. Members of *Longidorus* and *Xiphinema* (family Longidoridae) transmit the polyhedral nepoviruses (type member : tobacco ringspot virus) while *Trichodorus* and *Paratrichodorus* (family Trichodoridae) transmit the straight tubular tobraviruses (type member: tobacoo rattle virus).

Few examples of the nematodes as virus vectors are mentioned below:

Sl, No	Plant virus transmitted	Nematode species involved as vector
1.	Arabis mosaic	*Longidorus caespiticola, Paralongidorus maximus,Xiphinema index, Xiphenema* spp.
2.	Brome mosaic	*L. macrosoma, X. coxi, X. diversicaudatum*
3.	Carnation ringspot	*L. elongatus, X. diversicaudatum*
4.	Cowpea mosaic	*X. basiri*
5.	Grapevine fan leaf	*X. index* and *X. italiae*
6.	Grapevine vein banding	*X. index*
7.	Mulberry ringspot	*L. martini*
8.	Tobacco ringspot	*X. americanum, X. coxi*
9.	Tomato ringspot	*X. americanum, X. brevicolle*
10.	Tobacco rattle	*Paratrichodorus minor, Trichodorus cylindricus,T. primitivus*

Plant parasitic nematode management

Nematode management should be multifaceted. Since eliminating nematodes is not possible, the goal is to manage their population, reducing their numbers below damaging levels. Common management methods used include planting resistant crop varieties, rotating crops, incorporating soil amendments, and applying pesticides. In some cases, soil solarization also may be practical.

Disease-resistant varieties

Resistant varieties should be used whenever possible to reduce yield loss. It is important to have multiple disease resistance genes when more than one important pathogen is present in a field, such as with tomatoes where root-knot nematodes, *Verticillium,* and *Fusarium* can interact.

Crop rotation

Plant parasitic nematodes survive overwinter in the soil or in association with plant material. Crop rotation and weed control are very important in managing plant parasitic nematodes. Root-knot spp. have a very wide vegetable, field crop, and weed host range. Soybean cyst nematodes have a much narrower host range, but when both nematode species are present a rotation ideal for soybean cyst nematode reduction may favor buildup of root-knot spp.

Other cultural practices

Plant parasitic nematodes reduce the plant root system's ability to take up water and nutrients, especially when nematode population density is high at planting. Adequate water and fertilizer does not reduce the nematode density but reduces plant stress and thus the symptoms of nematode damage. Anything that moves soil can spread plant parasitic nematodes within fields and to other fields.

Soil Solarizarion

Solarization, the heating of soil by using clear plastic tarps to increase and trap the sun's heat, can be an effective means of controlling nematodes in the soil. The soil needs to be moist, well tilled, and heated to at least 140 ^{o}F (60 ^{0}C) for several days, preferably several weeks. This method can be practical for home gardens, but it should be done during the hot months of mid-summer. Similarly, other heat and steam-based pasteurization methods can be used to prepare potting soil. Healthy plants grown in nematode-free media have a better chance to survive after being transplanted to the soil.

Biological control—Another nonchemical approach to controlling nematodes is biological control—using other organisms against the pest organism. A high level of natural biological control is ordinarily present in the soil. This natural control probably keeps the nematode populations at 10–20 percent of what they would be in its absence. Nevertheless, the level of natural control is seldom adequate to prevent plant damage from nematodes.

The strategy for biological control of nematodes is to incorporate soil amendments such as manures (particularly chicken manure) and compost. Such additions of organic matter contribute to biological activity in the soil and enhance the natural activity of organisms antagonistic to nematodes. Many nematophagus fungi have been reported. *Pseudomonas* is antagonistic to the nematodes. Virus infection in *Meloidogyne incognita* has been reported. Amoeboid organisms attack larvae of potato cyst nematode

Chemical Control

Seedling diseases, root diseases, and vascular wilts caused by soil borne fungi and nematodes can be destructive problems in the field and greenhouse. Soil-applied fumigants or nematicides may help prevent serious losses to soil borne disease when used in conjunction with long-term management practices. Soil fumigants are chemicals that, when injected into the soil, emit toxic fumes that penetrate air spaces in soil in sufficient concentration to kill microorganisms. They must be sealed into the soil with water or a plastic tarp to ensure that a lethal concentration and exposure time are reached. Many fumigant are available to eradicate nematodes. Mehyl bromide @ 400-900 kg/ha, dichloropropene at 500-900 kg/ha, dibromochloro-propane (Nemagon) at 120 kg/ha are injected into the soil to eradicate nematodes. Because fumigants are harmful to all living plants, a period of 2 weeks to 2 months must be allowed between treatment and planting in order to avoid crop damage. Some of the granules also reduce nematode populations. Aldicarb @ 11 kg/ha and Oxamyl at 11 kg/ha effectively control nematode. Carbofuran 0.75-1.0 kg/ha also reduces nematodes. Several non fumigant nematicides are available for several vegetable crops. These generally are systemic compounds that also may provide good insect control. Seed treatment with chemical is also beneficial. Fumigation with methyl bromide controls stem nematode (**Ditylenchus dipsaci**) which is carried on onion and lucerne seeds. Sodium hypochlorite solution containing 1% available chlorine destroys the cysts of **Globodera rostochinensis**, the potato cyst nematodes found contaminated with potato tubers. A number of different factors affect the performance of these products, including soil temperature, soil moisture, soil tilth, organic matter, soil type, and time of application. Consult the product label for specific details on safe handling and application methods.

Quarantine

Potato cyst nematode is a quarantine objective and strict quarantine prevents the movement of the nematode from one country to another.

CHAPTER - 18

The Pathogens-Phanerogamic Parasites

Fungi, nematodes, bacteria, and viruses are probably the first things that come to mind when thinking of plant pathogens. These organisms certainly do cause damage to plants of economic importance, but it may surprise you to know that parasitic flowering plants are also important pathogens.There are few seed plants, which are parasitic on living plants and are called parasitic higher plants or **Phancrogamic parasites.** These parasitic higher plants attack some valuable crops and trees causing considerable losses. They produce flowers and seeds and belongs to several widely separated botanical families they differ to each other on their dependency on host plants. These parasites have haustoria as absorbing organ, which sent deep into the vascular bundle of the host to draw water and nutrients. More than 2500 species of higher plants are known to live parasitically on other plants.

Classification of flowering plant parasites:

i) Complete Parasite (Holoparasites)

a. Root Orobanche (Broom rape)

b. Stem Cuscuta (Dodder, Amarvel)

ii) Partial Parasites (Semi Parasites)

a. Root Striga (Sandle wood, witch weed)

b. Stem Loranthus (Banda or Dendrophae)

COMPLETE ROOT PARASITE - BROOM RAPE

Family : Orobanchaceae

Genus : *Orobanche*

1. Orobanche spp. are total root parasites affecting Tobacco, Brinjal, Tomato, Cauliflower, Turnip and many other solanaceous and cruciferous plants. In some areas of the world, broom rape cause losses varying from 15 to 70 % of the crop.

2. The parasite consists of a stout, fleshy stem 15 to 50 cm long. This stem is yellow or brownish red in colour and is covered by small thin and brown scaly leaves.
3. The flower appearing in the axil of the leaves are white and tubular. Seeds are very small and black in colour and many remain viable in soil for several years.
4. The haustoria of the parasite penetrate into the root of the hosts and draw it nourishment.
5. When the host is carefully uprooted, the parasitic roots are seen intertwined with the host root systems; the growth of the host is retarded and remains stunted.

Management

1. Long crop rotation.
2. Destroy the parasite before flowering.
3. Drenching of the soil with 0.25% copper sulphate solution has been reported to be successful in destroying the parasites.
4. Fumigating the soil with methyl bromide.
5. Broom rapes is also effectively controled after treatment with the herbicides "Glyphosate".

COMPLETE STEM PARASITE - DODDER

Family : Cuscutaceae

Genus : *Cuscuta*

1. These are non-chlorophyll bearing leafless, twining parasitic seed plants, they attach to the host.
2. They are yellow, pink or orange in colour.
3. The initial appearance of parasite in field is noticed as small masses of branched, thread like, leafless stem, which are devoid of green pigment and twice around the stem or leaves of the hosts.
4. The leaves are represented by minutes functionless scales.
5. When the stem of parasites comes in contact with the hosts, the minute root like organs, haustoria penetrates into the host cortex and serves as an organ of food absorption.
6. When the relationship with the host is firmly established, the dodder

plant losses the contact from soil.

7. The flowers are found in clusters, they are tiny, white, pink or yellowing in colour.
8. The seeds are formed in capsule. A single plant may produce as many as 3000 seeds.
9. The common dodder *Cuscuta granovil* attacks clovers, berseem flag and many other oilseed crops. It also attacks ornamental and hedge plants. It is fast developing parasites and within 2-3 seasons may destroy a complete plant.
10. The dodder perpetuates through seeds which remain dormant in the soil unitl favourable seasons returns, stem portion of parasite is also meant of perpetuation.

Management

1. Selection of dodder free seeds for sowing.
2. Crop rotation with non host plants.
3. Restriction of flow of irrigation water through infected field.
4. Dodder can be controlled by the use of soil herbicides, such as chloropropham, donoseb, DCPA, glyphosate, these chemicals kills the dodder plant upon its germiantion from seed.
5. Preventing the movement of grazing animals from infected field to clean field.

PARTIAL ROOT PARASITE - STRIGA

Family : Scrophulariaceae

Genus : *Striga* (Witch weed)

1. Striga is well known partial root parasite of sugarcane, cereals, jawar, maize, and millets in India.
2. There are four species of Striga reports in the country on sugarcane, rice , sorghum and other millets like *S.lutee S.densiflora , S. quphrasioldes, S.asiatica.*
3. These plants although obligate parasites do not obtain all of their nutrient material from their host root. They posses' chlorophyll bearing leaves.
4. Striga can be found on light as well as heavy soil in rabi and kharif season. The seeds of Striga are very minute and produced in great

abundance 50,000 to 1, 00,000 seeds /pl/yr.

5. One flower / capsule contains 1200-1500 seeds.
6. Viability of those seeds has been reported to be from 12-40 years.
7. For germination of seeds of Striga species, stimulant provided by the root executes of specific host is essential.
8. Seed starts germination after 7-10 days. After germination, the parasites grow below the soil surface for about 4-8 weeks and produces underground stem and root.
9. The underground portion of the stem contains bud in the axil of leaf.
10. Stem of parasite forms haustoria which penetrates the root of hosts plants and also water and nutrient eventually wasting and destroying the host.

Management of Striga

1. Deep ploughing after harvest reduces the vialibility of seed.
2. Complete eradication of parasite before flowering.
3. Regular Interculture should be followed.
4. Crop rotation with Cotton-Jowar- Groundnut.
5. Weedicides are used to control Striga before flowering.
   - 2-4-D @ 2.5 lit/500 lit of water per ha.
   - Attrazine @ 2 kg / 500 lit of water per ha.

PARTIAL STEM PARASITE - LORANTHUS OR BANDGUL

1. Loranthus is common parasites of mango trees.
2. In Northern India, 60-90% of mango trees and large no of other trees are heavily or moderately infected by these parasites.
3. Loranthus (*Dendrophthae falcate)*, the most common species in India is the semi parasitic of the tree trunk and branches. Their leaves posses chlorophyll and synthesize carbohydrate constituent of their food requirement.
4. The parasite attacks, the aerial parts of the host trees, by developing haustoria and obtain its nourishment directly from the vascular system of the host plant. The continuous sucking of the food material by parasite resulting the host to die.

5. Since the parasite attacks the aerial part of host tree, situated far above the soil level and as such devoid of root system of its own.
6. The flowers of parasites are borne in clusters. They are long tubular in shape and usually greenish, red or white in colour according to species.
7. The fruit is fleshy and contains a solitary seed. It is sweet eaten by birds and animals.
8. The parasite is spread by dispersal of its seed, mostly through birds and to some extent by other animals.
9. The damage done by the parasite is most marked in production of new growth of the host. Leaves are reduced in size and show unhealthy green colour. The quantity and yield of fruit is considerably lowered.

Management

1. Injection of $CUSO_4$ or 2-4-D into the infected branches has been found effective in eradicating the parasite from mango.
2. Scrapping of parasite before seedling from the infected bunches.

CHAPTER - 19

Physiological Disorders

DEFINITION

Plant disease in which no pathogens or parasites is associated with the cause is known as **Non-parasitic** disease. They are also called as **non-infectious** or **physiological disorders**. When no pathogen is found, cultured from or transmitted from a diseased plant, then the disease is said to be caused by a non-living or environmental factor. These diseases occur because of disturbances in the plant system by the improper environmental conditions in the air or soil or by mechanical influences.

GENERAL CHARACTERISTICS

1. Physiological disease occurs in the absence of pathogen and therefore, cannot be transmitted.
2. Physiological disorder of plants is caused by the lack or excess of something that supports life from diseased to healthy plants.
3. Non infectious disease may effect plant in all stages of their lives, such as seeds, seedlings, mature plants or fruits.
4. Symptoms may range from slight to severe and affected plants may even die.
5. These disease cause damage in field in storage or at the market.

FACTORS RESPONSIBLE FOR PHYSIOLOGICAL DISORDER OR NON PARASITIC DISEASE

1. Unfavourable Temperature

i) Effects of low temperature

1. Low temperature causes greater damage to crops than high temperature.

2. The frost injuries involved killing of buds of peach, cherry, killing of flowers, young fruits and sometimes succulent twigs of most trees.
3. Blotch type necrosis in potato is due to freezing injury.
4. Low winter temperature may kill young roots of trees such as apple and may also cause canker development and bark splitting.

ii) Effects of high temperature

1. Plants are normally injured quicker and to a greater extent when temperature becomes higher than maximum for growth.
2. High temperature are by and large responsible for sun scald injuries appearing the sun exposed sides of fleshy fruits and vegetables. For example. Sun scald of apple, tomato, onion- bulbs, peppers, potato tubers, canker of linseeds.

2. Effects of Moisture

i). Effects of low moisture

Plant suffering from lack or sufficient soil moisture generally remain stunted are pale green to light yellow, have hardly any small dropping leaves and finally in absence of moisture plant dry and wilt.

ii). Effects of high moisture

Excessive moisture by flooding in the field may cause decay or rotting of fibrous root of plants resulting into wilting. Primarily due to accumulation of toxic materials around the root and base of stem and also due to non availability of nutrients. For example. Tip burn of paddy.

3. Inadequate Oxygen

When there is too much respiration in closed atmosphere the entire oxygen supply may be exhausted resulting in disintegration of cells due to enzymic action. For example. Black heart of potato.

4. Unfavourable Light

Absence of light or lack of sufficient light retards chlorophyll formation and promotes slender growths with long internodes, thus leading to pale green leaves, spirally growth and premature drop of leaves and flower. This condition is known as "**Etiolation**".

5. Atmospheric Impurities

Presence of injurious gases in the atmosphere may cause definite injury to plant and plant parts. More severe and wide spread damage is caused to plant in the fields by chemicals such as hydrogen fluoride, nitrogen dioxide, ozone, sulphur dioxide, peroxyacetyl nitrates.

For example. Black tip of mango . Fruit on trees in close proximity to brick kilns may bear necrotic lesions and become useless for sale and consumption. The smoke of kilns polluted the air with toxic gases like sulphur dioxide which caused necrosis of tissues.

6. Soil Mineral Toxicity and Toxic effects of Decomposition Organic Matter in Soil

Excessive amount of sodium salt especially sodium sulphate, sodium chloride, and sodium carbonate raise the PH of the soil and cause alkali injury i.e chlorosis, stunting etc. Boron, copper and manganese have been most often implicated in mineral toxicity disease. Excess manganese is known to cause crinkle leaf disease in cotton. Excess boron is toxic to many vegetable and trees, Crop residue decomposing in soil produce toxic substances such as fatty acids which produce symptoms of damping off, root rot, wilt and nutritional deficiency.

7. Herbicidal Injury

Several of the most common plant disorder seems to be the result of extensive use of herbicides. Increasing number of herbicides in use for general or specific weed control has created problems.

8. Nutritional Deficiencies or Disorder in Plants

i) Deficiency of minerals *viz*, Nitrogen, Phosphorus, potash, manganese, zinc, copper, iron, magnesium, boron, etc. results in disorders in plant metabolism and cause **hunger signs** in the crops.

ii) Excess of minerals disturbs nutritional balance needed for good metabolism in the plant, hence hindering the effect of essential element.

iii) The deficiencies and excess of minerals also reduce the resistance of plant to fungal, bacterial and other diseases.

iv) The kind of symptoms produced by deficiency of a certain nutrient depend primarily on the functions of that particular element in the plant.

Table 4 : Plant disease due to lack of minerals

Sr.No	Deficient Nutrient	Disease
1.	Nitrogen (N)	Red leaf of cotton.
2.	Phosphorus (P)	Dwarfening of cotton.
3.	Potassium (K)	Cotton rust, Leaf spot of alfa alfa.
4.	Magnesium (Mg)	Sand drown disease in tobacco.
5.	Boron (B)	Internal cork of apple Cracked stem of celery, Black tip of mango, Heart rot of sugarbeed, Brown heart of cabbage and turnip, Internal brown spot of sweet potato, Terminal bud breakdown of tobacco, Fruit pitting and dieback of olive, Hollow stem of brassica.
6.	Copper (Cu)	Reclamation disease of oats, Diebacks of citrus, Wither tip of apple.
7.	Manganese (Mn)	Pahala blight of sugarcane, Marsh spot of garden pea, Grey speck of oats.
8.	Zinc (Zn)	White bud of corn, Little leaf of apple, Bronzing of twigs, Rosette of fruits trees, Mottle leaf of citrus, Khaira disease of rice.
9.	Iron (Fe)	Green netting of citrus.
10.	Molybdenum (Mo)	Whip tail disease of cauliflower.
11.	Calcium (ca)	Blossom end rot of tomato, Black heart of celery. Wither tip of flax.

CHAPTER - 20

Basic Terminology and Definitions in Plant Pathology

For the accurate identification and diagnosis of plant disease and plant problems a foundational knowledge of terms and definitions is vital for developing concepts, doing research, discussing and communicating issues and providing clarity to your work. The following terms and definitions are basic to the study of plant pathology. They are, however, just a brief introduction to the vocabulary of the science. If you have limited or no background in the subject and you are just getting started, the concepts and terminology of plant problems can seem somewhat daunting. However, your vocabulary and skill will develop through exposure to diagnostics, experience and correct use of the appropriate terms.

Plant pathology is the study of plant diseases and the abnormal conditions that constitute plant disorders. **Etiology** is the determination and study of the cause of disease. A pathogen can be living or non-living, but usually refers to a live agent. A **pathogen** is an organism which causes a disease. **Pathological** is a condition of being diseased. **Pathogenic** is having the characteristics of a pathogen and **pathogenicity** is the capability of a pathogen to cause a disease.

A **plant disease** is an abnormality in the structure and/or function of the host plant cells and/or tissue as a result of a continuous irritation caused by a pathogenic agent or an environmental factor. A disease is not static; it is a series of changes in the plant. All plants, to some extent, are subject to disease. Plant disease is the result of an infectious, or biotic agent or a noninfectious, abiotic factor. **Plant injury** is an abrupt alteration of form or function caused by a discontinuous irritant. Plant injury includes insect, animal, physical, chemical or environmental agents.

A causal agent is a general term used to describe an animate or inanimate factor which incites and governs disease and injury. A **causal organism** is a pathogen of biotic origin. When a pathogenic agent is virulent it can cause disease and if the agent is avirulent it is a variant of a pathogen that does not cause severe disease.

A **parasite** is an organism which lives on or in another organism and obtains its nutrition there from. An **obligate parasite** is an organism which is wholly dependent for its nutrition on another living entity. Obligate parasites are **biotrophs** which also depend entirely on a living host for its nutrition. An **autotroph** is a plant that can make its own food through photosynthesis. A **facultative parasites** has the ability, or "faculty" to adapt to an alternative mode of living, **saprophytes** are organisms that gain their nourishment by digesting dead organic material. Keep in mind that a **parasite** is defined by how the organism secures its nutrients and a **pathogen** is defined on the basis of causing abnormalities. Environmental disease includes such factors as extremes in weather, nutrient deficiency or excess, toxic chemicals and other nonliving agents.

A **host** is an organism (eg. a plant) that is harboring a parasite or pathogen from which it obtains its nutrients. The **host range** refers to the various kinds of host plants that a given pathogen may parasitize. A host is considered **resistant** when it has the ability to exclude, hinder or overcome the effects of a given pathogen or other damaging factor. A plant may be resistant to one pathogen or condition but not others. **Tolerance** is the ability of a plant to be colonized by a pathogen or exposed to an abiotic factor without dying or demonstrating disease symptoms. **Susceptibility** is the antithesis of resistance.

Symbiosis is the mutually beneficial association between two or more different kinds of organisms. The organisms in this association are referred to as **symbionts**. An example of symbiosis is demonstrated in the beneficial relationship between mycorrhizal fungi and the roots of over 85% of the plants in nature. The relationship between mycorrhizal fungi and the host roots of the plant result in increased surface area for absorption of nutrients and water. In return the fungi gain carbohydrates (simple sugars) from the plant. Other examples are the nitrogen-fixing nodules on the roots of legumes caused by bacteria of the genus Rhizobium and the symbiotic relationship of certain fungi and a photosynthetic partner, either an alga or a cyanobacterium, as in **lichens**.

The **signs** and **symptoms** of plant disorders are the appearance or manifestation of changes in the normal form and/or function of the plant. Signs and symptoms are usually the first indication you will notice in plant problems. **Signs** are the appearance and/or physical evidence of the causal factor of the plants abnormality. **Signs** are the physical evidence of damage caused by biotic or abiotic agents such as the pathogen itself, pests, spores, fruiting bodies, chemical residue, bacterial ooze and so forth. **Symptoms** are the visible response of a plant to biotic and/or abiotic factors that result in a change or abnormality in the plant. Symptoms can take form as galls, chlorosis, ring-spots, wilt, rot and so on. A **syndrome** is the totality of the effects demonstrated in a host by one disease, whether simultaneously or successively, and whether visible to the unaided eye or not. **Diagnostics** is the determination of the nature and/or cause of a disease or disordered condition.

For a biotic disease to occur, the environmental conditions must be conducive to the survival of the pathogen. This is especially true with moisture and temperature. Environmental factors can encourage or discourage the susceptibility of the host and the pathogenicity of the pathogen. The environmental conditions can also effect the interaction between the host and the pathogen. Environmental diseases are caused by persistent unfavorable environmental conditions. These conditions include temperature, moisture, wind, light, soil pH, soil structure, host nutrition, herbicides, chemicals and air pollutants. Nutrient deficiency and excess also can greatly affect the susceptibility of plants to disease and disorders. The four fundamental elements required for disease in plants are: a **susceptible host,** a **pathogen** capable of causing disease, a **favorable environment** and **adequate time**. This is referred to as the **"disease quadrangle**".

The **life cycle** of an infectious disease is the sequence of distinct events, such as sexual reproduction, that occur between the appearance and reappearance of the causal organism. The stages of the disease cycle are the appearance, development and perpetuation of a pathogen and the effect of the disease on the host. Because advancement of the disease involves the host, the pathogen and in some cases biological vectors, the life cycle of the pathogen as well as environmental factors are involved in the disease cycle. **Propagules** are any structure, fragment or part of an organism that can propagate the organism. The propagules, such as spores, sclerotia etc. that overwinter or oversummer and initiate an infection are referred to as **primary inoculum**. **Secondary inoculum** is produced by infections that take place during the same growing season. **Inoculation** is the process of applying inoculum to a host. Inoculum must be on a part of the host that can be invaded, this is the **infection court**. A **repeating cycle** is a series of secondary infections that continue for a specific period of time during the growing season. A **polycyclic** disease is one that completes two or more life cycles in one year. A **monocyclic** disease is one that has one life cycle in one year.

Pathogens are transmitted, disseminated and spread by many factors, which include biotic, abiotic and environmental factors. **Transmission** usually implies active transfer by means of grafting, insects, mechanical factors, animals and so on. To disseminate or spread means to disperse or distribute. **Disseminate** usually refers to long-distance distribution, and **spread** usually refers to local distribution. **Vectors** are active agents of transmission such as insects, mites, nematodes and other animals. The dissemination of pathogenic organisms can also be accomplished by wind, rain, irrigation, contaminated seeds and transplants. A few pathogens have the ability to move short distances on their own. Nematodes, zoosporic fungi, oomycetes and some bacteria can move from host to host if they are close enough to one another and the conditions are favorable.

Infection is the establishment of a parasite on or within a host cell or tissue. The **infection court** is a certain part of a given plant that is susceptible to a particular pathogen or pathogens. Successful infections usually result in the appearance of disease symptoms. **Colonization** of a host results from the establishment, growth and reproduction of the pathogen on or in infected plant. **Infestation** refers to the establishment (or "running over") on the surface of a host by a large number of insects or other animal pests. With infestation there is no implication that infection has occurred.

An **epidemic** is the unarrested, widespread increase of an infectious disease, usually limited in time. An epidemic may extend over a single season or many years and over a wide or relatively small area. An **endemic** disease is one that is permanently established in a moderate or severe form within a defined area. Endemic diseases usually become indigenous following initial introduction of the pathogen. **Epidemiology** is the study of factors affecting the outbreak and spread of infectious disease. The **epidemic rate** is the increase or decrease per unit or time in a given plant population.

The classification of a disease can be categorized by the pathogen, the host, the age of the host, the name of the disease, a plant part, symptoms, location, causal agent, geography or by order of importance within a given location. **Taxonomic classification** is the systematic ordering of plants and animals.

There is a very impressive and extensive number of terms and definitions used in plant science, many of which you will not come in contact with. With interest, study and practice, terms and names will come to light and become familiar to you. When you start out, don't worry too much about the scientific names of pathogens and diseases; but also don't be afraid of them. The more exposure you have to the subject the more comfortable you will be when dealing with your peers and the public. In time you will start to notice patterns in both nomenclature and in the biology of pathogens and diseases. These patterns will give you an overall appreciation of this science and a foundational knowledge on which to build your expertise. The feeling of being overwhelmed with new information is a common theme among all of us.

Chapter - 21

Classification of Plant Diseases

There are thousands of diseases, which attack crop plants. Classification can be made based on several criteria. The various ways of classifying diseases of plants are given below.

A. Based on Type of Infection

1. ***Localized disease***- affecting only a part of the plant; leaf spots and anthracnoses caused by different fungi.

2. ***Systemic disease-*** affecting the entire plant.

B. Based on Symptoms

Rusts, smuts, wilts, blights, cankers, mildews, rots, damping-off, die-back, scab etc.

C. Based on the Host Plant

1. ***On the basis of host***. e.g. disease of apple, diseases of wheat, diseases of rose, diseases of coconut, diseases of coffee, diseases of cotton.

2. ***On the basis of host group***- e.g. cereal crop disease, diseases of pulses, diseases of oilseed, root crop disease, forage crop disease, plantation crop disease etc.

D. Based on Their Occurrence

1. ***Endemic disease***: The word endemic means prevalent in, and confined to, a particular country or district and is applied to disease. These diseases are natural to one country or part of the earth. When a disease is more or less constantly present in one form or other or less constantly present form year to year in a moderate to severe form, in a particular country or part of earth, it is classed as endemic.

2. ***Epidemic or epiphytotic diseases***: The term 'epidemic' is derived from a Greek word meaning 'among the people' and in true sense applies to

those diseases of human beings which appear very virulently among large section of the population. To carry the same sense in the case of plant diseases, the term epiphytotic has been coined. An **epiphytotic** disease is one which occurs **widely** but **periodically**. It may be present constantly in the locality but assumes severe form only on occasions. A given disease may be endemic in one region and epidemic in another.

3. ***Sporadic diseases***: Sporadic diseases are those diseases which occur at very irregular intervals and locations and in relatively few instances.

4. ***Pandemic diseases***: When a disease is prevalent throughout the country, continent or the world it is known as a pandemic disease.

E. Based on the Cause

1. ***Infectious or Biotic disease*** *:*These are diseases which are incited by biotic or mesobiotic agents under a set of suitable environments. Example, fungal disease, bacterial disease, viral disease.

2. ***Non-infectious or Abiotic disease****:* These are the diseases with no biotic or mesobiotic agents associated, remain noninfectious and cannot be transmitted from one diseased plant to another healthy plant. Example. Disease caused by nature-frost, rain, wind, sun, hail storm etc.

F. Based on the Production of Inoculum

1. ***Single cycle disease (Simple interest disease)*****:** When the increase of disease is mathematically analogs to simple interest of money, it is called simple interest disease. There is only one generation of disease in the course of one epidemic. Such diseases develop from a common source of inoculums i.e the capital is constant, and often there is one generation of infection in a season. Example. Loose smut of wheat

2. ***Multiple cycle Disease (Compound interest disease*****):** When the increase in disease is mathematically analogues to compound interest of money, the disease is called compound interest disease. There are several or many generations of the pathogen in one life cycle of the crop, i.e the capital is increased by the amount of interest. Example. Late blight of potato.

G. Type of Perpetuation and Spread

1. ***Soil-borne diseases***: The causal agents perpetuate and spread through soil. Example. Damping off caused by fungi like *Pythium* sp. and root rot caused by *Rhizoctonia* spp.

2. ***Seed-borne diseases***: Seed or seed materials help in the perpetuation and spread of this disease. The disease causing agents may be internally seed-

borne or externally seed-borne e.g. Loose smut of wheat caused by *Ustilago nuda tritici* (internally seed borne) and blast of rice caused by *Pyricularia oryzae* (externally seed-borne).

3. ***Air-borne diseases***: In these type of diseases the causal agents are spread by wind (air). Example. Early leaf spot and late leaf spot of groundnut caused by *Cercospora arachidicola* and *Phaeoisariopsis personata,* respectively.

H. Based on Sugar Requirement of the Pathogen

Based on the sugar requirements of the pathogen, diseases can be grouped into high sugar diseases or low sugar diseases. Diseases such as rusts and powdery mildews increased when the crops were sprayed with chemicals like DDT or maleic hydrazide which inhibit the outflow of sugars from the leaf and termed these diseases as **'high sugar diseases'**. On the other hand when the crops were sprayed with chemicals like 2,4 D which increase the outflow of sugars e.g. the disease like spots increased and termed these diseases as **'low sugar diseases'**.

I. Iatrogenic Diseases

The diseases which appear on the plant while managing major diseases are called **iatrogenic** diseases e.g. when zineb is sprayed on grapes for the management of downy mildew, the crop suffers losses from grey mold which otherwise do not cause any disease. This happens owing to the effects of the chemical on microclimatic and microbial flora on the leaf surface. The chemical may affect the structural composition or chemical composition of the sugars or the leaf exudates or the phylloplane microflora resulting in conditions favorable for the new pathogen.

CHAPTER - 22

General Symptoms of Plant Diseases

INTRODUCTION

Plant pathogens induce diverse reactions in the body of their hosts. This result in creation of abnormalities which become visible on the plants. A visible or otherwise detectable expression of abnormal physiology, development, or behaviour in a plant resulting from disease is called **symptoms**. Normally, a distinction is made between symptoms and signs A **symptom** of disease is expressed as a reaction of the host to a causal agent, where as, a **sign** is evidence of disease other than that expressed by the host. **Signs** are usually the structures of the pathogen.A disease is first noticed by the presence of symptoms and /or signs, and recognition of specific type of symptoms or sign aid in the eventual diagnosis of the disease.

SYMPTOMS

Symptoms are classified into three general categories-

A. **Necrotic symptoms:** Those symptoms that results from termination of function leading to death.

B. **Hypertrophy/Hyperplasia symptoms: Hyperplasia**; An abnormal increase in number of cells in a particular tissue or organ. **Hypertrophy**; An abnormal increase in the size of a plant or plant part generally due to an abnormal increase in the size of the cells.

C. **Hypoplastic:** Under development; An abnormally small number of cells in a particular tissue or organ.

A. Necrotic Symptoms

1. **Anthracnose:** It is a sunken ulcer like lesion of necrotic cells on the infected parts of the host plant.

2. **Blasting:** The failure to develop fruit.

3. **Blight:** The sudden drying and browning of whole leaves, shoots or branches.
4. **Blotch**: Large, irregular lesions on leaves, shoots and stems.
5. **Canker**: Necrotic, often sunken lesions in the bark or cortex of the stem and roots of especially woody plants.
6. **Damping-off:** A symptom complex characterized by rapid dying, browning, and rotting of germinating seedlings. Shoots may be killed before emergence, stems may be attacked in the root collar region causing shoots to fall over, roots may be destroyed, or cotyledons may be attacked.
7. **Decay:** Disintegration of dead tissues.
8. **Dieback:** The progressive drying, shrivelling, and browning of twigs or branches from the tips inward toward the trunk.
9. **Hydrosis ;** A water soaked, translucent appearance of leaves, fruits and green stems due to the extrusion of water from the cells into the intercellular spaces.
10. **Scald:** Blanching of the epidermis and adjacent tissues.
11. **Scorch :**A sudden drying and browning of large, indefinite areas on leaves and fruits. Also damage to bark resulting in drying and death.
12. **Shot hole**: Circular hole, in leaves resulting from the dropping out of the central necrotic areas of spot.
13. **Spot:** Circular, areolate, or irregular discolored and dead areas on leaves, fruits, or green stems.
14. **Streaks or stripes**: They are prominent symptoms consisting of an elongated but relatively narrow lesions. These streaks or stripes are usually some shade of brown colour.
15. **Ring Spots**: are characterized by appearance of sometimes chlorotic but mostly necrotic rings on the leaves or also on the fruits and stem.Ring spots are common type symptoms produced by viral pathogens.
16. **Rot :** The disintegration and decomposition of dead tissues.
17. **Wilting;** A flaccid appearance of leaves and shoots resulting from a temporary or permanent loss of turgor due to excess transpiration by the leaves and shoots.
18. **Yellowing ;**The loss of green color from chlorophyllous tissues, due

to the destruction of the chlorophyll and/or degeneration of the chloroplasts, which unmasks yellow pigments.

B. Hypertrophy/Hyperplasia (Overdevelopment) Symptoms

1. **Anthocyanescence:** A reddish or purplish coloration of leaves resulting from abnormal development of anthocyanin pigments.
2. **Callus:** Tissue overgrowth produced in response to injury or other irritation and which tends to cover a wound, canker, etc.
3. **Enations:** Enations are outgrowths generally occurring in veins or midrib on the lower surface of leaves. They may be small, large, papillate, or spin like in shape and also vary in number.
4. **Leaf Curl** ; Abnormal bending or curling of leaves or shoots due to localized overgrowth on one side or in certain tissues.
5. **Fasciation :** Flattening or cohering of organs such as stems, flowers, and roots. The cause is unknown, but in some cases the condition can be propagated.
6. **Witches' broom ;**A type of overgrowth in which there is an abnormal bush like development of many weak shoots or roots.
7. **Sarcody:** Abnormal swelling of tissues above girdled branches or stems.
8. **Scab:** A limited, more or less circular, raised, and sometimes roughened lesion on fruits, tubers, leaves, and stems.
9. **Tumor;** Local swelling on any part of the plant, usually woody roots, stem, or branches, usually resulting from stimulation of the plant meristem by the pathogen.
10. **Virescence;** The process in which a normally white or colored tissue develops chlorophyll and becomes green.
11. **Warts:** Warts are protuberance developed on tubers and stems generally giving warty or discolored cauliflower like appearances.

C. Hypoplastic (Underdevelopment) Symptoms

1. **Chlorosis:** Yellowing of green tissue due to chlorophyll destruction or failure of chlorophyll formation.
2. **Dwarfing:** Subnormal size of a plant or some of its organs.
3. **Etiolation:** A symptom complex in which the major symptoms are

dwarfing of foliage and inflorescence, spindly stem growth, and chlorosis.

4. **Mosaic:** Pale green mottling of leaves.

5. **Russeting :**Rough or corky surfaces formed where they do not normally occur.

6. **Suppression:** The complete prevention of organ development.

7. **Leaf narrowing:** The infected leaves generally become narrow due to reduced growth of laminar tissue but the veins and midrib remain normal in growth.

8. **Leaf curling:** These symptoms represent irregular and extensive wrinkling and furrowing of leaves due to reduced growth of vein in comparison to the growth of laminar tissue resulting in sunken veins and raised plaminar tissue leading to the curling of the leaves.

SIGNS

Signs are divided into three general categories: (A) vegetative structures, (B) Reproductive structures, and (C) disease products.

(A) Vegetative Structures

Mycelium, haustorium, pathogen cells, rhizomorph, sclerotia, etc are structures generally observed.

(B) Reproductive Structures

Apotheica, Acervuli, asci, basidium, cleistothecium, conidiophores, mildews, perithecia, pycnidia, sporangium, spores, sporodochium etc are the structures commonly observed. Some major symptoms based on presence of reproductive structures are :

1. **Bunt:** A disease caused by fungi in which the grain contents are replaced by odorous smut spores.

2. **Mildew**: Mildews are plant diseases in which the pathogen is seen as a growth on the surface of the host. They appear as white, gray, brownish, or purplish patches of varying size on leaves, herbaceous stems, or fruits. In downy mildews the superficial growth is a tangled cottony or downy layer, while in the powdery mildews enormous numbers of spores are formed on superficial growth of the fungus giving a dusty or powdery appearance. Black minute fruiting bodies may also develop in the powdery mass.

3. **Rusts**: These are diseases with rusty symptoms. The rusts appear as relatively small pustules of spores, usually through the host epidermis. The pustules may be either dusty or compact, and red, brown, yellow, or black in colour.

4. **Smuts**: The word smut means a sooty or charcoal-like powder. The affected parts of the plant show a black or purplish-black dusty mass. These symptoms usually appear on floral organs, particularly the ovary but they can also be found on stems, leaves and roots.

5. **Sooty Mold**: A sooty coating on foliage and fruits formed by the dark hyphae of fungi that live on the honey dew secreted by insects.

(C) Disease Products

In various bacterial diseases *viz,* bacterial blight of rice, masses of bacterial ooze out to the surface of the affected organs where they may be seen as drops of various sizes or as thin smeer over the surface. In some cases some what raised, black coated fungus bodies appearing as a flattened out drop of tar on leaves.

CHAPTER - 23

Dispersal of Pathogens

To make a healthy plant sick or diseased, primary requirement of a pathogen is spread of its inoculums from the source of survival to the susceptible host. The spread of a plant pathogen within the common area in which it is already established is called **dispersal** or **dissemination**. Moving the inoculum only a few inches and transporting it for hundreds of kilometers both represent its dispersal. Nevertheless, the pathogen dispersal is not necessarily only for spread of diseases but also for continuity of the life cycle and development of the pathogen. A detail knowledge of pathogen dispersal is necessary to find out effective control measures for diseases because the possibilities of preventing dispersal and thereby breaking the infection chain always exist.

Plant pathogen dispersal generally occurs through two key groups:

A. **Direct (Autonomous) dispersal:** - Disease dispersal where the pathogen is carried through soil, seed or planting material like cuttings, sets, tubers, bulbs etc.

B. **Indirect (Passive) dispersal:-** The pathogen spreading itself or by natural agencies like wind, water, animals, insects, mites, nematodes, birds etc.

DIRECT DISPERSAL

1.Through seed: Infected/infested seed is one of the most important means of autonomous dispersal.Dispersal of inoculums through seeds is accomplished as

a. mixture and contaminant dormant structure of pathogens viz., galls, sclerotia, cysts and smut sori. etc. The oospores of the downy mildew pathogen of pear, millet, ergot pathogen of pearl millet and rye, bunted grains containing spore ball of the wheat blunt pathogen etc. found mixed with the seed as contaminats.

b. through presence of propagules on the seed coat e.g. Covered smut of barley.

c. or as dormant mycelium in the seed e.g. Loose smut of wheat, Ring rot and brown rot of potato, Whip smut and red rot of sugancane, Mosaic and leaf roll of potato.

2. Through soil: A big number of plant pathogens survive in soil. Their survival in soil depends on many factors including soil characteristics, soil environment, crop grown and other cultivation practices. In soil dispersal takes place in two ways

a. *Dispersal in soil* (when the soil remains static but the pathogens grow or move). Many pathogens survive in soil as facultative parasites or facultative saprophytes. Some of the fungi produce spores which are motile (Zoospores) and can move some distances in soil and infect their hosts. Nematodes can move some distances in soil infect their hosts.

b. *Dispersal by soil* - the contaminated soil is transported to other places along with planting material, seedlings or implements etc. while adopting agronomic practices.

3. **Through vegetative planting materials :** Dispersal of large number of plant pathogens takes place through the vegetative parts of the plants used as planting materials, such as tubers, cuttings, runners, rhizomes, grafts, etc. Over 40% of the bacterial plant pathogens are transmitted on vegetatively propagated materials. Among the important examples are *X. campestris pv.citri* (citrus canker) and *A. tumifaciens* (crown gall).Viruses are invariably transmitted by vegetative propagules; thus viral diseases are mainly severe in vegetative propagated horticultural crops.

Table 5 : Examples of autonomous dispersal of plant pathogens

Autonomous dispersal	Examples
Through seed	
Seed contamination	*Anguina tritici* (seed gall nematode), *Tolyposporium penicillariae* (Smut of bajra), *Claviceps , Cuscuta*
Internally seed borne	Loose smut of wheat *(Ustilago tritici)*
Externally seed borne	Covered smut of barley (*Ustilago hordei*), Stinging smut of wheat (*T. caries* and *T. foetida),* Black arm of cotton *(Xanthomonas campestris pv. malvacearum*
Through vegetative planting materials	
Seed tubers	Late blight of potato (*Phytophthora infestans*)
Sugarcane setts/cutting	Red rot of sugarcane(*Colletotrichum falcatum*)
Propagative materials	Citrus *tristeza* and greening
Rhizome	Rhizome rot of ginger

INDIRECT DISPERSAL

1. **Wind dispersal: -** Extensive and severe epidemics of plant diseases are mostly the results of wind dispersal of the pathogens. Wind dispersal involves four stages relating to the spores viz. Production of countless spores, their liberation in the wind currents, dispersal along with the wind and deposition on new susceptible host surfaces where they cause infection under favourable climatic conditions. This is the most dangerous mode of transmission of plant pathogenic fungi like those causing powdery and downy mildews, leaf spots, blasts, blights and rust diseases.

2. **Water dispersal:** Disease dispersal through the agency of water in different ways is comparatively less important as compared to the wind dispersal. Splashing rain drops generally transmit the foliar diseases from leaf to leaf, from shoot to shoot and even from plant to plant in case of closely spaced crops. Plant pathogens requiring high humidity conditions like the fungi causing downy mildew diseases or bacteria causing canker of citrus are well adapted to this kind of short distance water dispersal. Certain soil inhabiting pathogenic fungi and bacteria causing root and collar rots, wilts, foot, rots, etc are likely to be transmitted to much longer distances through the agencies like irrigation water, streams and rivers, etc. It is also an important agency in transmission of seeds of higher flowering parasites like dodder and striga.

3. **Insects dispersal:** Most of the viral diseases of plants are transmitted through the agency of different insects. Both types of insects viz. sucking and chewing or/biting are capable of transmitting viral diseases. The transmission may be simply 'mechanical' or it may be 'biological'. In case of mechanical transmission the pathogen is simply carried externally or internally by the insect. In the biological case the specific insect and the specific viral pathogen have some kind of association or relationship between the two. Insects in such cases are called the 'vectors' for the particular viral pathogen. Viruses carried 'biologically' by the insect vectors are of two types:

   1. **Non-persistent**-viral pathogen requiring no latent or incubation period in the insect body.

   2. **Persistent:** viral pathogens requiring certain incubation period inside the vector body before they are inoculated or transmitted to healthy host. The insects responsible for transmission of viral diseases belong to the species of aphids, jassids (leaf hoppers),

white flies, mealy bugs, etc. Certain bacterial viz, Fire blight of potato (*E. amylovora*),Citrus canker (*X. citri*) and several fungal pathogens viz, Dutch elm (*Ceratostomella ulmi*), Anthracnose of cucumber (*Colletotrichum lagenarium*) are also known to be carried by insects.

4. **Mites:** The mites are the only non insect arthropod vectors of plant viruses.The ability to transmit virus is restricted to a few species of eriophyd mites. Diseases transmitted by Eriyophyd mites include fig mosic, sterility mosaic of pigeon pea, wheat streak mosaic and wheat spot mosaic.

5. **Nematodes:** Nematodes have been observed to transmit viral, bacterial and fungal plant diseases. Nematodes feeding externally on host plant roots cause injuries to roots which become the avenues for entrance of fungal and bacterial pathogens infecting plant roots. Members of genera *Longidorus* and *Xiphinem*a transmit polyhedral nepoviruses such as the arabis mosaic, grapevine fan leaf, tomato ring spot. *Trichodorus* and *Paratrichodorus* transmit the netuviruses such as tobacco rattle and pea early browning.

6. **Animals:** Farm animals serve as disease transmitting agents in some cases. They are likely to carry the pathogen externally on their body surface, particularly on legs and hoofs, etc. or internally through their intestinal tract. Commonly, the soil inhabiting fungi causing rots and wilts are carried externally while certain smut fungi causing diseases to grain crops are transmitted through the intestinal tract.

7. **Birds:** Birds can fly and cover long distances than insects. The spores of fungul pthogens may adhere to the feathers of birds and may be carried to distant places and dispersed. *Loranthus* sp. parasitising certain trees like mango. Birds transmit loranthus both externally and internally.

8. **Implements and Tools:** Farm implements used for cultivation of soil are often likely to transmit plant pathogens from one place to another. The pathogens in this case are usually carried in the form of bits of plant disease debris lying in the soil. Similarly tools used for carrying out operations like cutting, pruning, budding, grafting, thinning,etc. also help in the transmission of certain diseases from plant to plant. Several viral diseases are disseminated through the budding and grafting operations.

9. **Human dispersal**: Man is often responsible for transmission of plant diseases in two ways viz.

1. Workers handling seedlings, other planting material or fruits are likely to get personally in contact with plant pathogens like fungi or bacteria. While handling the diseased material and unknowingly and indirectly transmit the pathogens to healthy seedlings or plant parts through his contaminated hands. This is a kind of 'continuous' mode of transmission.

2. The other or'discontinous' mode of transmission for which only man is responsible is the most efficient and equally dangerous phenomenon of transmission of plant diseases between distant geographical areas often separated by physical barriers like oceans, mountains or deserts, etc. Such long distances transmission of a disease to an area or country hitherto free from the disease is usually accomplished by the transport of infected seed, nursery stock or timber, etc. Thus it is a kind of direct transmission through propagating material.

Table 6 : Examples of passive (indirect) dispersal of plant pathogens

Passive dispersal		Examples
Through water	Water splash	Bacterial leaf blight of rice *(Xanthomonas campestris pv. oryzaecola),*
		Bacterial streak disease of paddy *(Xanthomonas oryzaecola)*
		Coffee rust *(Hemileia vastatrix)*
	Water flow dispersal	Club root of cabbage (*Plasmodiophora brassicae*)
		Late blight of potato (*Phytophthora infestans*)
		Red rot of sugarcane(*Colletotrichum falcatum*)
Through air		Scab of apple (*Venturia inaequalis*)
		Black stem rust of wheat (*Puccinnia graminias tritici*)
		Late blight of potato (*Phytophthora infestans*)
Through insects	Bees and wasp	Fire blight of apple (*Erwinia amylovora*)
	Beetle (*Scolytus)*	Dutch elm disease (*Ceratocystis elmi*)
	Leaf minor	Citrus canker (*Xanthomonas citri*)
Through nematodes	*Anguina tritici*	Yellow ear rot of wheat *(Coryne bacterium tritici*)

Contd...

	Aphlenchoidea	Leafy gall (*Corynebacterium tritici)*
	Xiphinema index	Grapevine fan leaf virus
Through fungi	*Synchitrium endobioticum*	Potato virus X, Potato mop top virus
	Olpidium brassicae	Tobacco necrosis virus, Letuce big vein virus
Through birds		Loranthus (*Dendrophthoe*), Mistletoe (*Viscum*) , Chestnut blight (*Endothea parasitica*)
Through man		Wart of potato (*Synchitrium endobioticum*)
		Flag smut of wheat (*Urocystis tritici*)

CHAPTER - 24

Survival of Plant Pathogens

The availability of a plant pathogens in given area presupposes its ability to survive not only during its parasitic relations with hosts but also during those seasons in which the hosts are not growing. The latter part of continued existence of plant pathogens in which they remain in dormant condition to overcome the unfavourable condition of non availability of hosts is called **"survival"**. Pathogens may survive between crop seasons by means of specialized resting structures, by functioning as saprophyte in or on the soil or in diseased plant debris, or by living in some intimate association with living plants or other organism.

Modes of Survival: The modes of survival of plant pathogens are described below:

1. Parasitic Survival

Organisms, parasitic on perennial plants (fruits, plantation and forest trees) survive in or on their hosts actively or passively depending on the environmental conditions. Certain bacterial pathogens viz, *X. campestris pv citri, X. campestris pv jugalandis, X. campestris pv. Pruni* and *Erwinia amylovora* are known to be carried over perennially in holdover cankers or blighted twigs, which may produce bacterial ooze in favourable weather to fresh inoculums. Similarly several fungal plant pathogens like *Colletotrichum gloeosporioides* (anthracnose of mango), *Oidium mangiferae* (powdery mildew of mango), *Podosphaera leucotricha* (powdery mildew of apple), etc survive on infected organs of the plants. Along with cultivated crops, several undesirable plant (weeds, etc) both annual and perennial, grow independently in the nature. Such plants which belong to the same botanical family to which cultivated hosts belong , are known as collateral hosts. Some important examples include the survival of three Puccinia spp. causing wheat rusts in Indian subcontinent . These fungi survive in active sporulating stage on wild species of *Triticum, Aegilops, Horedeum* and *Agropyron repens*. Similarly, Rice tungro virus survive actively on *Oryza* spp., *Echinocloa* spp. and *Leersia hexandra* .

Heterocious rust fungi require two kinds of host plants to complete their life cycle. The other host does not belong to the botanical family of cultivated host, is reoffered to as alternate host.Fungal pathogens *Rhizoctonia solani*, *Sclerotium rolfsii* and *Sclerotinia sclerotium* are known to have wide host range (plants belonging to different families).

2. Saprophytic Survival

Many plant pathogens adopt survival ability in the absence of their hosts. They grow saprophytically either in or on the soil, or in dead plant debris during this phase. Pathogens that can survive in or on the soil by growing saprophytically are generally considered to be of two types: **soil inhabitants** and **soil invaders**. **Soil inhabitants** are those facultative parasites that are able to survive indefinitely as saprophytes in the soil, and have a wide host range. *Pythium, Rhizoctonia* and *Fusarium* are good example of soil inhabitant fungal pathogens. **Soil invaders (soil transients)** are those that are rather more specialized parasites generally living in close association with their hosts but may survive in soil for relatively short periods of time as saprophytes. Most of the bacteria and fungal pathgoens of facultative saprophytic nature represent soil invaders.

3. Survival through Dormant Structures

Dormancy is the reversible interruption of phenotype development of an organism. It is an adaptation on part of biological organisms to ensure their survival. Dormant structures , due to less nutrient requirements and hardy structures, have better chance of survival under unfavourable conditions.Fungi, nematodes and phanerogams survives through their resting or dormant structures; phanerogams produce seeds, which can live in dormant stage, sometimes for years. Majority of phytophagous nematodes, survive through their dormant structures (cysts, galls, eggs). Plant parasitic fungi produce a variety of resting /dormant structures such as thickened hyphae, chlamydospores, sclerotial bodies, oospores, peritheicia, cleistotheica etc. Plant pathogenic bacteria do not form resting structures . They live in or on the host tissues in living or decaying rate.

4. Survival through Seeds

Seed can harbor a wide range of microflora, viruses and other causal agents of plant pathogens.The longevity of seed borne pathogens can be independent of the seeds they inhibits and depends on the capability of the pathogen to remain viable and ineffective from one season to next , in or on their seeds. Pathogen may live even longer than the seeds that they colonize. For instance, *Colletotrichum lindemuthianum* remained active even after the bean seeds it colonized lost their viability. Flax seeds retain germianbility for 18 to 24 months, whereas *Botrytis cinerea*, *Colletotrichum linicola* and *Aureobasidium lini* survived for more than four years in seeds. The tobacco ring spot virus remained viable in soyabean seeds for five years at 16 t o32 °C. even most seeds failed to germinate.

5. Survival through Insects

Survival of plant pathogens in association with insects is not uncommon in the nature. Some vectors such as aphids, and mites carry non persistent viruses externally on or near the mouth parts. Viruses are known to pesist between crops within vectors , which are themselves inactive. while in case of persistent viruses the vectors remain infective much longer , some times throughout life or infectivity is passed to next generation. This provides an opportunity to virus to manage continuity of infection cycle. Barley yellow mosaic virus can persist up to ten years in resting spores of its vector (*Polymyxa gramin's*) and tobacco rattle virus in dormant nematodes for about a year. The bacterium associated with corn wilt (*E. stewartii*) is present in the intestinal tract of its vector. Nematodes play vital role in survival and dispersal of many important plant viruses.

6. Survival through Nematodes

At least twenty plant viruses have been found perennating with soil inhabiting ,ectoparasitic nematodes. Nematodes of the genera *Longidorus* and *Xiphinema* aquire the viral pathgoens of tobacco ring spot, tomato ring spot, wheat spindle streak mosaic etc, diseases while those of genera *Trichodorus* and *Paratrichodorus* aquire viral pathogens of diseases like tobacco rattle and pea early browning.

7. Survival through Fungi

Some viral pathogens have been found surviving in association with certain fungi. *Olpidium*, is the source of survival and transmission of viral pathogens causing tobacco mosaic, cucumber necrosis, lettuce big vein, and tobacco stunt diseases. Viruses causing wheat mosaic and beet necrotic yellow vein diseases survive in a fungus, namely *Polymyxa* while those causing disease potato mop top survive in *Spongosproa*..These viruses are borne internally in or externally on the resting spores and the zoosproes of their respective fungi. Such resting spores and zoosproes introduce viruses in host plants when they infect the latter.

CHAPTER - 25

The Infection Process

A parasitic must establish an intimate relationship with the host tissues to absorb the desired nutrients. Successful establishment of this relationship is called **infection**. The chain of events that takes place in the causation of disease is called **pathogenesis** or **infection process**. It encompasses the germination or multiplication of an infective propagule in or on a potential host through to the establishment of a parasitic relationship between the pathogen and the host. The process of infection is influenced by properties of the pathogen, the host and the external environment. If any of the stages of the infection process is inhibited by any of these factors, the pathogen will not cause disease in the host. While some parasites colonise the outside of the plant (ectoparasites), pathogens may also enter the host plant by penetration, through a natural opening (like a stomatal pore) or via a wound. The symptoms of the diseases produced by these pathogens result from the disruption of respiration, photosynthesis, translocation of nutrients, transpiration, and other aspects of growth and development. The "infection process"can be divided into three phases:

1. Pre-penetration stage
2. Penetration
3. Post-penetration stage

PRE-PENETRATION STAGE

Before a pathogen can penetrate a host tissue, a spore must germinate and grow on the surface of the plant. Several pathogens develop specific penetration structures, such as appressoria, while others utilize pre-existing openings in the plant's surface, such as stomatal pores or wounds. In the case of motile pathogens, they must find the host and negotiate its surface before entering the host. Plant viruses are often transported and introduced into the plant via vectors such as fungi or insects. The initial contact between infective propagules of a parasite and host plant is called **inoculation**. Pathogens use a variety of stimuli to identify a proper entry point. Numerous fungi use topographical cues on the plant surface to guide them towards a likely stomatal site. Once the hypha reaches a stoma, volatile compounds escaping from the pore appear to provide a signal for the formation of a specialized penetration structure, the appressorium. Amino acids, sugars, and minerals secreted by plants at the leaf surface can non-specifically trigger spore germination or provide nutrition for the pathogen. Various pathogenic spores will not germinate in the absence of these substances. Pathogen development is influenced by temperature, moisture, light, aeration, nutrient availability and pH. The conditions obligatory for survival and successful infection differ between pathogens.

PENETRATION

Pathogens exploit every possible pathway to enter their host, although individual species of pathogen tend to have a preferred method.

Pathway for pathogen entry

1.**Direct penetration:** Fungal pathogens frequently use **direct penetration** of the plant surface to enter the host. This requires adhesion to the plant surface, followed by the application of pressure and then enzymatic degradation of the cuticle and cell wall, in order to overcome the physical barriers presented by the plant's surface. During the degradation of the cuticle and wall, a succession of genes are switched on and off in the pathogen, so that cutinase, followed by cellulase, then pectinase and protease are produced, attacking the cuticle, cell wall, and middle lamella in the order that they are encountered. The pressure needed for the hypha to penetrate the cell wall is achieved by first firmly attaching the appressorium to the plant surface with a proteinaceous glue. The cell wall of the apressorium then becomes impregnated with melanin, making it watertight, and capable of containing the high turgor pressure that builds up within the appressorium. The point of the appresorium that is in contact with the cuticle is called the penetration pore, and the wall is thinnest at this point. The increasing turgor pressure causes the pore to herniate, forming a penetration peg, which applies huge pressure to the host cuticle and cell wall.

Table 7 : Direct modes of penetration by plant pathogens

Mode of penetration	Pathogen
Cuticle	*Erysiphe graminis, Perenospora* spp., *Puccinia graminis.*
Epidermal cells	*Ustilago maydis, Puccinia graminis, Phytophthora infestans, Venturia inaequalis*
Cuticle and epidermal cells	*Erysiphe graminis*
Stigma and young ovary wall	*Ustilago scitaminea, Ustilago tritici, Claviceps* spp.
Young seedlings	*Tilletia caries and Tilletia foetida*
Root tips	*Fusarium oxysporum f. sp. lycopersici*
Seed coat and emerging tissues	*Pythium* spp.

2. Through pre-existing opening: The alternative pathway for pathogen entry is via a **pre-existing opening** in the plant surface. This can be a natural opening or a wound. Pathogenic bacteria and nematodes often enter through **stomatal pores** when there is a film of moisture on the leaf surface. Fungi can also penetrate open stomata without the formation of any specialized structures. Some fungi form a swollen **appressorium** over the stomatal aperture and a fine penetration hypha enters the airspace inside the leaf, where it forms a sub-stomatal vesicle, from which infection hyphae emerge and form haustoria in surrounding cells. Also vulnerable to pathogen invasion are **hydathodes**, pores at the leaf margin that are continuous with the xylem. Under particularly humid conditions, droplets of xylem fluid can emerge at the surface of the leaf where they can be exposed to pathogenic bacteria, which then enter the plant when the droplet retreats back into the hydathode as the humidity decreases. **Lenticels** are raised pores that allow gas exchange across the bark of woody plants. They exclude most pathogens, but some are able to enter the plant via this route. Some specialized pathogens can also use more unusual openings, such as **nectaries**, **styles** and **ectodesmata**. Entry through a wound does not require the formation of specialized structures, and many of the pathogens that utilize wounds to enter the plant are unable to penetrate the plant surface otherwise. Most plant viruses enter through **wounds**, such as those made by their insect vectors.

Table 8 : Indirect modes of penetration by plant pathogens

Mode of penetration	Pathogen
Natural openings	
Stomata	**Bacteria:** *Xanthomonas campestris pv. phaseoli, Xanthomonas campestris pv. malvacearum, Xanthomonas campestris pv. phaseolicola, Pseudomonas tabaci, Erwinia amylovora* **Fungi:** *Stemphylium solani, Cladosporium fulvum, Cladosporium cucumenrinum, Phoma herbarum var. medicaginis*
Hydathodes	*Botrytis cinerea, Erwinia amylovora ,Xanthomonas campestris*
Lenticels	*Streptomyces scabies, Erwinia amylovora, Armillaria mellea, Spongospora subterranean, Phytophthora infestans, Pencillium expansum*
Nectrothodes	*Erwinia amylovora*
Buds	*Fusarium oxysporum* f.sp.*pidi.,Taphirina cereasi,Uromyces pisi, Taphirina deformans*
Trichomes	*Corynbacterium michiganenses*
Root hairs	*Fusarium oxysporum* f.sp.*lini, Fusarium oxysporum f.sp conglutinas, Rhizobium, Plasmodiophora brassicae, Phymatotricum omnivorum*
Wounds	
Nematodes Fungi	*Pseudomonas solanacearum,* by *Meloidogyne incognita var acrita. Corynbacterium tritici* by *Anjuina tritici, Fusarium oxysporum f.* sp. *vasinfectum by Meloidogne* spp.

POST-PENETRATION STAGE

Infection and Colonization

A successful infection requires the establishment of a parasitic relationship between the pathogen and the host, once the host has gained entry to the pathogen. There are two broad categories of pathogens are **necrotrophs** (those that kill plant cells before parasitizing them) and **biotrophs** (those that establish an infection in living tissue). The toxins produced by necrotrophs can be specific to the host or non-specific. Non-specific toxins are involved in a broad range of plant-fungus or plant-bacterial interactions, and will therefore not usually determine the host range of the pathogen producing them. Necrotrophs often enter the plant through wounds and In the case of motile pathogens, they must find the host and negotiate its surface before entering the host. cause immediate and severe symptoms. An intermediate category of parasite is the

hemibiotrophs, which start off as biotrophs and eventually become necrotrophic, employing tactics from both classes of pathogen.

Pathogens that colonize the surface of plants, extracting nutrients through haustoria in epidermal or mesophyll cells are termed **ectoparasites**. The **haustoria** are the only structures that penetrate the host cells. Some parasites colonize the area between the cuticle and the outer wall of the epidermal cells, penetrating host epidermal and mesophyll cells with haustoria. These are called **sub-cuticular infections**. Pathogens can also form colonies deeper in the plant tissues. These are mesophyll and parenchyma **infections,** and can be biotrophic, hemibiotrophic, necrotrophic, or relationships. Necrotrophs do not produce specialized penetration structures. In its place, they kill host cells by secreting toxins, then degrade the cell wall and middle lamella, allowing their hyphae to penetrate the plant cell walls and the cells themselves. In hemibiotrophic infections, intercellular hyphae can form haustoria in living mesophyll cells, but as the lesion expands under favourable conditions, those greatly parasitized cells at the inner, older part of the colony collapse and die. A alike sequence of events can take place in plants infected by burrowing nematodes. **Viruses**, **rusts** and **mildews** develop specialized **biotrophic** relationships with their hosts. Intercellular hyphae of downy mildew colonize host mesophyll cells and form haustoria. The mildew sporulates and the infected cells eventually die, although necrosis is delayed and contained, compared to that caused by necrotrophic pathogens. Rust fungi can also delay senescence in infected cells while they sporulate. **Vascular infections** usually cause wilting and discoloration as a result of the physical blockage of infected xylem vessels. True vascular wilt pathogens colonize the vascular tissue exclusively, although other pathogens can cause the same symptoms if they infect the vascular system as well as other tissues. There are a few pathogens that manage to achieve **systemic infection** of their host. For example, many viruses can spread to most parts of the plant, although not necessarily all tissues. Some downy mildews can also systemically infect their host by invading the vascular tissue and growing throughout the host, causing deformation, rather than necrosis. Finally, there are some pathogens that complete their entire life cycle within the cells of their host, and may spread from cell to cell during cytokinesis. These are **endobiotic infections.**

Disease Physiology

While necrotrophs have little effect on plant physiology, since they kill host cells before colonizing them, biotrophic pathogens become incorporated into and subtly modify various aspects of host physiology, such as photosynthesis, **respiration**, transpiration and growth and development.

Photosynthesis: Pathogens affect photosynthesis, both directly and indirectly. Necrotrophs reduce the photosynthetic rate by damaging chloroplasts and killing cells while pathogens that cause defoliation deprive the plant of photosynthetic tissue, while Biotrophs affect photosynthesis in varying degrees, depending on the severity of the infection. A biotrophic infection site becomes a strong metabolic sink, changing the pattern of nutrient translocation within the plant, and causing net arrival of nutrients into infected leaves to satisfy the demands of the pathogen. The reduction, diversion and withholding of photosynthetic products by the pathogen stunts plant growth, and further reduced the plant's photosynthetic efficiency.

Respiration: The respiration rate of plants invariably increases following infection by fungi, bacteria or viruses. The higher rate of glucose catabolism causes a measurable increase in the temperature of infected leaves. An early step in the plant's response to infection is an oxidative burst, which is manifested as a rapid increase in oxygen consumption, and the release of reactive oxygen species, such as hydrogen peroxide (H_2O_2) and the superoxide anion (O_2^-). The oxidative burst is involved in a range of disease resistance and wound repair mechanisms to rapid active defense. In resistant plants, the increase in respiration and glucose catabolism is used to produce defence-related metabolites via the pentose phosphate pathway. In susceptible plants, the extra energy produced is used by the growing pathogen.

Transpiration: Pathogens affect water relations in the plants they infect. Biotrophs have modest effect on transpiration rate until sporulation ruptures the cuticle, at which point the plant wilts rapidly. Pathogens that infect the roots directly affect the plant's ability to absorb water by killing the root system, thus producing secondary symptoms such as wilting and defoliation. Pathogens of the vascular system similarly affect water movement by blocking xylem vessels.

Growth and development : Growth and development in general are affected by pathogen infection, as a result of the changes in source-sink patterns in the plant. Many pathogens upset the hormone balance in plants by either releasing plant hormones themselves, or by triggering an increase or a diminish in synthesis or degradation of hormones in the plant. This can cause a variety of symptoms, such as the formation of adventitious roots, gall development, and epinasty.

Exit of the Pathogens

In order to continue the infection chain and to escape death due to over crowding after the host is not left with healthy tissues to support the increasing population, the pathogens exist from the host. Fung produce various sporulating or the structures and the bacteria ooze out of the host. These propagules are further disseminated to new areas or host plants.

CHAPTER - 26

Pathogenesis: Role of Enzymes, Toxins, Growth Regulators and Polysaccharides

Pathogens are different from parasites, **Parasites** penetrate into the host and obtain nutrients from the host. They live inside the host without causing any other damage. They may be at times symbionts also i.e. they may be beneficial to the host. The examples for parasites are *Rhizobium* spp. which form nodules in leguminous plants and mycorrhizal fungi. **Pathogens** not only take nutrients from the host but also damage the host severely. They induce numerous symptoms of the disease and even kill the plants.

Pathogens in their life cycle enter into two distinct phases. One is **biotrophic** and the other is **necrotrophic** phage. In the biotrophic phase they invade the host cells inter and intracellularly and establish themselves in the living cells. In the second phase, they kill the cells and obtain nutrition from the dying cells. This phase is called necrotrophic phase. In case of **obligate pathogens** the biotrophic phase may be much longer while in case of **facultative saprophytes**, long biotrophic phase may be followed by necrotrophic phase. In case of **facultative parasites** necrotrophic phase will be much longer with short biotrophic phase. However in case of all pathogens, both the phases may exist either as a short or long spell.

In the biotrophic phase the pathogens establish themselves in the host cells. The first barrier between host plant and the attacking pathogen is the cuticle. Host cells have cell wall, structure surrounding the protoplast. Cell wall is divided into three regions: middle lamella, primary wall and secondary wall. Below the cell wall membranes are found. The membrane provides a semi permeable barrier between the cell and its external environment. The membrane consists of lipids and proteins. During the biotrophic phase, the pathogen invade the cells by degrading cuticle, middle lamella,cell walls and cell membranes, by producing a series of enzymes. After the biotrophic phase, the pathogens produce toxins which kill the cell and enter into the necrotrophic phase. Thus, **enzymes, toxins, growth regulators** are important tools of the pathogens for their pathogenesis.

ENZYMES

Different types of enzymes are produced by phytopathogenic fungi, bacteria and nematodes which are important in degrading cell wall structures and play an important role in penetration and infection process. Enzymes are the major weapons employed by necrotrophs for ingress and colonization. Biotrophs also employ such enzymes but their deployment is highly localized mainly to facilitate their penetration. Pectin degrading enzymes, produced either constitutively or inductively are responsible for tissue maceration. Recent studies have established that pectinases determine the pathogenicity in soft rot caused by *Erwinias. Erwinina chrysanthemi* was found to produce five pectate lyase isozymes (PLa,PLb,PLc,PLd and PLe). It is observed that bacterial mutants lacking genes for PL isozymes a, d and e are avirulent on *Saintpaulia ionantha.* This indicates involvement of these isozymes in pathogenesis.

The importance of cellulases, hemicellulases, and enzymes in pathogenesis have received scant attention. However, isolation and cloning of cellulose gene (cel gene) from *E. chrysanthemi* has opened up the possibilities for realistic assessment of these enzymes in pathogenesis. It is not only the production but release of wall degrading enzymes from concerned pathogens in the host tissues is essential for pathogenesis. Secretion deficient mutants of *E. chry snathemi* and *Xanthomons campestris* are nonpathogenic.

Plant cell wall constituents may serve as effective inducers of wall degrading enzymes in plant pathogens. Some pathogens may produce different types of wall degrading enzymes. Sequence of production and dominance of a particular enzymes may influence the nature of the symptoms. In soft rots predominant enzymes are pectinases, while cellulases and hemicellulases play important role in brown rots. Lignin degrading enzymes are reported to be employed by the white rot pathogens.

Table 9 : Cell wall and membrane degrading enzymes produced by certain plant pathogens

Enzymes	Substrate	Pathogen
Cutinases	Cutin	*Fusarium solani, Colletotrichum gloeosporioides*
Cellulases	Cellulose	*Erwinia carotovora, Ralstonia, Aschochyta pisi, Rhizoctonia solani*
Hemicellulases	Hemicellulose	*S. rolfsii, E. carotovora, Penicillium expansum*
Proteinases	Protein	*R. solani, S. rolfsii,*
Ligninases	Lignin	*B. cinerea, Heterobasidium annosus*
Esterases	Suberin	*F. solani f. sp. pisi*

Role of Important Enzymes in Pathogenesis

Cutinase

- The cutinase enzyme produce by pathogens degrades cutin layer.
- The amount of cutinase released by germinating spores of *Fusarium solani f.sp.pisi*, the pea rot was correlated with the degree of virulence of various isolates.
- The avirulent isolate did not produce cutinase.
- All these observations suggest the importance of cutinase in disease development.

Pectic Enzymes (*Pectinmethylesterase* (PME) and Polygalacturonases)

- These enzymes degrade middle lamella and cell wall and facilitates free movement of pathogens from cell to cell.
- Pectic enzymes release peroxidases from cell walls. Peroxidase induces browning of vascular tissues, a typical wilt syndrome in many plants.
- Pectic enzymes release endogenous ethylene from host cells. These ethylene causes loss of turgor, chlorosis and necrosis of leaves.
- Pectic enzymes causes vascular plugging producing gels. Swelling of gels leads to occlusion of vascular lumina. It leads to wilting of plants.
- Pectic enzymes in some cases cause cell death. *Erwinia carotovora* produces endo polygalacturonate trans –eliminase and this purified enzyme induces leakage from potato cell membrane and cell death.

Cellulase

- Plant pathogens produces cellulotic enzymes.
- These enzymes become activated only after the action of pectic enzymes.
- Cellulases quickly degrade cell walls and facilitate the invasion of host cells by the pathogens.

Hemicellulases

- Hemicellulases degrade hemicellulosic substances present in plant cells.

- The most important hemicellulasic enzymes are endoglucanase, β-xylosidase, endoxylanase, endomannanase, β-mann nosidase and α-galactosidase.
- *Sclerotium* rolfsii and *Fusarim* spp. are known to produce these enzymes.

Galactanase and Arabansae

- These enzymes are also produced by pathogens.
- Degradation of galactan is accomplished by exo- and endo galactansases while araban is degraded by exo-arabanase.

Phospholipases

- Phospholipases decompose cell membrane and kill the cells.
- Only very pathogens produce these enzymes.

Proteolytic Enzymes

- Many pathogens produce these enzymes.
- They hydrolyze peptide bonds in proteins found in cell walls.

TOXINS

'Toxins' can be defined as low molecular weight , non enzymatic microbial products toxic to the higher plants. These are differs from other microbial products like 'mycotoxins' and 'antibiotics' which are toxic to the animals and microbes (except producers).

Toxins are classified as phytotoxins, vivotoxins and pathotoxins.

Phytotoxins: Toxins produced by pathogens , which are toxic to plants but not considered as of primary importance during pathogenesis, is called as phytotoxin. Non specific toxins are considered as phytotoxins.

Vivotoxins: The toxin produced in vivo (in infected tissues) which function in disease development but not as the initial inciting agent, is termed as vivotoxin.

Pathotoxins: Pathotoxins are the toxins which are major determinants of disease and pathogenicity. Pathotoxin induces all the typical symptoms in reasonable concentration and is co-related with pathogenicity. Host specific toxin can be considered as pathotoxins.

In recent classification, toxins are divided into two categories.

1. **Host non specific toxin**: A toxin which may affect many unrelated plant species in addition to main host of the pathogen producing toxin; it includes phytotoxin and vivotoxin.
2. **Host specific toxin**: A toxin which affects only the specific host of the pathogen; it includes pathotoxins.

Toxins in general , interact with cell membrane or organelles (chloroplast or mitochondria) and alter their permeability. Major host specific and host non specific toxins are listed in table is :

Table 10 : Host specific and non host specific toxins

Toxins	Pathogen	Host	Chemical nature
Host Specific toxins			
AK-toxin	*Alternaria kikuchiana*	Pear	Altenin (furanose ring)
HV- toxin	*Helminthosporium victorae*	Oats	Victoxinine
HC-toxin	*H. carbonum*	Corn	Cyclic peptide
AM- toxin	*A. mali*	Apple	Alternariolide
AB-toxin	*A. brassicae*	Brassica spp.	
Destruxin B			
PC-toxin	*Periconia circinata*	Sorghum	Proteinaceous
Host Non specific toxins			
Tentoxin	*Alternaria alternata*	Mustard	Cyclic tetrapeptide
Tabtoxin	*Pseudomonas tabaci*	Tobacco	Aminoacid derivative
Alternatic acid	*Alternaria solani*	Potato	Hemiquinone derivative
Cerato-ulmin	*Ceratocystis ulmi*	Oak	Large M. carbohydrate
Pyricularin compound	*Pyricularia oryzae*	Rice	Nitrogen containing
Fusaric acid	*Fusarium spp.*	Pigeonpea	5-n-butypicolinic acid

Primary determinant: The toxin required for **pathogenicity** is called primary determinant. It is essential for colonization by the producing pathogens and disease development in the host. The primary determinant is otherwise called **pathogenicity factor**.

Secondary determinant: Thoe toxin required for **virulence** is called secondary determinant. Secondary determinant accounts for certain symptoms or contribute to virulence, but are not essential for colonization. The secondary determinant is otherwise called **virulence factor**.

Virulence is a quantitative term denoting relative disease inducing ability of a microorganism. **Pathogenicity** refers to the capacity of an organism to induce disease. A change in host range indicates a change in pathogenicity while a change in severity of disease indicates a change in virulence. But a question arises, when does pathogenesis begin and how much must the pathogen spread for colonization to be successful. Toxin is not required for penetration. Both toxin produced and no produced penetrate the host tissues. It is most likely that toxins play important role only as virulence factor rather than pathogenicity factor. In other words toxin is important in necrotrophic phase rather than in biotrophic phase. All the toxins isolated so far are from **saprophytic pathogens**. No toxin has been isolated from **obligate parasites** like powdery mildews, downy mildews and rusts.

GROWTH REGULATORS

Plant growth is regulated by a small numbers of groups of naturally occurring compounds that act as hormones and are generally called **growth regulators**. The most important growth regulators are **auxins**, **gibberellins**, and **cytokinins**, but other compounds, such as **ethylene** and growth inhibitors. Alternation in concentration of growth regulators have been found to be associated with several plant diseases particularly in those resulting in abnormal plant/organ/ cell growth like, galls, tumors, knot, stunting, curling , hypertrophy , hyperplasia, etc. Increase in level of a growth regulator may be either owing to its induced production (by pathogen or host) or inhibited degradation. Decrease in concentration is due to the enhanced degradation by the host's or pathogen's enzymes. Biotrophs like powdery mildews employ these hormones to draw their nutrients from the host cells.

Alternations in the level of growth regulators seems to be a consequence of pathogenesis. However, at least in three diseases hormones have been demonstrated to be determinant of pathogenicity. These are crown gall caused by *Agrobacterium tumefaciens,* (cytokinin and auxin), oleander and olive knot caused by *Pseudomonas syringae* sp. *savastanoi* (auxin), fasciation disease caused by *Corynebacterium fasciens* (cytokinin). In all these three bacteria genes have been identified and cloned which are responsible for the hormonal production. Deletion of these genes result in conversion of virulent strains into avirulent.

Table 11 : Certain Plant diseases involving altered concentration of growth regulators

Growth Regulators	Disease (Pathogens)
Auxins	**Increased concentration**: crown gall (*A. tumefaciens*), wheat stem rust (*Puccinin a graminis tritici*), downy mildew of rucifers (*Peronospora parasitica*), tomato wilt (*Verticillium albo-atrum*), banana wilt (*F. oxysporum f.* sp. *cubense*), bacterial wilt of solanaceous crops (*Pseudomonas solanacearum*)
	Reduced concentration: potato leaf roll (PLRV), curly top of sugarbeet (SBCTV), tobacco mosaic (TMV)
Gibberellins	**Increased concentration:** Bakanae disease of rice (*Gibberella fujikuri*), creeping thistle rust *(Puccinia punctiformis*)
	Reduced concentration: anther smut of sea campion(*Ustilago violacea*)
Cytokinins	**Increased concentrations**: club root of crucifers (*Plasmodiophora brassicae*), crown gall (*Agrobacterium tumefaciens*), white rust of crucifers (*Albugo candida*), root knot of tobacco (*Meloidogyne incognita*)
	Reduced concentrations: root knot of tomato (*M. incognita*), verticillium wilt of tomato and cotton
Ethylene	**Increased concentration:** tomato wilt (*F. oxysporum f.* sp. *lycopersici*), verticillium wilt of cotton (*V. albo-atrum*), wilt of tulip (*F. oxysporum f.* sp. *tulipae)*

POLYSACCHARIDES

The role of polysaccharides in plant disease appears to be mainly important in wilt diseases caused by pathogens that invade the vascular system of the plant. In the vascular wilts, large polysaccharide molecules released by the pathogen in the xylem may be sufficient to cause a mechanical blockage of vascular bundles an thus wilting. Even though such an effect by the polysaccharides alone and may occur rarely in nature, when it is considered together with the effect caused by the macromolecular substances released in the vessels through the breakdown of host substances by pathogen enzymes, the possibility of polysaccharide involvement in blockage of vessels during vascular wilts becomes evident.

CHAPTER - 27

Plant Defenses

Resistance to disease in a host plants is a condition in which the plant conquer the pathogen's attack and thus suffers small or no injury. Resistant hosts prevent or slow the development and reproduction of the majority of pathogen propagules that they come into contact with. Different plants defend themselves in different ways. Each kind of plant, probably, employ different defense mechanism against each of the pathogens that attack it. The defense barriers erected by plants are a co-ordinated system of molecular, cellular and tissue-based responses to pathogen attack.

There are various mechanisms of defense used by plants. For convenience, such mechanisms can be considered under two broads heads;

1. Pre existing or passive defense (Defense present on or inside the plant since beginning)

   a. Pre existing structural defense

   b. Pre existing biochemical defense

2. Post infection or active defense (Defense in response to attack by the pathogen)

   a. Post infection structural defense

   b. Post infection biochemical defense

PRE EXISTING OR PASSIVE DEFENSES

a. Pre existing structural defenses: The external or internal structural barriers existing before pathogen attack are called preexisting defense structures or passive or static or anti infection structures. Initiating from periphery, the following barriers occurring in different host plants are described.

Wax and cuticle: The cuticle covers the epidermal cells of plants and consists of cutinized layer, pectin layer and a wax layer. Cutin is composed of fatty acids. Waxes are combination of long chain aliphatic compounds which prevents the withholding of water on plant surface crucial for spore germination.

A negative charge generally develops on leaf surfaces owing to fatty acids. This charge repels various air borne spores/propagules which acquire negative charge during liberation. Thus, the cuticular wax reduces the chances of infection by many pathogens.

Epidermal layer: Thick and tough wall of epidermal cells may directly prevent the entry of pathogen completely or make it difficult. The toughness is due to polymers of cellulose, hemicelluloses, lignin, mineral substances, suberin etc. For instance, most outer wall of epidermal cells of rice plants are lignified and are seldom penetrated by *Magnaporthe grisea* that causes blast diseases of rice while the walls of motor cells are proteinaceous rather than lignified and the pathogens enter the host mainly through them. Potato tuber resistant to *Pythium debaryanum* contain higher fibre content in their epidermal cell walls in comparison to susceptible ones.

Natural openings: Natural opening such as stomata, lenticels, hydathodes, nectarines etc. allow many plant pathogenic fungi and bacteria to enter plants through them, but in some cases the structures of these openings prevent pathogen –entry. For instance, Mandarin orange is resistant to *Xanthomonas axenopodis pv. citri* because of broad cuticular lips covering the stomata. Similarly, the size and internal structure of lenticels may play a defensive role against the pathogens. The varieties having large size lenticels on fruit surfaces easily allow *Pseudomonas populosum* to cause spot disease in apple but the varieties having small lenticels prevent the entry of the pathogen. Hydathodes are natural openings on the edges of leaves and serve to excess water from the interior. They are easy entry points of bacterial pathogens such as *X. campestris pv. campestris* (black rot of cabbage). Similar to hydathodes are the nectarthodes in inflorescence of many plants. They secrete sugary nectar and this serves as barrier to those organisms that cannot tolerate high osmotic pressure. High hairiness of leaves and pods in chickpea is resistant character against *Aschochyta rabei.*

Internal structures: There are many pre existing structures inside the plant that prevent the entry of pathogen beyond them. For example, environmental conditions sometimes make cell walls of certain tissue thick and tough and these wall make the invasion of the pathogen quite difficult. In wheat varieties containing sclerenchymatous tissues in relatively high proportion in stem possess certain degree of resistance to *Puccinia graminis f. sp. tritici*. *Pythium* spp. invade only juvenile tissues, seedlings become resistant as they advance in age and secondary thickenings are formed.

Table 12 : Pre-infectional morphological and structural defense mechanisms against plant pathogens.

Sl.No	Defense barrier	Pathogen	Host
1.	Waxes and Cuticle	*Albugo candida*	Brussels sprout
		Puccinia graminis	Berberries
		Melampsora lini	Linseed
		Colletotrichum coffeanum	Coffee
2.	Structure of natural opening		
	Broad cuticular ridge projection over the stomata	*Xanthomonas campestris pv.citri*	Mandarins citrus
	Mechanical (Sclerenchymatous) tissues	*Entyloma oryzae*	Rice
	Late openining of stomata	*Puccinia graminis tritici*	Wheat
3.	Thick and tough outer cell wall (Presence of silicic acid and lignified epidermal cells)	*Pyricularia oryzae*	Rice

Pre existing biochemical defense :

Plants possess certain metabolic processes in their cells which imparts resistance to them against pathogen attacks. This type of defense adopted by the plants is called "biochemical defense". When biochemical defense exist in the plant even before the attack of the pathogen. This is called pre existing biochemical defense.

Release of antimicrobial compounds

Plant commonly exude organic substances from above ground parts and roots, containing amino acids, sugars ,organic acids, enzymes, glycosides etc. Some of the compounds occurring in exudates are inhibitory. These inhibitory substances directly affect the micro organism or encourage certain group to dominant the environment and function as antagonists of the pathogen. For instance, certain varieties of linseed resist infection of *F. oxysporum f. sp. lini* because of the presence of **HCN** in their root exudates. Presence of HCN in roots of sorghum and maize is also reported. HCN in sorghum root exudates might be responsible for reduction of pigeonpea wilt caused by *Fusarium udum* in plots where sorghum is grown as mixed crop with pigeonpea. Red scale of onion (red varieties) conatin **protocatechuic acid** and **catechol**, which may exude in drops and impart resistance to attack of *Colletotrichum circinanas* (onion smudge disease).The root exudates favor development of plant growth promoting rhizobacteria (PGPR), which suppresses the plant pathogens and induces resistance.

Inhibitor present in plant cells: The plant cells contain certain pre-existing inhibitory substances which mainly play a defensive role against the particular pathogen. Phenols and quinones are two classes of antimicrobial compounds produced by some plants. Inhibiting compounds may be excreted into the external environment, accumulate in dead cells or be sequestered into vacuoles in an inactive form. The young fruit of numerous plants (e.g. mangoes, avocado) contain antifungal or antimicrobial compounds that are gradually metabolised during fruit ripening, making unripe fruit less susceptible to disease than ripe fruit. Lactones, cyanogenic glucosides, saponins, terpenoids, stilbenes and tannins are also plant-produced compounds associated with pathogen resistance. Saponins are a class of phytoanticipins that destroy membrane integrity in saponin-sensitive parasites, and which are stored in an inactive form in the vacuoles of the plant cell, becoming active when hydrolase enzymes are released following wounding or infection. Some pathogens are able to release enzymes that detoxify plant saponins, making them insensitive to this line of defence. Conversely, resistance of some plants to specific pathogens is the result of an insensitivity to pathogen-produced host specific toxins. Resistance genes may encode an enzyme that converts the toxin into a non-toxic derivative or the absence of a receptor to the toxin. Another group of defensive compounds are the plant **defensins**, which interfere with pathogen nutrition and retard their development. Secreted defensins can create an antimicrobial microenvironment for germinating seeds and accumulated defensins can provide defence against insect-transmitted viruses in flowers, leaves and tubers. There are also proteins, both constitutive and induced that play a role in plant defence.

Lack of Essential Factors

Recognition factors

The first step in infection process is cell to cell communication between pathogens and host. Plant of species or varieties may not infected by a pathogen if there surface cells lack specific recognition factors. If the pathogen does not recognize the plant as one of its hosts it may not adhere to the host surface or it may not produce infection substances such as enzymes or structures like appresoria and haustoria. These recognition molecules are of various types of oligosaccharides, polysaccharides and glycoproteins.

Essential nutrients and growth factors

The majority of the obligate parasites and some of the facultative saprophytes, particularly among the fungi, are usually host specific and grow only on their specific variety of host. This is thought to happen because of host specialized pathogens need certain specific substances and these substances are only available in adequate quantities in the host they infect. Hence, absence of these specific substances makes the other varieties inappropriate host for such a pathogen. For instance, in seedling disease of several crops caused by *Rhizoctonia solani*, successful infection depends on formation of infection cushion from which infection peg develops and causes penetration. Formation of these cushions is induced by certain essential nutrients in the host. In resistant plants, lack of such nutrients results in resistance to *R. solani*.

Sometimes, a particular race of pathogen loses its ability to synthesize a certain substance owing to mutation and this makes the pathogen race non specific. For instance, A fungus , namely , *Venturia inaequalis* causes apple scab disease. Certain races of this pathogen recovered have lost their ability to synthesize a growth factor in them due to mutation. Races so mutated prove to be non pathogenic to apple.

Common antigen in host plant

Presence of common antigen (protein) in both host and pathogen determines disease occurrence in the host. But, if, the antigen is absent in the host and present only in the pathogen, it makes the host resistant to that particular pathogen. For instance, the varieties of linseed which have an antigen common to their pathogen *Melampsora lini* prove to be susceptible to rust disease. In contrary, the linseed varieties not having the antigen in them but occurring in the pathogen are resistant to the pathogen. Similar is the case with leaf spot disease of cotton caused by *Xanthomonas compestris pv. malvacearum.*

Table 13 : Pre-infectional biochemical defense mechanisms against plant pathogens

Sl.no.	Defense barrier	Pathogen	Host
1.	Inhibitors released by the plant in the environment		
	Glucoside	*Fusarium* spp.	Flax
	Malic acid	*Ascochyta rabiei*	Gram
	Catechol and protocatechuic acid	*Colletotrichum circinans*	Red scale onion
	Cutin acid	*Gloesporium limetticola*	Citrus
2.	Phenolic substances		
	Polyphenols	*Venturia inaequalis*	Apple
		Pyricularia oryzae	Rice
		Venturia pirina	Pear
3.	Inhibitory substances present in the plant cells		
	Chlorogenic acid	*Streptomyce scabies*	Potato
	Tuliposide	*Fusarium oxysporum f.sp. tulipae*	Tulip
	Avenacin	*Ophiobolus graminis*	Wheat
	Arbutin	*Erwinia amylovora*	Pear
4.	Absence of nutrients required by the pathogen		
	Histidine	*Erwinia amylovora*	Potato
	Sugar	*Ceratocystis ulmi*	Elm
		Alternaria solani	Potato
		Cochliobolus sativus	Barley
	Choline	*Venturia inaqualis*	*Apple*
	Myoinositol	*Rhizoctonia aurecina*	Plum

POST INFECTION OR ACTIVE OR INDUCED DEFENSES

a. Post infection or Induced structural defense

After the pathogen successfully penetrates the pre-existing defense barriers of the host, the latter, some how, generally develops definite defense structures inside them in response to the reaction taking place between host and pathogen. These structures so developed are generally of four types:

- Induced histological defense.
- Induced cellular defense.
- Induced cytoplasmic defense.
- Induced hypersensitive defense.

Induced histological defense : Certain defense structures are developed inside the host as a result of tissue differentiation or chemical substance deposition in tissues ahead of or around the pathogen. These defense structures are called induced histological defense.These may be at various levels:

Cork layer formation: The ability to repair wounds can help protect the plant from further infection by other, opportunistic pathogens. A secondary meristem in fleshy tissues, fruits, roots and bark, the cork cambium, can produce cork cells, which have thick, suberised walls/ layers. These cells can create a barrier to further colonization by the pathogen. Cork layer formation is a part of natural healing system of plants. Cork layers blocks the flow of nutrients and water from the healthy to the infected area and this deprives the pathogen of nourishment resulting in its weakness or , sometimes, death. Further more, it also block inward flow of toxic substances produced by the a pathogen so that such toxic substances could not damage the underlying healthy tissues of the host. Example. Common scab of potato (*streptomyces scabis*) and *Rhizophus* rot of sweet potato.

Tyloses formation: The tyloses are formed by protrusion of xylem parenchymatous cell walls, through pits into xylem vessels. The formation of tyloses can also restrict the spread of pathogenic propagules in the xylem, although they also tend to reduce the movement of water through the vessels, causing water stress in the plant. Examples: sweet potato: *Fusarium oxysporum f. sp. batatas*

Gum deposition: Wounded tree trunks often secrete protective gums that seal the wound from further infection. Example: Blast disease of rice (*Magnaporthe grisea*), Leaf spot of rice (*Helminthosporium oryzae)*

Abscission layers: It is the gap between host cell layers and devices for dropping-off older leaves and mature fruits. Plant may use this for defense mechanism also, i.e. to drop –off infected or invaded plant tissues or parts, along with pathogen. Shot holes in leaves of fruit trees is a common characteristic.

Induced cellular defense: The cellular defense structures, i.e. changes in cell walls, have only a restricted role in defense. Following types are generally observed:

- Carbohydrate apposition (synthesis of secondary walls and papillae formation).
- Callose deposition (hyphal sheathing just outside plasma lemma around the haustorium, which delays contact of pathogen (*Phytophthora infestans*) with host cells.
- Structural proteins

Induced cytoplasmic defense: When the hyphae of a pathogen succeed in penetrating a particular cell, the cytoplasmic content of such cell becomes organized in such a way that the cytoplasm beomes granular and dense and certain organelle like structures develop in it. As a result, the penetrating hyphae disintegrate into small granular bodies and further development of the hyphae is stopped. Cytoplasmic defense structures are, perhaps, the very last line of structural defense and are effective against some slow growing pathogens, weak parasites or some symbiotic relationships.

Table 14 : Post-infectional morphological and structural defense mechanisms against plant pathogens

Sl.No	Defense barrier	Pathogen	Host
1.	Formation of cork layer	*Rhizoctonia solani*	Potato
		Coccomyces prunophorae	Plum
2.	Formation of tyloses	*Fusarium oxysporum f.sp. batatas*	Sweet potato
		Verticillium- alboatrum	Tomato
3.	Formation of abscission layer	*Xanthomonas arboricola pv. pruni*	Sour cherry
		Clsterosporium carpophilum	Peach
4.	Sheathing of hyphae	*Phytophthora infestans*	Potato
5.	Gum deposition	*Pyricularia oryzae*	Rice
		Drechslera oryzae	Rice
		Physalopora cydoniae	Apple

Hypersensitivity: Hypersensitive **cell death** is another widespread mechanism used by hosts to prevent the spread of a pathogen. Infected cells and those surrounding them "suicide", preventing further spread, and in some cases, killing the pathogen. It is often associated with the initiation of other responses, such as lignification and the synthesis of anti-microbial compounds. The success of hypersensitive cell death as a resistance mechanism depends on the nutritional requirements of the specific pathogen and the timing, magnitude and location of the host response.

b. Post Infection or Induced biochemical defense

These mechanisms restrict the spread of the pathogen after infection is established and contain the damage to host tissues.

Role of Phytoalexins: Phytoalexins are low molecular weight antibiotics produced by many (but not all) plants in response to infection. There are several biotic elicitors of phytoalexin production, such as cell wall components, as well as abiotic elicitors, such as heavy metals and ultraviolet light. Phytoalexins inhibit the growth of bacteria and fungi *in vitro* and *in vivo*, and production of these antibiotics during an infection can induce resistance to consequent infections by that pathogen. Over 350 phytoalexins are known in over 100 plant species. They include **pterocarpans**, **cryptophenols isocoumarins**, **isoflavenoids, sesquiterpenes**, and others. Phytoalexins may be produced by any part of the plant, although different phytoalexins can accumulate in different organs. Normally, related plant species produce structurally-related phytoalexins, and many produce more than one, enabling the plant to present a toxic cocktail to invading pathogens. Phytoalexins are produced in cells surrounding an infection site and delivered to the infected cell packaged in lipid vesicles, creating a toxic micro-environment in the infected cell and, hopefully, preventing disease establishment. Phytoalexin accumulation is often associated with hypersensitive cell death, although only living cells can synthesise phytoalexins. Some plants can also sequester phytoalexins into vacuoles as stores of inactive sugar-conjugates, which can be cleaved and released quickly if initial defence responses are unsuccessful.

Table 15 : Some important phytoalexins

Sl. No	Phytoalexins	Producer Plant	Chemical nature
1.	Resveratrol	*Vitis viifera*	Stilbene
2.	Trifolirhazin	*Trifolium pratens*	Isoflavonoid
3.	Isocoumarin	Carrot root	Isocoumarin
4.	Orchinol	*Orchis militaris*	Dihydrophenanthrene
5.	Isomeamarone	*Ipomea batata*	Sesquiterpene
6.	Rishitin	Potato tuber	Sesquiterpene
7.	Lubimin	Potato tuber	Sesquiterpene
8.	Camelexins	*Aradiopsis thaliana*	Thiazoyl substituted indole camalexin
9.	Brassinins	*Brassica rapa*	Indole ring linked to a dithiocarbamate
10.	Pisatin	*Pisum sativum*	Isofalvonoid
11.	Maackiain	*Cicer arietinum*	Isofalvonoid
12.	Phaseollidin	*Phaseolus vulgaris*	Isofalvonoid

Role of Phenol Compounds

Phenolics are the common compounds found in plants and possess an aromatic ring bearing a hydroxyl substituent. Phenolics are toxic to fungi, bacteria and viruses. They inhibit:

- Mycelia growth
- Spore germination
- Producion of cellulotic and pectic enzymes
- Activity of cellulotic and pectic enzymes and
- Production of toxins by the fungi

The phenolic compounds are main toxic chemicals produced to inhibit pathogen or its activities. Some of these are preformed toxic chemicals while others may be *de novo* synthesized or modified to more toxic forms, viz., conversion of **phenols** to more toxic **quinines**.When a pathogen infects the plant, the latter either accelerates the synthesis of these compounds adjacent to infection site or accelerates the flow of pre- existing amount from healthy tissue towards the infected one and plant defend itself.Some of the individual phenolic substances have been identified as the key defense chemicals in plants. They are:

Phenolic substances	Crop
Chlorogenic acid	Potato
Catechol and Pyrocatechic acid	Onion
Avenacin	Oats
Hordatine	Barley
Tomatine	Tomato
Tuliposides	Tulip
Catechin and Isoquercitin	Cotton
Umbelliferone and Scopoletin	Sweet potato

Role of Pathogenesis-Related Proteins

There is a variety of novel proteins synthesized in response to infection, several of which have b- chitinase, glucanase, or lysozyme activity. Some pathogenesis-related proteins disrupt pathogen nutrition. The presence of low levels of these proteins in healthy plants suggests that they might have other roles in plant growth and development aside from disease resistance. Chitinase and glucanase accumulate in the vacuoles, and glucanase is also sometimes secreted into the intercellular space. They dissolve the fungal cell wall, fragments of which then elicit hypersensitive cell death. The breakdown of the vacuole during decompartmentalisation of the cytoplasm results in a flood of hydrolytic enzymes, which have antifungal, antibacterial and antiviral, activity. The accumulation of pathogenesis-related proteins peaks around 7-10 days after initial infection. The presence of these proteins *before* infection increases the plant's resistance to pathogens, as in the case of systemic acquired resistance.

Table 16 : Faimilies of pathogenesis –related proteins (PRPs)

Sl. No	Protein family	Protein activity	Targeted pathogen sites
1.	PRP-1	Unknown	Active against oomycetes
2.	PRP-2	A-1,3 glucanase	Cell wall glucan of fungi
3.	PRP-3	Endochitinase	Cell wall chitin of fungi
4.	PRP-4	Endochitinase	Cell wall chitin of fungi
5.	PRP-5	Taumartin-like	Active against oomycetes
6.	PRP-6	Proteinase inhibitor	Active on nematodes and insects
7.	PRP-7	Endoproteinase	Microbial cell wall dissolution
8.	PRP-8	Endochitinase with lysozyme activity	Cell wall chitin of fungi, and mucopeptide wall of bacteria
9.	PRP-9	Peroxidase	
10.	PRP-10	Ribonuclease activity	Viral RNA
11.	PRP-11	Endochitinase	Cell wall chitin of fungi
12.	PRP-12	Defensin	Antifungal and antibacterial activity
13.	PRP-13	Thionin	Antifungal and antibacterial activity
14.	PRP-14	Lipid transfer proteins	Antifungal and antibacterial activity
15.	PRP-15	Oxalate-oxidase	Produces H_2O_2 that inhibits microbes and also stimulates host defense
16.	PRP-16	Oxalate-oxidase-like with superdismutase	Produces H_2O_2 that inhibits microbes and also stimulates host defense

Inactivation of enzymes and toxins: The role played by enzymes and toxins of pathogens during pathogenesis is well established. The hemibiotrophs and necrotrophs employ more of these substances for causing host tissue damage as compared to biotrophs. The defense strategy of resistant plants, through activity of phenols, tannins, proteins as enzymes inhibitors. the phenolics are not anti –fungal but make pathogen ineffective by neutralizing their enzymes. In immature grape fruits catechol- tannin is known to inhibit enzymes produced by *Botrytis cinerea*

In resistant varieties of plants, which get diseased as a result of toxins produced by the pathogens, the pathogenic toxins released are detoxified by the ability of metabolic processes of plants. For example, *Pyricularia oryzae*, while causing blast disease of rice, releases picolinic acid and pyricularin toxin inside the host. Though, susceptible varieties get affected by these toxic substances, the resistant varieties convert 40-60% of picolinic acid into its methylester and N-methylpicolinic acid, pyricularin into other compounds. These resistant compounds are non toxic to rice plants.

Table 17 : Defense through detoxification of pathogen toxin

Detoxifying compound	Pathogen toxin	Disease	Pathogen
Chlorogenic acid	Piricularin	Blast of rice	*Pyricularia oryzae*
Dehydroascorbic acid	AK toxin	Black spot of pear	*Alternaria kikuchiana*
High concentration of cysteine Fusaric acid		Wilt of cotton	*Fusarium oxysporum f. sp. vasinfectum*
		Wilt of tomato	*Fusarium oxysporum f. sp. lycopersici*

Systemic acquired resistance and Induced systemic resistance

Systemic acquired resistance (SAR) or induced resistance, is characterised by the increased resistance of a plant to a wide range of pathogens following infection by one pathogen. It is therefore fundamentally different from the specific antigen-antibody mechanism of resistance seen in the immune response of mammals. Rather than providing immunity *per se*, systemic acquired resistance reduces the severity of later diseases. The development of systemic acquired resistance usually requires the development of a slowly expanding necrotic lesion and other localised responses to infection, the release of a phloem-translocated signal originating from the infection site, and the subsequent priming of the plant against further attacks, allowing a more rapid response in the case of future infections. The nature of the signal that triggers systemic acquired resistance is as yet unknown, and is likely to be a complex signal transduction pathway mediated by a number of stress signals. **Salicylic acid** plays a key role, via interaction with salicylic acid-binding proteins that can cause build-up of reactive oxygen species or activate gene expression. The levels of salicylic acid increase around necrotic lesions and remain high in plants that have acquired resistance. It is not, however, salicylic acid itself that acts as the signal that is translocated systemically throughout the plant.

Induced Systemic Resistance (ISR)- ISR functions independently of SA and PR gene activation. Jasmonic acid (JA) and ethylene have been shown to act in concert in activating genes encoding defensive proteins, such as proteinase inhibitors and plant defensins. JA –dependent ISR pathway is triggered by non pathogenic *Pseudomonas fluorescens* (rhizobacteria). In Arabidopsis, ISR is active against the fungal root pathogen *Fusarium oxysporum f.sp. raphani*, the oomycetous leaf pathogen *Peronospora parasitica*, the bacterial leaf pathogens *Xanthomonas campestris pv. campestris* and *Pseudomonas syringae pv. tomato.*

Significance of ISR and SAR

- Induce a set of defense gene expression.
- Dramatically accumulated after infection.
- Both have been recognized as inducers of plant defense for many years.
- Exogenous application evokes the protection against pathogen attack.
- Deficient mutants exhibit reduced defense gene expression and enhance disease management.

Difference between ISR and SAR

Features	ISR	SAR
Activation of resistance	Resistance activated in response to artificial application of non pathogenic strains of pathogen, PGPR, and abiotic stresses etc.	Resistance activated in response to pathogenic infection.
Pathway	Jasmonic acid dependent pathway	Salicyclic acid dependent pathway
Signalling molecule	Jasmonic acid	Salicyclic acid
Defense gene involved	CHIB, HEL,PDF1,2	PR-1 and PR-2
Pathogen associated	Operates against biotrophic pathogens	Operate against necrotrophic and facultative parasite

CHAPTER - 28

Variation in Plant Pathogens

INTRODUCTION

Variability in different organisms is common feature and is an important process for the continuity of life under stress conditions. Plant pathogens especially fungi, bacteria, virus and nematode show variations in their pathogenic potential (virulence) and physiological functions that support their survival and perpetuation in different environmental conditions. These variations may be largely due to genetic factors that may be conditioned by environmental factors. Various studies on genetic variability of microbial plant pathogens have shown that variations may occur in characters which affect their ability to infect host plants and also other characters that do not alter the pathogenic potential, but they may be concerned with their survival. Knowledge of variation in pathogenic characteristics is valuable in planning effective measures for disease management. In addition, development of resistant to fungicides has been a serious concern to growers, researchers as well as the administrators, since the decision to continue application or withdrawal of a fungicide can affect both the growers and industry.

TERMINOLOGY

Variability: It is the property of an organism to change its characters from one generation to the other.

Variation: When progeny of an individual show variation in characters from parents such a progeny is called a variant.

Physiological specialization: Within the species of a pathogen there exist certain individuals that are morphologically similar but differs with respect to their physiology, biochemical characters and pathogenicity and are differentiated on the basis of their reaction on certain host genera or cultivars.

Physiologic race:– Individuals within the species of a pathogen that morphologically similar but differ with respect to their pathogenicity on particular set of host varieties.

Forma specialis (f. sp.):– Individuals within the specie of a pathogen that morphologically similar but differ with respect to their pathogenecity on particular host genera • E.g. *Puccinia graminis f.sp. tritici.*

Pathotype: A pathotype is a population of a parasite species in which all individuals have a stated pathosystem character (pathogenicity or parasitic ability) in common.

Biotype: Progeny developed by variant having similar heredity is called a biotype or a subgroup of individuals within the species, usually characterized by the possession of single or few characters in common.

MECHANISMS OF VARIABILITY IN FUNGI

1. Mutation

Mutation is one of the major causes of variability in the absence of sexual process. It is a more or less abrupt change in the genetic material of an organism i.e. DNA and the change is heritable to the progeny. Mutation represent change in sequences of the bases in DNA either by substitution or by deletion or addition or may be by amplification of particular segment of DNA to multiple copies by insertion or excision of a transposable element into coding or regulatory sequences of the gene.Mutations in single cell organisms , are expressed immediately after their occurrence. Most mutant factors, however, are usually recessive. Mutations in the extranuclear DNA are just as common as in the nuclear DNA. Mutations occurring in morphological or physiological characters can be induced by chemical and physical agents. Fungi can mutate on culture media or on host plant. The frequency of mutation differs from biotype to biotype. Mutation factors are mostly recessive. Mutations for virulence occur in plant pathogenic fungi. Such mutants have been reported in *Phytophthora infestans, Puccinia graminis* and other fungi.Fungi of class ascomycetes are most suitable for mutation studies. Pahtogenic phase in these fungi is haploid and contains therefore, one of the each pair of homologus chromosomes. Mutation, if any, is immediately expressed unless suppressed by epistasis,. Usually, there is loss in pathogenicity by mutation.

2. Recombination

Most changes in the characteristics of pathogens are the result of recombination occurs during sexual processes. When two haploid nuclei (1N) containing different gnentic material unite to form diploid (2N) nucleus called a Zygote, when undergo meiotic division produce new haploid. Recombination of genetic factor occurs during meiotic division of zygote as a result of cross over in which part of chromatid of one chromosome of a pair are expressed with that of the other. Recombination can also occur during mitotic division of cell in the course of growth of the individual and is important in fungi. The majority of fungi being **haploid**, have only a very brief **diploid** phase, very often undergoing meiosis very soon after karyogamy. Some Oomycetes are predominantly diploid. Many Basidiomycetes are functionally diploid by virtue of their extended dikaryon phase. In case of homothallic fungi which are essentially self compatible and a single thallus. In these fungi the extent of out crossing will be close to zero and there will be little opportunity for recombination between different individuals. On the other hand , there are heterolhallic fungi with physiologic distinct mycelia upon which produced compatible male and female gametes. Here the extent of out crossing might reach 100%. A good example is the black stem rust fungus, *Puccinia graminis*

3. Parasexuality

Parasexuality was first demonstrated by **Pontecorvo (1956)** in *Aspergillus nidulans*. **Parasexuality** in fungi can be called **genetic recombination without meiosis**. In the absence of meiosis during the life cycle of imperfect fungi, recombination of hereditary properties and genetic variation still occur by a mechanism called parasexuality. It includes the production of diploid nuclei in a heterokaryotic, haploid mycelium that results from plasmogamy and karyogamy; multiplication of the diploid along with haploid nuclei in the heterokaryotic mycelium; sorting out of a diploid homokaryon; segregation and recombination by crossing over at mitosis; and haploidization of the diploid nuclei. Sexual and parasexual cycles are not mutually exclusive. Some fungi that reproduce sexually also exhibit parasexuality. However **imperfect fungi** reproduce **asexually** and exhibit **parasexuallity**. Parasexuality has been reported in many rusts, including *P.graminis tirtici, P. coronata* and in some smuts *Ustilago hordei* and *U. maydis*. In rust fungi as *P. graminis tritici*, mitotic recombination may represent a most important method of generating new races especially in countries such as India where sexual stage of the fungus is rare due to scarcity of the alternate host, the barberry. For other fungi with no known sexual stage such as *P.striiformis*, mitotic recombination is the only means of genetic assortment.

4. Heterokaryosis

The phenomenon of existence of different kinds of nuclei in the same individual is known as **heterokaryosis**. (Gr. *heteros* = other+ *karyon* = nucleus). The individual which exhibit heterokaryosis is called heterokaryon or heterokaryotic. It has been demonstrated in numerous Ascomycetes,

Basidiomycetes and Fungi Imperfecti. In a heterokaryotic individual, each nucleus is independent of all other nuclei, but the structure and behaviour of the individual appear to be controlled by the kinds of genes it contains and the proportion of each kind. Heterokaryosis may arise in a fungal thallus in four ways:

1. By the germination of a heterokaryotic spore, which will give rise to a heterokaryotic soma.
2. By the introduction of genetically different nuclei into homokaryon (Gr. homo=same + karyon = nut, nucleus), a soma in which all nuclei are similar.
3. y mutation, in a multinucleate homokaryon. The mutant nuclei subsequently survive, multiply and spread among the wild-type nuclei.
4. By fusion of some nuclei in a haploid homokaryon to form diploid nuclei which subsequently survive, multiply and spread among the haploid nuclei.

Thus in some fungi it is possible to have different kinds of haploid nuclei in the same soma and a mixture of haploid and diploid nuclei. In most fungal individuals, the haploid and diploid phases of the life cycle are clearly distinguishable. **Hansen and Smith** (1932) first suggested **heterokaryosis** as a means of variation in *Botrytis cinerea*. The even pathogenicity is influenced by heterokaryosis, has been demonstrated in *Fusarium oxysporum f. pisi*, the incitant of pea wilt. Heterokaryosis is known to occur in wheat rust fungus.

5. Heteroploidy

Heteroploidy is the existence of cells, tissues or whole organisms with numbers of chromosomes per nucleus that are different from the normal 1N or 2N complement for the particular organism. Heteroploids may be haploids, diploid, triploid, tetraploids or aneuploids, i.e. have one or more extra chromosomes or are missing one or more chromosomes from the normal euploid number e.g. N+1. This represents a normal situation in the development of eukaryotes. Heteroploidy has been repeatedly observed in fungi and has been shown to affect the growth rate, spore size and rate of spore production , hyphal color, enzyme activities, and pathogenicity.

6. Adaptation

When a pathogen acquires ability to carry out a physiological process that it could not carry out before or could not carry out efficiently, it is said to have adapted and this phenomenon is known as **adaptation**. It may be for utilization of some substances for tolerance to toxic material or for change in virulence to host plants. The exact mechanism of adaptation is not clearly known. Adaptive changes may be temporary or permanent and may be heritable. Adaptations in pathogenicity have been reported in *Fusarium, Phytophthora* and *Helminthosporium* spp.

7. Satation

Saltation is expressed by morphologically distinct areas or sectors in a fungal colony. These sectors may be remain stable or saltate again. Saltants have been reported in *Fusarium, Helminthosporium, Alternaria, Phoma* and *Sphacelotheca* spp. Mechanism of saltation is not clearly understood.

VARIABILITY IN BACTERIA

The genetic recombination processes (transformation, conjugation, and transduction) lead to the variability in pathogen's population.

1. Conjugation

Conjugation is a mating process involving bacteria. It involves transfer of genetic information from one bacterial cell to another, and requires physical contact between the two bacteria involved. The contact between the cells is via a protein tube called an **F** or **sex pilus**, which is also the conduct for the transfer of the genetic material. Basic conjugation involves two strains of bacteria: **F+** and **F-**. The difference between these two strains is the presence of a **Fertility factor** (or F factor) in the F+ cells. The F factor is an **episome** that contains 19 genes and confers the ability to conjugate upon its host cell. Genetic transfer in conjugation is from an F+ cell to an F- cell, and the genetic material transferred is the F factor itself. Recombination rarely occurs with this kind of conjugation. This is because the F factor is not homologous to the DNA in the bacterial chromosome. As we will see, however, there are variations of this basic conjugation process that allow recombination to occur. Conjugation increases the genetic variability of bacterial populations and facilitates the emergences of antibiotic resistance.

2. Transduction

Transduction involves the exchange of DNA between bacteria using bacterial viruses (bacteriophage) as an intermediate. There are two types of transduction, **generalized transduction** and **specialized transduction**, which differ in their mechanism and in the DNA that gets transferred.

Generalized Transduction: Sometimes, during bacteriophage replication, a mistake is made, and a fragment of the host DNA gets packaged into a viral capsid. The resulting phage would be able to infect another cell, but it would not have any viral genes, so it would not be able to replicate. The cell infected by this phage would survive, and would have an extra piece of bacterial DNA present, which could undergo recombination with the host chromosome, and perhaps cause a gene conversion event. Because it is a random fragment that gets packaged into the viral capsid, any segment of the bacterial DNA can be transferred this way (hence the name 'generalized').

Specialized Transduction: Specialized transduction occurs only with certain types of bacteriophage, such as phage **lambda**. Lambda has the ability to establish what is called a **lysogenic infection** in a bacterial cell. Only bacterial genes immediately adjacent to the prophage can be transferred. Example, In a population of *Escherichia coli* cells infected with lamda phage, a small portion of progeny virions may carry either *gal* or *bio* loci of the *E.coli* genes at the expense of certain phage genes at the opposite end of the prophage.

3. Transformation

Transformation is a process by which DNA released by the donor bacteria into a **environment** is acquired by the recipient bacteria. Frederick Griffith, and English bacteriologist in 1928, while searching for a vaccine against bacterial pneumonia, first time demonstrated this phenomenon in *Streptococcus pneumonia*. Griffith observed that a non virulent strain of *S. pneumonia* was transferred into a virulent one when mixed with heat killed virulent cells of *S. pneumonia*. However, the DNA as transforming principles was established in 1944 by *O. Avery, C. MacLeod* and *M. McCarty*. They showed that it is the genetic materials that was released into the media by heat killed cells and up taken by the non virulent cells. As a result of uptake, the non virulent one gets transformed into virulent one.

In ordinary circumstances, transduction, conjugation, and transformation involve transfer of DNA between individual bacteria of the same species, but occasionally transfer may occur between individuals of different bacterial species and this may have significant consequences, such as the transfer of antibiotic resistance. In such cases, gene acquisition from other bacteria or the environment is called **horizontal gene transfer** and may be common under natural conditions. Gene transfer is particularly important in antibiotic resistance as it allows the rapid transfer of resistance genes between different pathogens.

VARIABILITY IN VIRUSES

Virus also show variability. Variability in virus is due to recombination , mutation, selection pressure and pseudo recombination.

Recombination

Plant viruses have always been regarded to undergo recombination. When two strains of the same virus are inoculated into the same host plants, one or more new virus strains are recovered with properties (symptomatology, virulence and so on) different from those of either of the original strains combinants. For example. two tobravirus strains called N_5 and 16 are formed by natural recombination of RNAs $_2$ of tobacco rattle and pea early browning viruses. Formation of new strains also occurs in brome mosaic virus by genetic recombination.

Mutation

Mutation is also a important source of origin of mutants. Mutations can be base substitutions and deletion mutations. Base substitution results in point mutation whereby base of a nucleotide is changed so that encoded protein molecule of parent strain. Such base substitutions have been discovered in cauliflower mosaic viruses and tobacco mosaic. Deletion mutations occur when part of the genome is deleted so that the mutant has lost the character encoded by the deleted segment of genome. **Deletion mutations** were first reported by **Reddy** and **Black** (1974, 1977) in **wound tumor virus**. Since the deletion mutations have been discovered in several other viruses.

Selection Pressure

Selection pressure resulting in the selection of new strains under changed conditions. With a change in selection pressure , an earlier minor strain of the mixture becomes the new dominant strain which seemingly leads to origin of new strains. **Temperature** and **host** are the two most common and important selection pressure operative in nature leading to the selection of new strains.

Pseudo Recombination

RNA genome of multicomponent viruses exists as more than one segments. In vitro experiments have established that RNA segments of closely related plant viruses can be exchanged to create new viable strains, called **pseudorecombinants** and the process as **pseudorecombination**. It appears that cucumber mosaic virus Q strain is a pseudorecombiannt.

Variability in Nematodes

Individual produced as a result of sexual reproduction are expected to be different from each other and from their parents in a number of characteristics which can be expressed morphologically or physiologically. The morphological characters like head shape, and scelrotisation, type of oesophagus, type of stylet and stylet knobs, position of vulva, number and types of ovaries, and neuroreceptors like amphids and phasmids , number of lateral lines, body dimensions and tail shape are important for the taxonomic identification of a specimen. The physiological variations may include preference of a host by a nematode species found in particular environmental and edaphic conditions where as the other members of the same species may not be host specific to that corp.

STAGES IN VARIATION IN PATHOGENS

Species

Species is one or more natural populations in which individuals are inbreeding and are reproductively isolated from other such groups of sexually reproducing organisms. For a fungal or bacterial pathogens, certain morphological and other phenotypic characteristics in common make up the species as *Puccinia graminis*

Varieties or special forms

Some individuals of the species attack only certain species of host plants, which make up formae specialis such as *Puccinia graminis f. sp. tritici.*

Race

Within the special form , some individuals attack a set of the host varieties but not the others, which make up a race such as *P. graminis f.sp. tritic* race 1,2, or 3.

Variant

Sometimes , one of the off springs of a race can suddenly attack a new variety that was not infected before, this individual is called a variant.

Biotypes

The identical individuals produced asexually by a variant make up a biotype (clone). Each race consists of one or several biotypes.

CHAPTER - 29

Plant Disease Epidemiology

CONCEPT

The word "**epidemic**" is derived from the greek word, epi= (on) and demons=(people) and in true sense applies to those disease of human being which appear very virulently among a large section of population. To carry the same sense in the case of plant diseases the term **epiphytotic** has been coined. an **epiphytotic** disease is one which occur **widely** but **periodically**. it may be present constantly in a locality but assumes severe form only on occasions. Of late, the term "**epidemiology**" has come to have a broad meaning within plant pathology. The term has been variously defined as the study of disease in populations; the study of environmental factors that influence the amount and distribution of diseases in population, and the study of either increase or decrease in the amount of disease in time, in space, or both.

Elements of An Epidemic

Generally, the elements of an epidemic are referred to as the "**disease triangle**": **a susceptible host, pathogen,** and **favorable environment**. For disease to occur all three of these must be present. Where all three items get together there is disease. As long as all three of these elements are present disease can commence, an epidemic will only arise if all three continue to be present. Sometimes a fourth factor of **time** is added as the time at which a particular infection occurs, and the length of time conditions remain viable for that infection, can also play an important role in epidemics If all of the criteria are not met, such as a susceptible host and pathogen are present but the environment is not conducive to the pathogen infecting and causing disease, disease cannot occur.

Factors that affect the development of epidemics

Pathogen	Host	Environment
Presence of pathogen	Type of crop	Temperature
Mode of dispersal of pathogen	Degree of genetic uniformity of host plants	Rainfall / Dew
High birth rate of pathogen	Genetic make-up	Leaf wetness period
Low death rate of pathogen	Host age	Soil properties
Survival efficiency	Host nutrition	Wind
Reproductive fitness	Host population structure	Fire history
Adaptibility of pathogen	Nature of propagation	

1. Host Factors

a. **Type of crop**: Epidemics generally develop much more rapidly in **annual crops** (cereal, pulses, oilseeds and vegetable crops) than **perennial crops** (fruit and forest trees). Some epidemics of fruit and forest trees, for instance, pear dcline, tristeza in citrus, dutch elm disease and chestnut blight , takes year to develop.

b. **Degree of genetic uniformity of host plants**: A severe plant disease epidemic may develop when genetically uniform plants are grown over large area, greater likely hood exists that a new pathogen race will appear that can attack their genome and result in an epidemic.This phenomenon has been observed in repeatedly, for instance,in southern corn leaf blight on corn carrying Texas male sterile cytoplasm. The **lowest rates** of epidemic development generally occurs in **cross pollinated crops**, **intermediate** rates in self **pollinated crops** and the **highest rates** in **vegetatively** propagated crops.

c. **Level of genetic resistance or susceptibility of the host**: **Vertical** and **horizontal** resistance have distinct bearing on development and progress of epidemic. Hosts plants carrying horizontal resistance will probably become infected, but the rate at which the disease and the epidemic will develop depends on the level of resistance and the environmental conditions, Host plants carrying vertical resistance do not allow a pathogen to become established in them, and thus no epidemic can develop. Susceptible host plants lacking genes for resistance against the pathogen provide the ideal substrate for establishment and development of new infections.

d. **Host age**: Plant change in their susceptibility to disease with age. For instance, Damping off and roots rots, downy mildews, peach leaf curl, rusts, smuts, bacterial blights and viral infections, the host plants are susceptible only during their growth period and becomes resistant during adult stage. In some other diseases such as flower or fruit blights caused by fungal pathogens like *Alternaria, Penicillium, Glomerella* and *Monilinia* and in all post harvest infections, plant parts (fruits) are resistant during growth and early adult stage but become susceptible near riepning.

e. **Host nutrition**: Balanced nutrition is required for proper growth and development of plants. The type and amount of fertilizers have influence on the development of plant diseases. Under good nutritional conditions, biotrophic fungi have a relative advantage; under poor nutritional conditions necrotrophic and perthotrophic fungi have a relative advantage.

f. **Host population structure:** Crop rotation and sequence and crop density have major bearing on the type and amount of plant diseases. High crop density will influence microclimate and will make infection and dispersal of inoculums more effective. Both these factors will help the development of disease.

g. **Nature of propagation**: Nature of propagation affects the development of disease. Chances of disease are more if plants are vegetatively propagated.

2. Pathogen Factors

There are certain important pathogen factors that affect the course of epidemic

a. **Level of virulence:** Virulent pathogens capable of rapidly infecting the host ensure faster production of larger amounts of inoculums and thereby, disease, than pathogens of lesser virulence.

b. **Mode of dispersal of pathogen**: Rapid and easy dispersal of the pathogen inoculums from its source to healthy hosts in the field may help frequent and wide spread epidemic. Epidemics of diseases like mildew, rusts and leaf spots occur usually as the spores of the pathogen are released into the air and get disseminated quickly by it over distances up to several miles. Contrary to it, soil borne pathogens like *Fusarium, Verticilium*, etc., and most nematodes usually have 2 to 4 reproductive cycles per growing season. Since, the dispersal of such pathogens is limited both in space and time, only localized and slower developing epidemics are caused.

c. **High birth rate of pathogen:** High birth rate or fast reproductive cycle of pathogen is key factor for establishment and development of epidemics. Some fungal pathogen have capacity to produce enormous quantity of spores asexually and these spores, if dispersed fast over long distances and favored by conducive weather conditions, can result in epidemics in their respective areas.

d. **Low death rate of pathogen**: Epidemics attributed to low death rate of pathogens are those in which the causal organism is systemic and protected by the plant tissues. Thus, the chances of high mortality are considerably reduced and ultimately greater chance of widespread infections in a given area exist.

e. **Adaptibility of pathogen:** This is another factor vital to development of epidemics. For pathogens having capacity to acclimatize to adverse conditions, the occurrence of epidemics is about certain. The units of propagules produced by the pathogen are dispersed by external agencies which must be available if epidemics are to develop.

3. Role of Environmental Factors

The presence of a pathogen against a particular plant will generally not cause serious disease unless the environmental conditions are favourable. This includes the **aerial environment** and the **soil (edaphic) environment**.

i) Aerial environment

Properties of the **aerial environment** that influence disease development include, temperature, moisture levels and pollution.

a) **Temperature** : **Temperature** affects the incubation, or **latent period** (the time between infection and the appearance of disease symptoms), the **generation time** (the time between infection and sporulation), and the **infectious period** (the time during which the pathogen keeps producing propagules). The disease cycle speeds up at higher temperatures, resulting in faster development of epidemics. The period of leaf wetness, combined with temperature information can be used to predict outbreaks of some diseases (infection periods) and be used to time preventative treatments, such as spraying.

b) **Moisture: Moisture** is mainly important to pathogenic fungi and bacteria. Rain splash plays a significant role in the dispersal of some fungi and nearly all bacteria, and a period of leaf wetness is essential for the germination of most air borne spores. By using water for dispersal, propagules are dispersed at a time when they are likely to be able to germinate as well. Because the process of germination and infection takes time, the duration of leaf wetness also influences the success of the infection. The duration necessary for infection varies with temperature. Generally, a longer period of leaf wetness is desired to establish an infection in cooler temperatures, as germination and infection are normally accelerated in warmer conditions.

c. **Pollution:** A lately recognised aspect of the aerial environment that can influence disease in plants is air **pollution.** A high concentration of pollutants can affect disease development and, in extreme cases, damage the plants directly by causing acid rain.

ii) Soil environment

The **soil environment** affects soil-borne diseases, largely by determining the amount of **moisture** available to pathogens for germination, survival and motility. Germination and infection success also rely on the temperature of the soil. The **fertility** and **organic matter content** of the soil can affect the development of disease. Plant defences are weakened by nutrient deficiency, although some pathogens, such as rusts and powdery mildews, thrive on well-nourished plants. Other diseases thrive in soils that are specifically low in organic matter.

4. Role of Humans Activities

Humans/farmers have a direct and indirect influence on plant disease epidemics. Human decide the kind, the time, the number, and the density of plants cultivated in a particular area. If these aspects are not decided with precision, they may lead to the occurrence of an epidemic in that area. Similarly continuous monoculture , use of high dozes of fertilizers, excess of irrigation, and poor field sanitation are certain cultural practices adopted by man which invite severe epidemic in a given area. The planting of certain variety or the use of certain chemical may lead to selection of virulent strains that either can attack the resistance of the variety or are resistant to the chemical and thus lead to epidemics.

MEASUREMENT OF PLANT DISEASE AND YIELD LOSS

While measuring disease, one is interested in measuring

- **Disease incidence**; the proportion of a plant community that is diseased.
- **Disease severity** ; as the proportion of plant area that is affected.

- **Yield loss**: the proportion of the yield that the grower will not be able to harvest because the disease destroyed it directly or prevented the plants from producing it.

Disease and crop loss assessments are essential for evaluating the economic impact of a disease and the benefit of particular control strategies. There is no point in implementing a management practices if it will cost more that the increased crop yield return. The growth of the crop, its yield potential, the development of the disease and its impact on yield all have to be measured to predict the impact on yield of particular levels of disease. This information can be combined with predictions of likely disease levels to determine whether preventative treatments should be applied or not.

Assessment of the effect of disease on crop yield normally involves five steps:

- Developing a descriptive growth stage key for the particular crop species.
- Developing methods to assess the incidence and severity of disease.
- Developing statistically sound methods of sampling crop populations for assessment of the amount of disease.
- Estimating the negative impact of particular levels of the disease on crop yield and quality, and
- Evaluating the economic benefit from various methods available for reducing the amount of disease.

Assessment of Crop Growth and Development

The initial step to quantify the effect of disease is to develop a key that describes the growth and development of healthy plants during the growing season. It should describe development, either from sowing to harvest, in the case of annual plants, or from season to season in perennial plants. Details drawings or photographs, showing characteristics of the various stages of development, including leaf formation, flowering, fruiting and senescence are needed. Standardized growth keys have been developed for a number of crop plants, enabling comparison between different countries and different conditions.

Assessment of Disease Incidence and Severity

Whether it is disease incidence, or disease severity, or both, that are measured, depends on the nature of the disease. An "all or nothing" disease, for example, that inevitably kills any plant it infects, could be measured just by counting the number of plants that infected (**disease incidence**). However, in the case of a disease that causes varying degrees of damage to plants throughout the crop, a more complex measurement is needed, that assesses **disease severity**.The disease incidence for biotrophic pathogens can be measured by counting the number of plants, leaves, flowers etc that are infected, but the disease severity is assessed by estimating the proportion of total photosynthetic area that is diseased. While this is generally less precise and less controllable than counting individual plants, it is usually a better predictor of crop loss. Because judging the proportion of diseased leaf by eye is unreliable, **disease assessment keys**, showing different disease severities as blackened areas, have been devised for various crops.

To produce a disease assessment key, the development of disease over the whole disease cycle and at diverse stages of plant growth must be studied to make prototype standard diagrams or descriptions. The precision of the key then required to be tested, by assessing disease severity in the field using the key, and then assessing the same samples using accurate measurement techniques in the laboratory. There are also computer-programs designed to train observers in disease severity assessment, by presenting images of diseased leaves, which the observer assesses, and comparing their result with the known level of disease in the diagram. This aims to lessen variation in results caused by different observers.

These disease assessment methods will only be precise if performed on a representative sample of the crop. Samples of crop units (plants, leaves, fruit etc) can be taken randomly from a crop, or standard quadrats can be placed in the crop and all plants within the quadrat assessed. In a test plot, a part of the plot is generally assessed for disease. Taking samples only from the edge of a plantation will not necessarily be representative of the bulk of the crop. To determine how many samples need to be taken, it is probable to sample a number of times with progressively more samples, and find the point at which the standard error is low. A disease that is uniformly spread all through a crop will need fewer samples for an precise assessment than a disease that has a patchy distribution throughout the crop.

Assessment of Crop Losses

Once the amount of disease has been determined, the subsequently step is to assess, either experimentally or statistically, the effect of different levels of disease on the crop yield. Experimental assessment involves setting up test crops in which the level of disease is controlled. Monitoring crops with different levels of disease allows the comparison of epidemic progress and crop yield under different disease conditions. A relationship between disease parameters and yield can then be formulated, allowing prediction of crop loss for a certain level of disease at a particular point in the crop's growth. This method is dependent upon the assumption that the treatments used to keep disease at a certain level have no effect on crop yield themselves. This might not always be the case. Likewise, assessments using susceptible and resistant cultivars rely on both cultivars having a similar yield to start with. Again, this might not be true, and must be determined first in a disease-free environment. All aspects of experimental design need to be cautiously considered in order to gain an accurate assessment of the effect of disease on crop yield. For instance, harvesting methods under experimental conditions are often more efficient than under field conditions, giving the appearance of a higher crop yield. From crop loss assessment studies, models can be devised. Crop loss models are usually based on one of three types of disease assessment: disease at a critical point in development, disease at multiple points in development, and disease throughout crop development.

The statistical approach to assessing disease involves statistical analysis of crop yields under different levels of disease that occur naturally in the field. The levels of disease and the crop yields are monitored, but not manipulated, and then yields from different seasons or areas with different levels of disease can be compared to determine the effect of disease on crop yield.

Types of Epidemics

Monocyclic epidemics: Monocyclic epidemics are caused by pathogens with a low birth rate and death rate meaning they only have one infection cycle per season. They are typical of soil born diseases such as *Fusarium* wilt of pigeonpea. Mathematical equations used to predict epidemic development in time is

$$dx/dt = r\,(x_a - x)$$

Where, dx/dt= rate of increase of disease; r =infection rate; x =number of infected individuals; t =time; x_a= total population size.

Examples: r for *Verticillium* wilt of cotton= 0.02 units/day, 'r' for *Phymatotrichum* root rot of cotton= 1.60 units per year.

Polycyclic epidemics: Polycyclic epidemics are caused by pathogens capable of several infection cycles a season. These are most often caused by airborne diseases such as powdery mildew. Mathematical equations used to predict epidemic development in time is :

$$dx/dt = xr\,(1 - x)$$

Where, dx/dt= rate of increase of disease; r = exponential rate of disease increase; x = amount of disease on a scale of 0-1 and t =time under consideration during which host and pathogen have interacted.

Examples: r for late blight of potato = 0.3 to 0.5 units per day 'r' for stem rust of wheat = 0.3-0.6 units per day. 'r' for *Phymatotrichum* root rot of cotton= 1.60 units per year.

Polyetic epidemics: Some diseases takes several years from the time of infection until symptom develop and pathogen reproduction. Epidemics that occur under these conditions are referred to as polyetic epidemics and can be caused by both monocylcic and polycyclic pathogens. Apple powdery mildew is an example of a polyetic epidemic caused by a polycyclic pathogen and Dutch Elm disease a polyetic epidemic caused by a monocyclic pathogen.

Differences between monocyclic and polycyclic plant disease epidemics

Characters	Monocyclic	Polycyclic
Birth rate	Low	High
Death rate	Low	High
Rate of increases	Like simple interest	Like compound interest
Survival	Long lived	Short lived
Reproduction	Reproduces only one generation per growing season	Reproduce new batches of propagules several times per growing season

Epidemiologists use specific terminology to accurately communicate magnitudes and potentials for disease.

Disease progress curve: Periodic observations on disease severity , in any field or area, when plotted against time on a graph paper gives curved lines representing progress of disease over time . These cumulative disease curves are known as disease progress curve (DPC).

A saturation curve-monocyclic disease

A sigmoid curve- polycyclic disease

A bimodal curve-polycyclic disease affecting different organs

Disease-gradient curve; A graph that plots disease vs. distance from an inoculum source.

Epidemic; A disease increase in a population; usually a widespread and severe outbreak of disease.

Epidemiology; The study of factors affecting the outbreak and spread of disease.

Course of Epidemic

The course of epidemic follows two distinct phases viz.,

i. Progressively destructive phase and

ii. the decline phase

i. Progressively destructive phase

Some epidemics develop rapidly while others develop slowly. Slow epidemics (or epiphytotics) generally occur among population caused by systemic pathogens. The pathogen multiplies slowly following the characters of simple interest disease. They belong to low death rate category and have less incubation period and sporulation period. On the other hand, the rapid epiphytotics are greatly influenced by environmental factors.

ii. Decline phase

During early stage, an epidemic spreads briskly causing diseases in new hosts. After development of a saturation stage it shows a decline by itself. No epidemics may be due to non-availability of susceptible stages of the crop, unfavourable weather conditions and reduction in aggressiveness of the pathogens. Normally the hosts are prone to the disease at a specific developing stage. Once this stage is crossed in a plant it's proneness to infections is reduced or completely lost. Under the conditions the epidemic declines. The decline in the epidemic may also be due to unfavourable weather conditions for disease development. As a result future spread of the disease will be checked and the epidemic will decline.

Slow and Rapid Epiphytotics

The form of epidemic is decided by the nature of the pathogen, host and the weather. Epidemic may develop slowly and is called **'tardive'**. In between these intermediate forms of Epidemic which develops rapidly is called **'explosive'** epidemic may occur.

i. Rapid epiphytotics

Rapid epiphytotics occur among **annual crops**. It is caused by non-systemic pathogens with high birth rate. Several generations of the pathogen is produced within a short time. Rapid epiphytotics are largely governed by environmental factors compared to slow epiphytotics. Disease increase is rapid and the disease rises to a peak in short time and then show sharp decline when the weather turns unfavourable or when the host becomes resistant due to maturity or due to restricted dispersal of propagules of pathogen. e.g.,apple scab. This type of epiphytotic is controlled by protective **spraying** or **dusting** with **chemicals**.

ii. Slow epiphytotics

Slow epiphytotics occur among **perennial** (tree) **populations**. Infected host survives for several years before dying. Most of the characters of a **simple interest** disease are found in slow epiphytotics. The causal agent is mostly systemic. The pathogen multiplies slowly. Their movement from plant to plant is much slower. They are low death rate pathogen. In slow epiphytotics, crop **sanitation** is the best method. e.g., Swollen shoot of cocoa. This disease spreads very slowly from tree to tree and still less from one garden to another garden

Modeling in Plant Pathology

Models are simple representation of otherwise more complex real systems. The model provide opportunity for better understanding and system management. Kranz (1974) stated that a model might be **verbal statement**, a **hypothesis**, a **theory** or a **law**. The selection of suitable model is determined by the purpose and goals which must be defined very precisely.

1. Conceptual Models: These models were conceived during early stages of introduction of models in Plant Pathology. They were fundamentally **qualitative**, without much quantification. The relationships and interactions were displayed in **diagrammatic** form or **flowchart** manner. examples, Disease pyramid, Components of pathogenesis, gene for gene hypothesis.

2. Analytical Models: Vanderplank (1963) used differential equations for calculation of pathogen population growth. Equation of single and multiple cycle diseases, threshold theorem and fitting curves to empirical data are common analytical models used in Plant Pathology.

3. Predictive Models: are those in which the emphasis is placed on those variables which have the greatest value in forecasting the likely course of events. These are generally used in **estimation of yields** and **forecasting diseases**. Regression and differential equations are generally employed. They are considered a boon to growers for bringing precision in management decisions. Examples, **BLITECAST** in USA and **PHYTOPROG** in West Germany in giving shot term warnings of potato late blight attacks. **FAST** is the computer model for forecasting early blight in tomato.

4. Simulation Models: The simulation models try to **simulate** or **mimic** the real life situations under study. When a computer is provided data describing the diverse subcomponents of the epidemic and measures of control at specific points in time, it then provides back the continuous information regarding not only the spread and severity of the disease over time, but also the final crop and economic losses likely to occur due to disease under the conditions of the epidemic as provided to the computer. The first computer simulation programme, called **EPIDEM**, was written in 1969 to simulate **early blight** epidemics of tomato and potato. Examples of other simulators are:

Name of the programme	Disease	Pathogen
EPIPRE	Cereal rusts and aphids	*Puccinia graminis tritici*
EPICORN	Southern corn leaf blight of maize.	*Helminthosporium maydis*
CERCOS	Leaf blight of celery	*Cercospora spp.*
MYCOS	Blight of chrysanthemum	*Mycosphaerella spp.*
EPIVEN	Apple scab	*Venturia inaequalis*
EPIDEMIC	Stripe rust	*Puccinia striiformis*
TOM-CAST	Early blight of tomato	*Alternaria solani*
BLIGHT-CAST	Late blight of potato	*Phytophthora infestans*
PLASMO	Downy mildew of grapes	*Plasmopara viticola*
SIMCAST	Late blight of potato	*Phytophthora infestans*
NEGFRY	Late blight of potato	*Phytophthora infestans*
EPIVET	Viral diseases of potato	Contact and aphid transmitted viruses

CHAPTER - 30

Plant Disease Forecasting

DEFINITION

Fore casting involves all the activities in ascertaining and notifying the grower of community that conditions are sufficiently favourable for certain diseases, that application of control measures will result in economic gain or on the other hand, and just as important that the amount expected is unlikely to be enough to justify the expenditure of time , energy and money for control. The above statement made explicit distinction between positive forecast and negative forecast and both have value for growers as well as society in general.

Positive forecast: Employs need based chemical sprays, provides adequate protection to crop and reduces damage to environment.

Negative forecast: Avoids unnecessary chemical sprays, no risk to the crop health and no disruption of environment.

Importance of Forecasting

- Forecasting informs the growers whether the conditions are not favourable and the disease is unlikely to be intense enough. This helps growers to save the expenditure in terms of energy, time and money by not applying unnecessary management measures.
- It informs the growers about when the conditions are going to be sufficiently favourable for economically important diseases of an agroclimatic zone. This help growers to apply disease management timely that results in economic gain.
- It helps growers to plan advance preventive measures against likely losses due to the occurrence of economically important severe diseases.
- Government and other organizations initiate necessary steps for the timely stocking of chemicals, equipments, etc. when they are timely warned by the possibility of an epidemic by the forecasting's.

Requirements for Disease Forecasting

The following requirements are necessary to make useful and successful disease forecasts

- The disease must cause economically significant damage in terms of yield loss or quality.
- Control measures must be available at an economically acceptable cost.
- Disease should not be regular feature.
- Reliable means of communication with farmers.
- Growers must have sufficient manpower and equipments to apply control measures when disease warning is given.
- Farmers should be adaptive and have purchase power.

Information's needed for Disease Forecasting

The information's required for forecasting are:

1. Host factors

a. Prevalence of susceptible varieties in the given locality.

b. Response of host at different stages of the growth to the activity of pathogen.

c. Density and distribution of the host in a given locality.

2. Pathogen factors

a. Amount of primary inoculum in the air, soil or planting material.

b. Dispersal of inoculums.

c. Spore germination.

d. Infection.

e. Incubation period.

f. Sporulation on the infected host.

g. Re-dispersal / Dissemination of spores.

h. Perennating stages.

i. Inoculum potential and density in the seed, soil and air.

3. Environmental factors

a. Temperature

b. Humidity

c. Light intensity

d. Wind velocity

Methods of Disease Forecasting

Disease forecasting requires field observations on the pathogen characters, collection of weather data, variety of the crop and certain investigations and their correlations. Usually the following methods are employed in disease forecasting.

1. Forecasting based on amount of initial inoculum

Amount of primary inoculum present in seed, soil or vector can be estimated and disease prediction can be made without much problem. This criterion is more important for **monocyclic** diseases where the secondary infection does not take place and the amount of primary inoculums is related to disease severity and damage. It is being used in case of loose smut of wheat and soil borne inoculums of *Rhizoctonia, Sclerotium, Verticillium*, nematodes can be estimated and disease can be forecast. Presence of loose smut of wheat, ergot of pearl millet and viral diseases of potato can be detected in the seed lots at random by different seed testing methods. Seed testing methods can be used to determine potential disease incidence and enable decision to be made on the need for chemical seed treatment.

2. Forecasting based on weather conditions

Prevailing weather conditions *viz.*, temperature, relative humidity, rainfall, light, wind velocity etc., have become a major criteria for diseases forecasting for **polycyclic** diseases where in addition to amount of primary inoculums, the multiplication and dispersal of secondary inoculums are weather dependent. Forecasting of late and early blight of potato, wheat rust, anthracnose, apple scab, powdery mildew of cucurbits and downy mildew of grapes are made considering the prevailing weather conditions which determine the amount of disease and damage of the crop.

3. Forecasting based on correlative information

Weather data of numerous years are collected and correlated with the intensity of the diseases. The data are compared and then the forecasting of the disease is done. Forecasting criteria developed from comparisons of disease observation with standard meteorological data have been provided for diseases like fire blight of apple and powdery mildew of barley.

4. Use of computer for disease forecasting

In some developed countries forecasting of disease is made by the use of computers. The computers are fed with weather data collected on the farm by individual farmers. The computer then processes the data, determines whether an infection period is imminent, likely to occur or can not occur, and a recommendation is made to the farmer as to whether or not to spray and what materials to apply. This system gives the results quickly. One such computer based programmes in the USA is known as **'Blitecast'** for potato late blight.

Examples of Plant Disease Forecast Symptoms

a. Late blight of potato

Late blight of potato had been instrumental in development of diverse fundamental concepts in plant pathology and disease forecasting is no exception. The potato growers in Europe were intelligent enough to recognize blight weather (Moderate temperature and lots of moisture: rain, dew or humidity) much earlier than **Van Everdingen** postulated **Dutch rules in 1926**. Followings are four conditions correlated with weather that could predict about appearance of late blight in Netherlands:

- Night temperature below dew point at least 4 hours.
- Minimum temperature of 10^0C or slightly above.
- Clouds on the next day.
- Rainfall during next 24 hours of at least 0.1 mm.

Notable contributions in late blight forecasting

Van Everdingen postulated Dutch rules in 1926

Krause, *et al.* (1970), BLITECAST

Singh , *et al.* (1980), JHULSACAST for Indi Gangetic plains

Fry and Apple (1983), Integrated host resistance and fungicide weathering in BLITECAST

Dommermuth (1988), Phytoprog I. late blight warning service.

Runno and Kopple (2002), NEGFRY

Grunwald (2002), Modified and validated SIMCAST

b. Southern corn leaf blight

'Epimay' is a system for forecasting, Southern corn leaf blight (*Bipolaris maydis*). It is based on conceptual model.

c. Rice blast

Forecasting of rice blast (*Pyricularia ozyzae*) in India is done by **correlative information** method. It is predicted on the basis of minimum night temperature 20 to 26°C in association with high relative humidity of 90% or above. Computer based forecasting system has also been developed for rice blast in India.

d. Wheat stem rust

Forecasting wheat stem rust epidemic is done by analysing therein samples which give precise data for inoculum present in the air. Moreover several wind trajectors are also prepared to survey the air-borne primary inoculums and its deposition. It has been observed that primary inoculum comes from South India, to the plains of Central and North India.

e. Early and late leaf spots of groundnut

A technique has been developed for forecasting early and late leaf spots of groundnut in the U.S.A. When the groundnut foliage remains wet for a period greater than or equal to 10 h and the minimum temperature is 21°C or higher for two consecutive days or nights, the disease development is forecasted.

A computer programme has been developed in the USA. This is accurate and is widely used in the USA. The data on hours for day with relative humidity (RH) of 95% and above and minimum temperature (T) during the RH observations for the period, for the previous 5 days are fed to the computer. Calculations are rounded to whole numbers. The T/RH index for each of the five days is calculated e.g., when hours of the RH 95% equal 10 and the minimum temperature during the period equals 21.1°C the T/RH index is 2.0 .The T/RH indices for days 4 and 5 are summed. If the total index exceeds 4 disease is forecasted. If the index is 3 or less no disease is forecasted.

f. Blister blight of tea

A system for predicting epidemics of blister blight of tea (*Exobasidium vexans*) has been developed based on the number of spores in the air in the tea plantation and the duration of surface wetness on the leaves. The duration of sunshine is negatively correlated with the duration of surface wetness. The following prediction equation has been developed. $Y = 1.8324 + 0.8439\ X1 +$

0.9665 X2 – 0.1031 X3where, X1 = log % infection t2X2 = log % infection t2 – log infection t1Y = log of the number of spores in the air and t1 – t2 three weeks X3 = mean daily sunshine for a 7 days period preceding t2.

Empirical vs Fundamental forecasting

Bourke (1955) designated two methods of disease forecasting. They are 'empirical' and 'fundamental'

Empirical methods: is a method in which correlation between the results of disease surveys and the corresponding weather conditions in a particular area or near the same area for as long a time as possible has to be related to the biology of the host plant and pathogen.

Fundamental methods: is a method which uses results obtained from laboratory research on weather factors affecting pathogen, host, and the disease process as the starting point, interpreted and applied according to conditions in the region concerned.

Neither method is more reliable than the other. Both need to be tested and evaluated in actual use. Each methods contains some elements of the other. The two methods naturally tend to merge in practice, because experimental results provide standards for judging the correctness of the assumptions underlying the empirical method, whereas field performance of the predictions is at least of the adequacy with which research is put to use in the fundamental method.

PROGNOSIS

Prognosis is characterized as the prediction of the outbreak, development and outcome of disease. The objective is to decide in advance whether expected damage is threatening and whether control measures are to be taken. Prognosis has been attempted at two levels: (a) Date prognosis and (b) Loss prognosis

(a) **Date prognosis**: mainly deals with the prediction of the out break of a disease. Following two criteria are considered for date prognosis:

- Estimate the initial population of pathogens and their antagonist, if feasible.
- Record weather parameters and their prediction over prognosis time span.

(b) **Loss prognosis:** is based on estimate of expected economic loss, in relation to disease intensity-crop damage, and constitutes the basis or the decision as to spray or not. In loss prognosis in addition to economic aspects, consideration of the biological and eco toxicological consequences of a plant protection measure are important factor.

Expert Systems in Plant Pathology

An Agricultural Expert System is a Decision Support System for agricultural extension agents who have to decide what advice to be offered to farmers who in turn decide about suitable action based on it. It is one of the most efficient extension tools to take the technology from scientists to the farmers directly without any dilution of content which normally creeps in because of the number of agencies involved in normal technology transfer systems.

Expert systems are the frontiers, which combines and integrate both **science of plant pathology** and **art of diagnosis** and **disease management**. These computer decision support systems were formally introduced in Plant Pathology in 1987. **Expert system are computer programs that emulate the logic and problem solving proficiency of human expert.** The computerized disease forecasting systems of 1970s (BLITECAST) and 1980s (apple scab forecaster) were the precursors to expert system. In principle the Expert system are an artificial intelligence application that uses encoded knowledge from a human expert. Expert system has the ability to use complete or incomplete data; accordingly it will assign certainty values to the solutions of the problems. The Expert system are programmed to review a consultation and provide user with an explanation. Three main areas involved in decision making are **pest risk estimation, current threat assessment** and **pesticide application**.

Expert System used in Plant Pathology

Expert System	Description
PLANT/ds	First expert system (1983) developed for diagnosis of 17 soybean diseases (USA)
EPIPRE	Epidemic prediction and prevention for spring and winter wheat
POTATOES	Late and early blight of potato
TOMEX	Diagnosis of 37 diseases of tomato
POMME	For management of disease and insects of apple
PSACO	For management of diseases and insects of apple
PRO-PLANT	For cereals, potato, sugarbeet and vegetables
More Crop	For management of rusts and other problems
TOMEx -UFV	For diagnosis of tomato diseases
SIMPHYT-III	For *Phytophthora infestans*

Chapter - 31

Principles of Plant Disease Management

INTRODUCTION

Plant diseases have caused severe losses to humans in several ways. Starvation and uprooting of families resulted from the Irish famine caused by potato late blight . A valued resource was lost with the virtual elimination of the American chestnut by chestnut blight. And direct economic loss such as the estimated one billion dollars lost in one year to American corn growers from southern corn leaf blight . Many plant diseases cause less dramatic losses annually throughout the world but collectively constitute sizable losses to farmers and can reduce the aesthetic values of landscape plants and home gardens.

The **goal** of plant disease management is **to reduce** the economic and **aesthetic damage** caused by **plant diseases.** Conventionally, this has been called **plant disease control**, but current social and environmental values believe **"control"** as being **absolute** and the term **too rigid**. More multifaceted approaches to **disease management**, and **integrated disease management**, have resulted from this shift in attitude. However, single, often severe, measures, such as pesticide applications, soil fumigation or burning are no longer in common use. Further, disease management measures are often determined by disease forecasting or disease modeling rather than on either a calendar or prescription basis. Disease management might be viewed as **proactive** whereas disease control is **reactive**, although it is often difficult to distinguish between the two concepts, especially in the application of specific measures.

Plant disease management practices rely on anticipating occurrence of disease and attacking vulnerable points in the disease cycle (i.e., weak links in the infection chain). Therefore, correct diagnosis of a disease is necessary to identify the pathogen, which is the real target of any disease management program. A thorough understanding of the disease cycle, including climatic and other environmental factors that influence the cycle, and cultural requirements of the host plant, are essential to effective management of any disease.

The many strategies, tactics and techniques used in disease management can be grouped under one or more very broad principles of action. Differences between these principles often are not clear. The simplest system consists of two principles, **prevention** (prophylaxis in some early writings) and **therapy** (treatment or cure).The first principle (prevention) includes disease management tactics applied **before** infection (i.e., the plant is protected from disease), the second principle (therapy or curative action) functions with any measure applied **after** the plant is infected (i.e., the plant is treated for the disease). An example of the first principle is enforcement of quarantines to prevent introduction of a disease agent (pathogen) into a region where it does not occur. The second principle is illustrated by heat or chemical treatment of vegetative material such as bulbs, corms, and woody cuttings to eliminate fungi, bacteria, nematodes or viruses that are established within the plant material. Chemotherapy is the application of chemicals to an infected or diseased plant that stops (i.e., eradicates) the infection. There are five general disease control principles, **avoidance, exclusion**, **eradication**, **protection** and **resistance** since plants do not have an immune system in the same sense as animals). These principles have been expanded or altered to some extent by others. They are still valid and are detailed

Principles of Plant Disease Management

Principles of plant disease management include

1. **Prophylaxis** (preventive)
   - Avoidance
   - Exclusion
   - Eradication
   - Protection
2. **Immunization**
   - Genetic resistance
   - Therapy (Physical therapy and chemical therapy)

I) **Avoidance of pathogen** :Avoiding disease by planting at times when or where inoculum is absent or ineffective due to unfavorable environment conditions.

- Choice of geographic area
- Selection of field
- Choice of time of sowing
- Disease escaping varieties

- Selection of seed and planting stock
- Modification of cultural practices

II) Exclusion of inoculum :Preventing the inoculum from entering or establishing in the field or area where it does not exist.

- Seed treatment
- Inspection and certification
- Quarantine
- Eradication of insect vectors

III) Eradication of pathogens :Reducing, inactivating, eliminating or destroying inoculum at the source, either from a region or from an individual plant in which it is already established.

- Biological control of plant pathogen
- Crop rotation
- Removal or destruction of diseased plant organs
- Rouging
- Eradication of alternate and collateral hosts
- Sanitation
- Heat and chemical treatment of diseased plants
- Soil treatments

IV) Immunization: It involves the modification of certain physical or physiological character(s) of the host such that it can repel infection or can reduce disease development or can minimize damage caused by the pathogen. The methods used are

- Use of resistant varieties
- Cross-protection

Cross protection: Refers to the protection of a plant by use of a mild strain of a pathogen against a virulent strain of the same pathogen that can cause more severe symptoms and damage. The method is generally used for viral disease management.

Disease resistance: Altering the effectiveness of the pathogen by selection or introduction of resistance genes in the plant.

- Selection and hybridization for disease resistance
- Resistance through chemotherapy

- Resistance through host nutrition

V) **Protection measures**: Preventing infection by creating a chemical toxic barrier between the plant and the pathogen is comes under protection measures

- Chemical treatment
- Chemical control of insect vectors
- Modification of environments

VI) **Therapy**: Reducing severity of disease in an infected individual

- Chemotherapy
- Heat therapy
- Tree surgery

Strategy of Disease Management

It is well accepted that complete eradication of a pathogen from the earth of the ecosystem is very difficult. They are also intimate part of the ecosystem as human beings, animals and plants Therefore; complete eradication is against the law of nature. The strategy for management lies on a amending the methods of cultivation through supplementary treatments, which can compensate for the upsetting of the natural ecosystem. The strategy should be to reduce the population of pathogen below permissible level so they do not cause damage. Keeping this in mind, the strategy of disease management should integrate all known methods taking into account the following factors.

1. Pathogen inhibition

As complete eradication of a pathogen is not possible, there should be more emphasis on management of its population. The pathogens will exist but control systems will have to be developed to **maintain their population** below the **damaging level**.

2. Tolerable losses

A few diseased seeds or plants are permissible in the field. If the loss is less, uprooting the diseased plants is more economical. In crops raised for seed two per cent disease infection is permissible, whereas in crops raised for consumption the permissible limit is 5 per cent.

3. Economical control

The strategy for disease management should be implemented after considering the **cost benefit ratio**. The return per unit of money spent must be sufficiently high.

4. Long term control

The strategy of disease management should attempt to utilize methods which have a long term effect so as to reduce the expenses and pollution of the environment.

5. Collective approach

Disease control cannot be achieved by a single farmer since pathogen can move from field to field. Hence, collective area wise approach is necessary for effective control.

One should always keep in mind that chemical control is a part of the strategy for disease management. Care should be taken not to accelerate the frequency of pesticide application. The use of **chemical** should be the **last resort** for controlling the diseases.

It is well known that any war cannot be won only on quantity of weapons available. Success only comes from a well planned strategy involving the best use of weapons in a coordinated manner at the right time and with proper methods. Similarly, the **war** against diseases can be won provided an **integrated approach** is **employed** and all the five basic factors discussed above are taken into account.

Chapter - 32

Physical Management

PRINCIPLES

The principles involved in thermotherapy is that the pathogens present in seed material are inactivated or eliminated at temperatures nonlethal for the host tissues.The exact mechanism by which heat inactivates the pathogen is not fully understood. However, it is universally accepted that **heat** causes **inactivation** and not **immobilization** of the pathogen by heat. Th rate at which the pathogen is inactivated is determined by temperature, the higher the temperature, the faster is the inactivation.

METHODS

Following physical methods are employed for reduction or elimination of primary inoculums that may be present in seed, soil or planting material.

i. Hot Water Treatment (HWT)

Hot water treatment is widely used for the control of seed borne pathogens, especially bacteria and viruses. A list of various important diseases claimed to have been controlled by hot water treatment is given in Table-18.

Table 18 : Control of seed borne pathogens through Hot –water treatment

Crop	Disease	Causal organism	Seed Treatment
Rice	White tip	*Aphluenchoides besseyi*	51-53°C for 15 min after dipping for 1 d in cool water.
	Udbatta	*Ehelis oryzae*	54°C for 10 min
Pearl millet	Downy mildew	*Sclerospora graminicola*	55°C for 10 min
Safflower	Leaf spots	*Alternaria spp.*	50°C for 30 min
Tomato	Black speck	*P. syringae pv. tomato*	52°C for 1h
Cauliflower & Cabbage	Black rot	*X. campestris pv. campestris*	50°C for 20 min
Tobacco	Hollow stalk	*E. carotovora pv. carotovora*	50°C for 12 min.
Cluster bean	Blight	*X. campestris pv. cyamopsidis*	56°C for 10 min
Sugarcane			**Setts Treatment**
	Red rot	*Colletotrichum falcatum*	54°C for 8 h
	Smut	*Ustilago scitaminea*	55 to 60°C
	Wilt	*Fusarium moniliforme*	50°C for 2 h
	Grassy shoot	MLO	54°C for 2h

The main drawback in the hot water treatment is that the seeds may be killed or loose its germinability, if the period of treatment exceeds the specified time. So this method is replaced by other physical methods like hot air and aerated steam treatment wherein the seeds are exposed only to hot air/aerated steam.

ii. Hot Air Treatment (HAT)

Hot air treatment is less effective than hot water treatment but less injurious to seed and easy to operate. It has been used against several diseases of sugarcane.It is employed for treating canes which are soft and succulent. Hot air treatment at 54°C for 8h, effectively eliminates RSD pathogen without impairing the germination of buds. Similarly, grassy shoot disease of sugarcane has also been controlled by hot air at 54°C for 8 h.

iii. Steam and Aerated Steam Therapy (AST)

The use of **aerated steam** is more effective than **hot air** and safer than **hot water** in controlling seed borne infections. The heat capacity of water vapour is about half that of water and 2.5 that of air, hence air temperature and time required may be higher than that of hot water and lower than that of hot air. The advantages of this method include easier drying of seeds, low loss in germination, easy temperature control and no damage to seed coat of legumes.Sugarcane setts are also exposed to aerated steam at 50°C for 3 hrs to eliminate mosaic virus.

iv. Moist Hot Air Treatment (MHAT)

This method is effectively used in sugarcane to eliminate grassy shoot disease. Initially the setts are exposed to hot air at 54^{0}C for 8 hrs, then exposed to aerated steam at 50 ^{0}C for 1 hr and finally to moist hot air at 54^{0}C for 2 hours.

v. Solar Heat Treatment (SHT)

Solar heat treatment is effective in controlling both seed borne and soil borne diseases

a. Seed Borne Diseases

Solar heat treatment has been devised in **India to** eliminate the pathogen of **loose smut of wheat. Luthra** in **1953** devised a method to eliminate the deep seated infection of *ustilago nuda.* The method is popularly known as solar heat or solar energy treatment. In this method the seeds are soaked in cold water for 4 hours in the forenoon on a bright summer day followed by spreading and drying the seeds in hot sun for four hours in the afternoon. Then, the seeds are again treated with carboxin or carbendazin at 2g/kg and stored. This method is highly useful for treating large quantities of the seed lots.

SOIL SOLARIZATION

i. Introduction

Soil solarization **is a soil disinfestations method** which aims to reduce or eradicate the inoculums existing in soil. It was the credit of **Israel** extension workers and growers who suggested that intensive heating that occurs in mulched soil might be used for the control of **soil borne pathogens**. Since then , this approach to control soil borne pathogens and weeds has been widely used in Israel and other countries.

ii. The Principles

Solar heating method for disease control is similar, in principles, to that of artificial soil heating by steam or other means, which are usually carried out at 60 to 100°C. There are, however, biological and technological differences with soil solarization there is no need to transport heat from its source to the field. Solar heating is carried at relatively low temperatures, as compred to artificial heating; thus, its effect on living and nonliving components of soil is likely to be less drastic. Of the four components of disease severity, **inoculums density** is the most affected component by solarization, either through the direct effect of the heat or by microbial processes induced in the soil. The other components except the host susceptibility which is genetically controlled, might also be affected

iii. How to solarize soil

Soil Preparation

Preparation of the soil begins by disking or turning the soil by hand to break up clods and then smoothing the soil surface. Remove any large rocks, weeds, or any other objects or debris that will raise or puncture the plastic. Solarization is most effective when the plastic sheeting is laid as close as possible to a smooth soil surface.

Types of plastic used

Transparent or **clear plastic** is most effective for solarization. The thinner the plastic, the greater the heating will be. **Polyethylene (PE) plastic 1mil (0.001 inch [0.025 mm])** thick is efficient and economical but not very resistant to tearing by wind or puncture by animals. Users in windy areas should consider plastic sheets that are 1.5 to 2 mils (0.038-0.050 mm) thick. If holes or tears do occur in the plastic they should be patched with clear patching tape. Users are encouraged to select plastic sheeting containing ITV inhibiting additives that prevent sheets from becoming brittle and difficult to remove from the field and extend the life of the plastic. Plastic sheets laid by hand can often be used more than once for solarization, although if the plastic is dirty or dusty reuse is less effective.

Laying the plastic

Plastic sheets may be laid by hand or machine . The open edges of the plastic sheeting should be anchored to the soil by burying the edges in a shallow trench around the treated area. Plastic is laid either in complete coverage, where the entire field or area to be planted is treated, or strip coverage, where only beds or selected portions of the field are treated.

Complete coverage

In complete coverage, plastic sheeting is laid down to form a continuous surface over the entire field or area to be planted. The edges of the sheets may be joined with an ultraviolet (UV)-resistant glue or anchored by laying adjacent strips of plastic and burying both edges in soil. If beds are formed after complete coverage, care must be taken to avoid deep tillage that could bring untreated soil to the surface. Complete coverage is recommended if the soil is heavily infested with pathogens, nematodes, or perennial weeds, since there is less chance of reinfestation by soil being moved to the plants through cultivation or furrow-applied irrigation water.

Strip coverage

In strip coverage, plastic is applied in strips over preformed beds . Strips should be a minimum of 75 cm wide; beds up to 1.5 m wide are preferred because several crop rows can be planted per bed. In some cases, strip coverage may be more practical and economical than complete coverage because less plastic is needed and it is not necessary to join the edges of the plastic sheets together. Strip coverage effectively kills most pests and eliminates the need for deep cultivation after solarization. It is especially effective against weeds, since the furrows are cultivated. With strip coverage, however, long term control of soil pathogens and nematodes may be lost because pests in the untreated soil in the rows between the strips can contaminate and reinfest treated areas.

Irrigation

The soil under the plastic sheets must be saturated to at least **70 percent of field capacity** in the upper layers and moist to depths of **24 inches** (60 cm) for soil solarization to be effective. **Wet soil** conducts heat better than **dry soil** and makes soil organisms more vulnerable to heat. Soil may be irrigated either before or after the plastic sheets are laid. Fields treated by strip coverage can be irrigated by drip lines on or in the bed. The soil does not usually need to be irrigated again during solarization, although if the soil is very light and sandy, or if the soil moisture is less than 50 percent of field capacity, it may be necessary to irrigate a second time. This will cool the soil, but because of the increased moisture the final temperatures will be greater.

Duration of treatment

The plastic sheets should be left in place for **4 to 6 weeks** to allow the soil to heat to greatest depth possible. To control the most resistant species, leave the plastic in place for 6 weeks. Soil in the Central Valley can be solarized for 4 weeks any time from **late May to September**. In coastal areas the best time may be **August to September** or **May to June**.

Removal of the plastic and planting

After solarization is complete, the plastic may be removed before planting.

Or, the plastic may be left on the soil as a mulch for the following crop by transplanting plants through the plastic. Clear plastic may be painted white or silver to cool the soil and repel flying insect pests in the following crop. A disadvantage of leaving the plastic on the soil is that it may degrade and be difficult to clean up in the spring. Treated soil can be planted immediately to a fall or winter crop or left fallow without the plastic until the next growing season. If the soil must be cultivated for planting, the cultivation must be shallow-less than 2 inches (5 cm)-to avoid moving viable weed seed to the surface.

Results of solarization

- Increased soil temperature.
- Improved soil physical and chemical features.
- Control of pests.
- Encouragement of beneficial soil organisms.
- Increased plant growth.

Table 19 : Pathogens and pests controlled by soil solarization

Disease	Crop	Causal organism
Wilt	Cucumber	*Fusarium oxysporum f. sp. conglutinans*
Wilt	Strawberry	*Fusarium oxysporom f. sp. fragariae*
Wilt	Tomato	*Fusarium oxysporum f. sp. lycopersici*
Wilt	Cotton	*Fusarium oxysporum f. sp. vasinfectum*
Club root	Cruciferous	*Plosmodiophora brassicae*
Phytophthora root rot	Many crops	*Phoma terrestris*
White rot	Garlic and onions	*Sclerotium rolfsii*
Bacteria		
Crown gall	Many crops	*Agrobacterium tumefaciens*
Canker	Tomato potato	*Clavibacter michiganensis*
Scab		*Streptomyces scabies*
Nematodes		
Common name		**Scientific name**
Ring nematode		*Criconemella xenoplax*
Stem and bulb nematode		*Ditylenchus dipsaci*
Potato cyst nematode		*Globodera rostochiensis*
Spiral nematode		*Helicotylenchus digonicus*
Sugarbeet cyst nematode		*Heterodera schachtii*
Root knot nematode		*Meliodogyne hapla Meliodogyne javanica*
Pin nematode		*Paratylenchus hamatus*
Lesion nematode		*Pratylenchus penetrans, Pratylenchus thornei*

Factors that limit effectiveness of solarization

- Location
- Weather
- Timing
- Duration of treatment
- Soil preparation
- Soil moisture content
- Soil color
- Orientation of beds

Advantages

- Nonpesticidal and simple.
- No health or safety problems associated with use.
- No registration is required.
- Crops produced are pesticide-free and may command a higher market price.
- Controls multiple soilborne diseases and pests.
- Selects for beneficial microorganisms.
- Tends to increase soil fertility.
- Increases soluble NO_3, NH, Ca, Mg, K and soluble organic matter.
- May improve soil filth.
- Can speed up in-field composting of green manure.

Disadvantages

- Is restricted to areas with warm to hot summers.
- May be less effective in cooler coastal areas.
- Land must be taken out of production for 4 to 6 weeks during the summer.
- May not fit in with some cropping cycles.
- May be difficult for those using a small amount of land intensively.
- Limited number of retail outlets for UV-inhibiting plastics.

- Disposal may be a problem.
- Large amounts of plastic cannot currently be recycled in California.
- Some pests are not controlled or are difficult to control.
- No pest control in the furrows between strips (if applied in strip coverage).
- High winds and animals may tear the plastic.

Refrigeration

The low temperature at or slightly above the freezing point checks the growth and activities of all such pathogens that cause a variety of post harvest diseases of vegetables and fruits. Therefore, most perishable fruits and vegetables should be transported and stored in refrigerated vehicles and stores. Cool chains refrigerated space from field to consumer table is becoming very popular. Regular refrigeration is sometimes preceded by a quick hydro cooling or air cooling to remove the excess heat carried in them from the field to prevent development of new or latent infections.

Radiation

Electromagnetic radiations such as ultraviolet (UV) light, X rays and Y rays as well as particulate radiations have been studied in relation to management of post harvest diseases of horticultural crops. Y rays controlled post harvest fungal infections in peaches, straw berries and tomatoes but doses of radiation required to kill pathogens, were found injurious to host tissues. Some plant pathogenic fungi sporulate only when they receive light in the ultraviolet range. It has been possible to control diseases on green house vegetables caused by species of these fungi by covering or constructing the green house with a special UV absorbing vinyl film that blocks transmission of light wavelengths below 390 nm.

CHAPTER - 33

Cultural Management

INTRODUCTION

The Cultural practices which includes manipulation /or adjustment of crop production techniques have been as old as possibly agriculture itself. In early stages of agriculture development, the growers through their experiences and observations had known that repeated cultivation of a particular crop species or variety on a piece of land often resulted in crop sickness. By proper crop rotations they had been avoiding such sickness. As a matter of fact, in the present day agriculture, cultural practices are being considered as essential backup methods for plant disease management. Cultural practices often offer the opportunity to alter the environment, the condition of the host, and/or the behavior of the causal agent, to achieve economic management of disease. Most cultural practices used to control plant disease are **preventive** in nature. Integration of cultural practices, host resistance and pesticides or biocontrol agents may be necessary to provide options for controlling economically important plant diseases

Concept and Applications

Katan (1996) has divided cultural practices into three categories:

- Practices which are usually applied for agricultural purposes not related to crop protection, such as fertilization and irrigation. They may or may not have a positive effect on disease incidence.
- Practices which are used solely or mainly for disease control, such as sanitation (for the eradication of infected plant residues) and flooding.
- Practices which are used for both agricultural purposes and disease control, such as crop rotation, grafting, and composting. Cultural practices may be employed, before or after planting. Deep ploughing and flooding are used before planting while irrigation and fertilization can be applied several times during the crop season for disease management.

Basic Principles of Cultural Practices for Disease Control

The basic principles of cultural practices for disease control are

- Any potential control method may be considered, providing that it is environmentally, technologically and economically feasible.
- Pesticide usage is minimized by combining with other non-chemical or chemical methods
- Diseases that are difficult to control or that involve problematic pesticides, e.g. methyl bromide, should be prioritized
- Economic aspects are taken into consideration.

The Procedures for Disease Management through Cultural Practices

The procedures for disease management through cultural practices are described under the following three heads:

a. Production and use of pathogen free planting material.

b. Adjustment of cultural practices to minimize disease.

c. Sanitation.

A. Production and use of pathogen free planting material

Many plant pathogens like bacteria, virus, fungi and nematodes are transmitted by diseased seed or other vegetative propagating parts. For successful disease control this source of primary inoculums must be destroyed. The following methods are followed to produce and use pathogen free seed material

1. Proper drying and storage of seeds

If the seeds are not dried properly before storage they loose their germination capacity and also harbor several types of plant pathogen in it. The fungus, causing downy mildew of maize is found to be present in the seed when it is fresh. But when the seed is thoroughly dried the fungus present in it dies. Prolonged storage of seed also helps in eliminating several pathogens. *Fusarium solani f. sp. cucurbitae*, infecting cucurbits, is eliminated if the seeds are stored for 2 years before sowing. Similar eradication of pathogen has been achieved in anthracnose of cotton. Proper conditions of storage must be maintained avoid any harm to the seed.

2. Cleaning of seed

In many cases the pathogen is present in plant parts mixed with the seed.

When such seed are used pathogen easily gets into the field. Thus, proper cleaning of seeds before sowing is essential. Common examples of diseases disseminated in this manner are ergot and smut of pearl millet, ear cockle of wheat, white rust of crucifers, ascochyta blight of chickpea, etc.

3. Adjustment of harvesting time

Disease incidence can be minimized by reducing spread of inoculums through adjustment of harvesting time and practice. For example, potatoes harvested when the tops are still green may easily get contaminated by late blight fungus present on the leaves. One of the practices to avoid tuber contamination or infection is to first remove the green tops and let them dry in the soil for 15 days before digging the tubers. When digging of tubers is prolonged the late blight fungus are killed and the produce becomes disease free.

4. Seed production areas

Seed should be produced in areas where the pathogens of major concerns are unable to establish or maintain themselves at critical levels during periods of seed development. Area with **low relative humidity** and **low rainfall** are favorable for production of high quality seeds. Some examples are bacterial blight of legumes, ascochyta blight of chickpea and anthracnose of cucurbits, etc. Such crops can be grown in **dry areas** with the help of irrigation.

5. Inspection of seed production areas

Periodical inspection of crops raised for seed production is an important procedure in the production of clean and healthy seeds. Destruction of diseased plants/organs at the time of inspection helps in reducing inoculums in the field and thus, the percentage of healthy seeds in the produce is increased. If disease incidence is high , the entire crop may be rejected for seed.

B. Adjustment of cultural practices to minimize disease

The main purpose of adjusting of cultural practices is to **seed healthy in healthy soil and to obtain a healthy crop stand.**

1. Crop rotation

In plant pathology, crop rotation means using plant to manage plant pathogens. If a particular crop is grown continuously on the same piece of land, the crop gets disease easily, because pathogens survive due to regular presence of susceptible host. Regular crop rotation can control the diseases in the following ways.

- The physical, chemical and biological effects of different crops cause unfavorable soil environment to the pathogens.
- The survival ability of pathogen in soil is limited. By changing the crop every year, their population can be reduced by starvation due to lack of host.
- Better growth of crop plants due to better nutrient availability also helps in avoiding disease.

Most of the soil-borne diseases can be reduced by adopting proper crop rotation. Its success depends upon proper selection of crops in the sequence and knowledge of the survival of the pathogen. The crops between two susceptible host crops should be resistant to the particular pathogen. Along with this the mode of survival and longevity of pathogen in soil should also be know. For example, if the pathogen can survive in the soil for two years, the interval between susceptible crops should be more than two years. Pigeon pea wilt causing fungus infects only pigeon pea crop but after harvesting the crop the pathogen remains in the dead roots of the plant. So there should be a gap of at least one year after growing pigeon pea in the field.

2. Fallowing

Fallowing, is the mode of preparing land, by ploughing it a considerable time before it is ploughed for seed. It is normally adopted in plant disease management for killing pathogens persisting in soil or in crop residues. For fallowing the field should remain weed free. Fallowing is of three types: (a) dry fallowing, (b) wet fallowing and (c) flood fallowing.

2.1. Wet fallowing : In wet fallowing frequent irrigation is given during the fallow period. It is usually practiced for some weeks. The main aim is to make the **pathogen germinate** in the soil which later **dies due** to lack of host plant. Wet fallowing reduced the pathogen population especially of sclerotia which retains viability in dry conditions for several years. It is also partly successful in reducing the population of *Pythium* and *Alternaria* .

2.2. Dry fallowing : Dry fallowing is generally used where other methods of dis-infestation of soil pathogens are not economical. In this method the field is kept as such for a period of one season to kill the pathogen **by starvation**.

2.3. Flood fallowing : In flood fallowing the land is kept submerged and the pathogens die due to **lack of oxygen**. Rotting of plant debris also releases materials toxic to pathogens.

3. Mixed cropping

Mixed cropping is growing of two or more crops simultaneously on the same piece of land. It reduces the economic loss from diseases. The reduction in disease incidence in a mixed crop can be attributed to following causes.

- Due to reduced number of host plants there is sufficient spacing between them and chances of contact between foliage or roots of diseased and healthy plants are greatly reduced.
- The roots of non host plants may act as a physical barrier obstructing the movement of pathogen in soil. They may also release toxic substances in their root exudates which suppress the growth of pathogens attacking the main crop. **HCN** in root exudates of sorghum is toxic to *F udum* attacking pigeon pea in the mixture.
- Due to reduced number of host pants in a mixed crop the susceptible area for an air borne foliar pathogen is decreased. Therefore, there is less primary infection and less production of secondary inoculums for spread of the disease. This slow down the rate of disease control.
- By proper selection of crops for the mixture, soil environment can also be changed to one that is not favorable for the pathogen. Control of root rot of cotton by growing cotton with moth is an example.
- The soil borne pathogens are not uniformly distributed in the field soil. Generally they are randomly present as dormant structures. Activation of these dormant structures is often dependent on contact with host roots. The chances of which are highly reduced in mixed crop due to spacing between plants.

4. Adjustment of sowing dates

The sowing time is adjusted in such a way that it reduces the infection period of a pathogen to meet the susceptible stage of the host plant to the minimum. It can be achieved by changing the date of sowing so that the susceptible stage of plant growth does not coincide with the environments highly favorable for the pathogen. Bunt of winter wheat can be controlled by either planting before mid September or after mid October. Early planting of potatoes enables the crop to reach tuberization stage before the insect viz. aphid, reaches it peak in the months of January.

But this sowing time adjustment also has some disadvantages. For example, **late sown** pea can reduce the extent of early root rot and wilt, but during pod formation stage in late sown pea, powdery mildew and rust will affect the crop. Therefore the farmer has to select the planting date according to the importance of a particular disease in his locality.

5. Sowing depth

Sowing depth can also be adjusted with due regard for soil type and moisture to shorten the period of emergence and to reduce the incidence of damping off disease in many crops. **In heavy soil**, seed should be placed **shallow** as compared to light soils. Similarly, in **dry soil** the seed should be placed **deeper** in the moist zone, while if water is available irrigate the field before sowing of the a few centimeters and then sow the seeds.

6. Spacing

Of late, the production technology emphasizes on high plant population for getting high yields. But it facilitates luxuriant plant growth, which can cause disease. Luxuriant vegetative growth due to high fertilizer dose, himidity and solar radiation combined with lack of aeration and light to plants, invites pathgen and favours their rapid growth. Damping off ,late blight of potato and mildew of grape vines are some of the diseases which spread fast in **close spaced plantings**.

But there are also examples where dense sowing help in disease reduction. For example, virus of leaf disease of tomato transmitted by white fly is less in crowded planting than in wide spaced planting. The same is true for cucumber mosaic and groundnut rosette transmitted aphids. Incidence of fungal disease of brown rot of soybean and wilt in cotton is reduced in close sown crop.

7. Plant nutrient management

The relationship between pathogen and crop can be affected by the application of nutrients, viz. nitrogen, phosphorus and potassium. Field applied with **potassium** fertilizer is **less** affected by **cereal rusts** as compared to the fields where no potash is applied. Deficiency of **calcium** promotes **wilt** disease in tomato. Similarly, downy mildew infects maize crop due to lack of zinc in the soil. The heavy dose of fertilizer also has some disadvantage. For example, late blight of potato in severe due to thick canopy resulting from high nutrition. In such cases, either reduce nitrogen dose or adjust plant spacing. In many crops, nitrogen dose is reduced if crop is already infected by any disease because nitrogen makes plant succulent.

8. Irrigation

The amount of water given in an irrigation should be enough only to wet the soil so that the roots easily get water. If water is in excess, it directly affects the activities of pathogen. As examples, **wet soil** favours club root of crucifers, silver scurf of potatoes and Cercosporella on wheat, while **dry soil** increases severity of white mold of onion, common scab of potato and Fusarium diseases of cereals. **Damping off** diseases caused by Pythium spp. can be decreased by maintaining a **dry soil** surface. The charcoal rot fungus *Macrophomina phaseolina* attacks potato when there is a **water stress**. So by irrigating the field stress is removed and the disease is suppressed.

Sprinkler irrigation increases diseases owning to enhanced leaf wetness and dispersal of propagules of the pathogens by water splashes as in the case of rain.At the same time, it has some advantages also such as washing off of inoculums from the leaf surface.

C. Sanitation

Field and plant sanitation is a main part of disease control through cultural practices. This step is essential even if disease or pathogen free seed or propagating material has been used and other recommended cultural practices have been followed. The inoculums present on few plants in the field may nullify in soil or on the plant and in due course of time may be sufficient to nullify the effect of other cultural practices. Therefore, plants bearing such pathogens or plant debris introducing the inoculums in the soil should be removed as early as feasible. For instance, wilt disease pathogen of banana remains in dead roots, rhizomes and upper portions of the plant. When these plant remains are removed there is rapid decline in the population of the pathogen in the soil. Similarly, the wilt of cotton and arhar and root rot of bean are also reduced to some extent by removal of diseased plant debris.

1. Removal of crop debris

The plant stubbles and roots, left in the field form most of the crop debris. The infected crop debris not only harbours pathogen but also provides media for their growth. The fungus of downy mildew of pea, jowar, bajara and maize, powdery mildew of pea and cereals are some of the diseases which remain in crop debris after harvesting the diseases crop. Destruction of crop debris by burning immediately after harvest reduces the amount of innoculum surviving through debris.

Deep ploughing during hot summer (after rabi crop) burries the debris to such depth where pathogen is destroyed easily. Turning of soil also exposes the pathogen present in the deeper zone, to hot temperature during day time and kills them. Letting the field fallow for some time also serves this purpose as pathogen die to starvation.

2. Rouging

Rouging means removal of unwanted crop plants. The removal of diseased plant is an effective measure in reducing the spread of many diseases. It is very effective against virus diseases of filed crops. Rouging not only checks the spread but also reduces the survival of pathogen. In the production of virus free potato tubers for seed and for the control of virus in soybean and other pulse crops, rouging is an effective control. But in large sized fields it becomes difficult to locate all the diseased plants and uproot them.

3. Removal of diseased parts of plant

In trees and vines, sometimes only a small part is affected by the disease. Powdery mildew of grapevine, apple scab, leaf curl of peach, fire blight of apple and pears are such infections which can be recognized and the infected parts can be removed by pruning with care. Pruning is always carried out after harvest and when the tree is reaching dormancy, a stage least susceptible to fresh infections. Pruning also enables the removal of infected fruits and debris for destruction by burning. The fallen leaves, twigs, etc. are removed from the orchard and destroyed. Similarly, during grafting, care should be taken to ensure that neither stock nor scion is affected by any diseases.

4. Crop free period and crop free zone

The pathogen attacking crops of secondary importance and having a narrow host range can be controlled by maintaining a crop free period of definite duration. When the growers in an area agree not to grow the crops susceptible to the pathogen for a definite period, depending on longevity of the pathogen without its host , the pathogen is automatically starved out. Similarly, when the host crop is not grown in a zone surrounding the infested area, spread of the disease is checked.

On this basis , for control of bunchy top of banana, it has been suggested that a crop free belt around the area affected by the disease checks it spread provided disease planting material is also quarantined and insect vectors are unable to cross crop free zone. This method is effective for those diseases which are not seed borne and either there is no insect vector or if insect vectors spread then their flight range is limited.

5. Creating barriers by non-host or dead hosts

The spread of majority of diseases from one plant to another in the same field depends on the proximity of healthy roots to infected roots. Growing of other crop in between as in mixed cropping creates barrier by the presence of roots of non-host crops in between.One of the control measure for bacterial wilt of banana and spreading decline of citrus is to destroy the healthy plants around the diseased plants. This checks the movement of pathogen from diseased to healthy plants that are left in the field.

6. Weed management

Weeds are the alternate host of many pathogens. They carry over the pathogen from one season to another and also provide a base from which pathogen is multiplied. For instance, powdery mildew of cucurbits persists on wild cucurbit plant during winter season. Kans grass is an alternate host of sugarcane smut and downy mildew of sugarcane.

7. Adjustment of harvesting time and other practices

The time and method of harvesting is chosen by considering sanitary precautions so that the quality of produce especially fruits and vegetables, does not deteriorate. It also reduces the chances of carrying over the pathogen from the current season to the next. The hill bunt and karnal bunt of wheat, cyst nematode of potato and parasite Orobanche are some of the examples of plant pathogens which are spread in the field during harvesting. Spores of many seed-borne smuts such as karnal bunt of wheat, covered smut of barley and grain smut of sorghum, reach the healthy seeds during harvesting also enables the smut balls, ergot of pearl millet, and ear cockle of wheat to get mixed with the seed lot and contaminate it for next season. To remove these diseases, the following measures should be practiced.

1. Removal of diseased plants and their affected heads as and when they are noticed.
2. Harvesting under conditions unfavourable to the pathogen; for example, digging out potatoes in dry warm weather reduces the infection of mobile spores called zoospores of late blight can check the bacterial disease transmission up to some extent.

CHAPTER - 34

Biological Management

Plant diseases need to be controlled to maintain the quality and abundance of food, feed, and fiber produced by growers around the world. Different approaches may be used to prevent, mitigate or control plant diseases. Beyond good agronomic and horticultural practices, growers often rely heavily on chemical fertilizers and pesticides. Such inputs to agriculture have contributed significantly to the spectacular improvements in crop productivity and quality over the past 100 years. However, the environmental pollution caused by excessive use and misuse of agrochemicals, as well as fear-mongering by some opponents of pesticides, has led to considerable changes in people's attitudes towards the use of pesticides in agriculture. Today, there are strict regulations on chemical pesticide use, and there is political pressure to remove the most hazardous chemicals from the market. Additionally, the spread of plant diseases in natural ecosystems may preclude successful application of chemicals, because of the scale to which such applications might have to be applied. Consequently, some pest management researchers have focused their efforts on developing alternative inputs to synthetic chemicals for controlling pests and diseases. Among these alternatives are those referred to as biological controls.

DEFINITION OF BIOCONTROL

Biological control is the reduction of inoculums density or disease producing activities of a pathogen or parasite in its active or dormant state, by one or more organisms accomplished naturally or through manipulation of the environment, host or antagonist, or by mass introduction of one or more antagonists.

MECHANISM OF BIOCONTROL

Because biological control can result from many different types of interactions between organisms. In all cases, pathogens are antagonized by the presence and activities of other organisms that they encounter. Here, we assert that the different mechanisms of antagonism occur across a spectrum of directionality related to the amount of interspecies contact and specificity of the interactions (Table 20). While many investigations have attempted to establish the importance of specific mechanisms of biocontrol to particular pathosystems, all of the mechanisms described below are likely to be operating to some extent in all natural and managed ecosystems.

Table 20 : Types of interspecies antagonisms leading to biological control of plant pathogens

Type	Mechanism	Examples
Direct antagonism	Hyperparasitism/predation	Lytic/some nonlytic mycoviruses
		Ampelomyces quisqualis
		Lysobacter enzymogenes
		Pasteuria penetrans
		Trichoderma virens
Mixed-path antagonism	Antibiotics	2, 4 diacetylphloroglucinol
		Phenazines
		Cyclic lipopeptides
	Lytic enzymes	Chitinases
		Glucanases
		Proteases
	Unregulated waste products	Ammonia
		Carbon dioxide
		Hydrogen cyanide
	Physical/chemical interference	Blockage of soil pores
		Germination signals consumption
		Molecular cross-talk
Indirect antagonism	Competition	Exudates/leachates consumption
		Siderophore scavenging
		Physical niche occupation
	Induction of host resistance	Contact with fungal cell walls
		Detection of pathogen-associated, molecular patterns
		Phytohormone-mediated induction

Direct competition: In this case, the biocontrol agent out-competes the target organisms for **nutrients** and **space**. This is typically a fungus or bacteria that grows very fast and overwhelms the target organism with sheer numbers. The target organism is suppressed due to lack of food and space. The target organism may not die out completely, but its population becomes so low it is no longer a legitimate threat to the host plant. In order for this type of biocontrol agent to be most effective, the environmental conditions must favor the growth and reproduction of the biocontrol agent. For instance. Competition for the same carbon source between *Pythium uttimum*, a common cause of seedling damping-off and rhizosphere bacteria has resulted in effective biological control of *P. uttimum* in several crops. One of the best documented examples of nutrient competition in biological control involves competition for **iron** between fluorescent pseudomonads and soilborne fungal pathogens such as *Fusarium oxysporum*. Strains of bacteria including *Pseudomonas fluorescens* and *P. putida* produce **siderophores**, metabolic products of micro-organisms that bind iron and facilitate its transport from the environment into the microbial cell. The siderophores **pyoverdine** and **pseudobactin** have a high affinity for the soluble ferric iron (Fe^{+++}) and inhibit the growth of pathogens by limiting the availability of **iron**. The usefulness of nutrient competition as a mechanism of biological control depends on the type of pathogen that is targeted. It may not be useful in suppressing **biotrophs** such as rusts and powdery mildews because they do not require exogenous nutrients to infect the host. On the other hand, a necrotrophic pathogen such as *Botrytis cinerea* is directly affected. Such pathogens require some exogenous nutrients during a definite saprophytic phase prior to infecting the host and are therefore vulnerable to nutrient competition. There are many examples of bacteria and yeasts effectively reducing spore germination or germ tube growth in **necrotrophic** pathogens by competing for nutrients

Antibiosis. With antibiosis, the biocontrol agent produces a chemical compound such as an **antibiotic** or some type of toxin that kills or has some sort of detrimental effect on the target organism. Many microorganisms produce antibiotics and toxins and are toxic to other micro-organisms (e.g. antibiotics and mycotoxins). They may be volatile or non-volatile. Among the known volatile substances, **hydrogen cyanide** and **ammonia** have been studied in most detail, mainly in soil ecosystems. Knowledge of non-volatile antimicrobial substances is extensive but their ecological significance on plant surfaces is uncertain. Unfortunately, most research on antibiotic production has been done in the laboratory under conditions of nutrient abundance. Many antibiotic substances are only detectable when the producer organism is cultured in a nutrient rich medium. They are difficult to find in the nutrient poor environment that often exists on plant surfaces. The detection and extraction of antibiotics from the rhizosphere is hindered by adsorption to clay colloids and humus and also because only small amounts are produced. Antibiotics are also easily lost to the atmosphere, particularly from aerial plant surfaces. In addition, enzymatic breakdown of antibiotics can occur in all situations due to the activity of micro-organisms that are insensitive to these compounds.There are very few examples of antibiotics being detected in natural environments and shown to play a role in suppressing a pathogen.

Table 21 : Some of antibiotics produced by BCAs

Source	Antibiotic	Target pathogen	Disease
Trichoderma virens	Gliotoxin	*Rhizoctonia solani* R	Root rots
Pseudomonas fluorescens F113	2, 4-diacetyl-phloroglucinol	*Pythium spp.*	Damping off
*P. fluorescens*2-79 and 30-84	Phenazines	*Gaeumannomyces graminis* var. *tritici*	Take-all
P. fluorescens Pf-5	Pyoluteorin, pyrrolnitrin	*Pythium ultimum* and *R. solani*	Damping off
*Bacillus subtilis*AU195	Bacillomycin D	*Aspergillus flavus* Contamination	Aflatoxin
Bacillus amyloliquefaciens FZB42	Bacillomycin, fengycin	*Fusarium oxysporum*	Wilt
B. subtilis QST713	Iturin A	*Botrytis cinerea* and *R. solani*	Damping off
B. subtilis BBG100	Mycosubtilin	*Pythium aphanidermatum*	Damping off
*Bacillus cereus*UW85	Zwittermicin A	*Phytophthora medicaginis* and *P. aphanidermatum*	Damping off
Agrocin 84	*Agrobacterium-radiobacter*	*Agrobacterium tumefaciens*	Crown gall
Xanthobaccin A	*Lysobacter* sp. strain SB-K88	*Aphanomyce scochlioides*	Damping off

Hyperparasites and Predation

In hyperparasitism, the pathogen is directly attacked by a specific BCA that kills it or its propagules. In general, there are four major classes of hyperparasites: **obligate bacterial pathogens**, **hypoviruses**, **facultative parasites**, and **predators**. *Pasteuria penetrans* is an obligate bacterial pathogen of root-knot nematodes that has been used as a BCA. Hypoviruses are hyperparasites. A classical example is the virus that infects *Cryphonectria parasitica*, a fungus causing chestnut blight, which causes **hypovirulence**, a reduction in disease-producing capacity of the pathogen. The phenomenon has controlled the chestnut blight in many places. However, the interaction of virus, fungus, tree, and environment determines the success or failure of hypovirulence. There are several fungal parasites of plant pathogens, including those that attack sclerotia (e.g. *Coniothyrium minitans*) while others attack living hyphae (e.g. *Pythium oligandrum*). And, a single fungal pathogen can be attacked by multiple hyperparasites. For example, *Ampelomyces quisqualis, Acrodontium crateriforme*, *Acremonium alternatum*, *Cladosporium oxysporum*, and

Gliocladium virens are just a few of the fungi that have the capacity to parasitize powdery mildew pathogens. Other hyperparasites attack plant-pathogenic nematodes during different stages of their life cycles (e.g. *Paecilomyces lilacinus* and *Dactylella oviparasitica*). In contrast to hyperparasitism, microbial predation is more general and pathogen non-specific and generally provides less predictable levels of disease control. Some BCAs exhibit predatory behavior under nutrient-limited conditions. However, such activity generally is not expressed under typical growing conditions. For example, some species of *Trichoderma* produce a range of enzymes that are directed against cell walls of fungi. However, when fresh bark is used in composts, *Trichoderma* spp. do not directly attack the plant pathogen, *Rhizoctonia solani*. But in decomposing bark, the concentration of readily available cellulose decreases and this activates the chitinase genes of *Trichoderma* spp., which in turn produce chitinase to parasitize *R. solani* .

Induction of Host Resistance

Plants respond to a variety of chemical stimuli produced by soil- and plant-associated microbes. Such stimuli can either induce or condition plant host defenses through biochemical changes that enhance resistance against subsequent infection by a variety of pathogens. Induction of host defenses can be **local** and/or **systemic** in nature, depending on the type, source, and amount of stimuli. Recently, phytopathologists have begun to characterize the determinants and pathways of induced resistance stimulated by biological control agents and other non-pathogenic microbes (Table-22). The first of these pathways, termed **systemic acquired resistance** (SAR), is mediated by **salicylic acid** (SA), a compound which is frequently produced following pathogen infection and typically leads to the expression of pathogenesis-related (PR) proteins. These PR proteins include a variety of enzymes some of which may act directly to lyse invading cells, reinforce cell wall boundaries to resist infections, or induce localized cell death. A second phenotype, first referred to as **induced systemic resistance** (ISR), is mediated by **jasmonic acid (JA)** and/or **ethylene**, which are produced following applications of some nonpathogenic rhizobacteria. Interestingly, the SA- and JA- dependent defense pathways can be mutually antagonistic, and some bacterial pathogens take advantage of this to overcome the SAR. For example, pathogenic strains of *Pseudomonas syringae* produce coronatine, which is similar to JA, to overcome the SA-mediated pathway. Because the various host-resistance pathways can be activated to varying degrees by different microbes and insect feeding, it is plausible that multiple stimuli are constantly being received and processed by the plant. Thus, the magnitude and duration of host defense induction will likely vary over time. Only if induction can be controlled, i.e. by overwhelming or synergistically interacting with endogenous signals, will host resistance be increased. A number of strains of root-colonizing microbes have been identified as potential elicitors of plant host defenses. Some biocontrol strains of *Pseudomonas* sp. and *Trichoderma* sp. were known to strongly induce plant host defenses . In several instances, inoculations with plant-growth-promoting rhizobacteria (PGPR) were effective in controlling multiple diseases caused by different pathogens, including anthracnose (*Colletotrichum lagenarium*), angular leaf spot (*Pseudomonas syringae* pv. *lachrymans)* and bacterial wilt (*Erwinia tracheiphila*). A number of chemical elicitors of SAR and ISR may be produced by the PGPR strains upon inoculation, including **salicylic acid**, **siderophore**, **lipopolysaccharides**, and **2,3-butanediol**, and other volatile substances. Again, there may be multiple functions to such molecules blurring the lines between direct and indirect antagonisms. More generally, a substantial number of microbial products have been identified as elicitors of host defenses, indicating that host defenses are likely stimulated continually over the course of a plant's life cycle.

Table 22 : Bacterial determinants and types of host resistance induced by biocontrol agents

Bacterial strain	Bacterial determinant	Plant species	Type
Bacillus mycoides strain Bac J	Peroxidase, chitinase and α-1,3-glucanase	Sugar beet	ISR
Bacillus subtilis GB03 and IN937a	2,3-butanediol	*Arabidopsis*	ISR
Pseudomonas fluorescens strains CHA0	Siderophore	Tobacco	SAR
Pseudomonas fluorescens strains WCS417	Lipopolysaccharide	Carnation, Radish *Arabidopsis*, Tomato	ISR
Pseudomonas putida strains WCS 358	Lipopolysaccharide	*Arabidopsis*	ISR
Pseudomonas putida BTP1	Z,3-hexenl	Bean	ISR
Serratia marcescens 90-166	Siderophore	Cucumber	ISR

Role of Biocontrol

1. **Disease Control** :*Trichoderma* is a Potential biocontrol agent and used extensively for post harvest disease control. It has been used successfully against various pathogenic fungi belonging to various genera, *viz, Fusarium*, *Phytophthora, Sclerotia.*
2. **Plant Growth Promoter**: Biocontrol agents solublize phosphates and micronutrients. The application of biocontrol *viz Trichodema/ Pseudomons* with plants such as grasses increases the number of

deep roots, thereby increasing the plant's ability to resist drought.

3. **Stimulation of plant resistance and plant defense mechanism**: Species of *Trichoderma* or *Pseudomonas* added to the rhizosphere protect plants against numerous classes of pathogens including viral, bacterial and fungal, which points to the induction resistance mechanisms similar to the hypersensitive response (HR), systemic acquired resistance (SAR), and induced systemic resistance (ISR) in plants.

4. **Transgenic plants**: Introduction of endochitinase gene from *Trichoderma* into plants such as tobacco and potato plants increased their resistance to fungal growth. Selected transgenic lines are highly tolerant to foliar pathogens such as *Alternaria alternata*, *A. solani,* and *Botrytis cinerea* as well as to the soil borne pathogen, *Rhizoctonia* spp.

5. **Bioremediation**: *Trichoderma* strains play an important in the bioremediation of soil that are contaminated with pesticides and herbicides. They have the ability to degrade a wide range of insecticides: organocholorines, organophosphates and carbamates.

Advantages and Disadvantages

Even though it appears as if these biocontrol agents are the cure-all, there are distinct advantages and disadvantages to using them, when compared to traditional chemical controls.

Advantages

- If used properly, they help to reduce the use of chemical-based fungicides. This is good for the environment and is one of the most important reasons to consider their use.
- In most cases, they are safer to use. Most biocontrol agents have very low or no toxicity to humans and other mammals. This is a tremendous benefit in this day and age.
- They help reduce the risk of developing pathogen resistance to traditional chemicals. Due to the overuse of certain chemical fungicides, some common plant pathogens such as Pythium sp. and Botrytis sp. have become resistant to these fungicides. This is less likely to happen with biocontrol agents because the beneficial organism co-evolves along with the target organism and adapts to the changes. Something a chemical cannot do.

- In most cases, they have lower re-entry interval (R.E.I.) times. This is a significant factor especially when it is necessary to enter the production facility immediately following application.
- They tend to be more stable than chemical pesticides if stored properly. These are living organisms and must be stored as such. If they spoil, they are no longer affective.
- Substantially reduced impact on non-target species
- In most cases, they are less phytotoxic. Because they are "natural" they are less likely to cause toxic effects on the host plant, especially if mistakes are made and rates are miscalculated.
- Can be cheaper than chemical pesticides when locally produced.
- When used as a component of Integrated Pest Management (IPM) programs, biocontrol can contribute greatly

Disadvantages

- Biocontrol agents tend to be more difficult to implement when compared to chemicals. Since most of these products have to be implemented prior to the onset of disease, greater preparation by the user is necessary. Biologicals work best in greenhouses that routinely scout for diseases and insects and detect problems early.
- In most cases, they have a narrower target range. Most are not broad-spectrum products. Identification of the correct target organism is imperative.
- These products do not eradicate the pathogen or rescue the host from infection. They have to be administered prior to the onset of disease, in most cases at preplant.
- They may not work as quickly as chemicals. Since their populations need to take time to build up they can take more time to be effective. That is why it is necessary to apply them prior to the onset of severe disease outbreak.
- In most cases, biocontrol products are more expensive to use. This includes both time and money. They may be a bit more expensive to purchase initially, and they take more time to initiate, if used properly.
- They may have a shorter shelf life if not stored properly. Remember, these are living organisms that don't take well to extreme temperatures.

- They may not be compatible with the use of other chemical fungicides and bactericides. The product label should be checked to see with what chemicals the product is compatible

The most commonly used biocontrol agents for control of plant pathogens are

1. Trichoderma.
2. Plant Growth Promoting Bacteria (PGPR).

What is *Trichoderma*?

Trichoderma, genus of asexually reproducing fungi, is present in nearly all tropical and temperate soils. The strains of *Trichoderma* spp. are strong opportunistic invaders, fast growing, prolific producers of spores and powerful antibiotic producers. These properties make these fungi ecologically very successful and are the reason for their ubiquitousness. They show a high level of genetic diversity, and can be used to produce a wide range of products of commercial and ecological interest The most common BCAs of the **Trichoderma** genus are strains of *T. viride*, *T. virens* and *T. harzianum*. Several plant diseases caused by fungi can be potentially controlled by *Trichoderma* species (Table-23).

Table 23 : Importamt plant diseases controlled by *Trichoderma* species.

Name of the Disease	Disease causing organism	Name of the Crop
Collar rot	*Sclerotium rolfsii*	Elephant foot yam
Damping off	*Pythium, Phytopthora, Fusarium*	Chilli, Tomato, Brinjal
Rhizome rot	*Pythium, Phytopthora, Fusarium*	Ginger , Onion
Wilt	*Fusarium oxysporum*	Tomato, Brinjal
Sheath blight	*Rhizoctonia solani*	Maize, Rice

General Characteristics

Colonies, at first transparent on media such as cornmeal dextrose agar (CMD) or white on richer media such as potato dextrose agar (PDA). Mycelium typically not obvious on CMD, conidia typically forming within **one week** in compact or loose tufts in shades of **green** or **yellow** or less frequently **white**. **Yellow pigment** may be secreted into the agar, especially on PDA. A characteristic sweet or 'coconut' odor is produced by some species.

Conidiophores are highly branched and thus difficult to define or measure, loosely or compactly tufted, often formed in distinct concentric rings or borne along the scant aerial hyphae. Main branches of the conidiophores produce lateral side branches that may be paired or not, the longest branches distant from the tip and often phialides arising directly from the main axis near the tip. The branches may re-branch, with the secondary branches often paired and longest secondary branches being closest to the main axis. All primary and secondary branches arise at or near 90° with respect to the main axis. The typical *Trichoderma* conidiophores with paired branches assumes a pyramidal aspect.

Phialides are typically enlarged in the middle but may be cylindrical or nearly subglobose. Phialides may be held in whorls, at an angle of 90° with respect to other members of the whorl, or they may be variously penicillate (gliocladium-like). Phialides may be densely clustered on wide main axis (e.g. *T. polysporum*, *T. hamatum*) or they may be solitary (e.g. *T. longibrachiatum*).

Conidia typically appear dry but in some species they may be held in drops of clear green or yellow liquid (e.g. *T. virens*, *T. flavofuscum*). Conidia of most species are ellipsoidal, 3-5 x 2-4 µm. Conidia are typically smooth but tuberculate to finely warted conidia are known in a few species.

Synanamorphs are formed by some species that also have typical *Trichoderma* pustules. Synanamorphs are recognized by their solitary conidiophores that are verticillately branched and that bear conidia in a drop of clear green liquid at the tip of each phialide.

Chlamydospores may be produced by all species, but not all species produce chlamydospores on CMD at 20° C within 10 days. Chlamydospores are typically unicellular subglobose and terminate short hyphae; they may also be formed within hyphal cells. Chlamydospores of some species are multicellular (e.g. *T. stromaticum*).

Teleomorphs of *Trichoderma* are species of the ascomycete genus **Hypocrea** Fr. These are characterized by the formation of fleshy, stromata in shades of light or dark brown, yellow or orange. Typically the stroma is discoidal to pulvinate and limited in extent but stromata of some species are effused, sometimes covering extensive areas. Stromata of some species (*Podostroma*) are clavate or turbinate. Perithecia are completely immersed. Ascospores are bicellular but disarticulate at the septum early in development into 16 part-ascospores so that the ascus appears to contain 16 ascospores. Ascospores are hyaline or green and typically spinulose. More than 200 species of *Hypocrea* have been described but only few have been grown in pure culture and fewer have been redescribed in modern terms.

Secret of Success of *Trichoderma* as BCAs

The success of *Trichoderma* strains as BCAs is due to their

- High reproductive capacity.

- Ability to survive under very unfavorable conditions.
- Efficiency in the utilization of nutrient.
- Capacity to modify the rhizosphere
- Strong aggressiveness against phyto pathogenic fungi
- And efficiency in promoting plant growth and defense mechanisms.

Method of Application of *Trichodema*

The biological control practices of the plant pathogens start with the definite principles and practices. There is no hazard to flora, fauna and life and also no disturbance to soil , water and air on account of biological control practices. The following practices are taken up in biological control of the plant diseases.

Seed treatment : Seed treatment with *Trichoderma* has tremendous potential to make the control a great success especially for seed and seedling diseases in vegetables, fruit forest and other plantation crop nurseries . *Trichoderma* seed treatment increased plant stand, reduced seedling mortality and were effective as the chemical fungicides. Generally seed treatment with talc based *Trichoderma* product @ 4gm/kg of seed is recommended for control of root diseases of crop plants.

Soil application: The talc based formulations of *Trichoderma* are used as soil application by mixing in well decomposed compost before application into soil. The quantity required is 2.5 kg/ha. It is mixed with 50 kg, FYM and broadcast on the soil and then incorporated into soil through harrowing. It is used to control *Fusarium* wilt , *Sclerotium* foot rots and *Macrophomina* root rots. Applied at least 2 weeks before sowing of crops.

Furrow application: It is comparatively economical to broadcasting and is followed in nurseries. The quantity required is 2.5 kg/ha. It should be applied in the open furrows and then covered with the soil. Applied 15 days before sowing of the seeds.

Root zone application: This is used in wide spaced crops such as plantation and fruit crops. The formulation is mixed in soil in the root zone upto one kg/plant.

Wound treatment: This is used to treat pruning wounds of forest and plantation crops. It is done in peach and plum against silver leaf disease.

Pot culture treatment: This treatment is generally applicable in nurseries .Application of bioagents @ 5gm/kg of soil is recommended.

Seedling treatment: The seedling are dispersed in the solution of *Trichoderma* and then they are taken for sowing to control the seedling blight diseases. Apply 2.5 kg of the formulation to the stagnated in an area of 25 sq m. The seedings, after pulling out from the nursery can be left in the stagnating water containing the bioagent.

Spraying: The liquid suspension prepared by mixing powder and water to get 10^6- 10^8 cfu /ml and sprayed on to the plant surface and soil surface 4g/ liter of water may prepared.

Plant Growth Promoting Rhizobacteria (PGPR)

The rhizosphere bacteria that can colonize the plant roots have been termed as **rhizobacteria** by **Kloepper** and **Schroth** (1978). The rhizobacteria that are strains of *Pseudomonas fluorescens* and *Pseudomonas putida*, have been regarded to have coevolved woth their host plants. The term rhizobacteria has been used to accentuate their intimate association with root. These naturaly occurring, non pathogenic , root colonizing bacteria , may be harmful or beneficial for growth of plants are called deleterious **rhizobacteria** (DRB) and **plant growth promoting rhizobacteria** (PGPR), respectively. PGPR, fall under genera *Pseudomonas, Bacillus, Arthrobactor, Achromobacter, Citrobactor, Enterobacter* and *Flavobacterium*.The PGPR besides enhancing growth and yields, are also potential biocontrol agents and are usually isolated from suppressive soils. Most of the PGPR are fluorescent pseudomonas (*Pseudomonas fluorescens* and *Pseudomonas putida)* but also include non fluorescent *Pseudomonas* sp., *Bacillus subtilis* and *Serratia* spp.

Plant growth promoting rhizobacteria are bacteria that colonize plant roots, and in doing so, they promote plant growth and/or reduce disease or insect damage. There has been much research interest in PGPR and there is now an increasing number of PGPR being commercialized for crops. Organic growers may have been promoting these bacteria without knowing it. The addition of compost and compost teas promote existing PGPR and may introduce additional helpful bacteria to the field. The absence of pesticides and the more complex organic rotations likely promote existing populations of these beneficial bacteria. However, it is also possible to inoculate seeds with bacteria that increase the availability of nutrients, including solubilizing phosphate, potassium, oxidizing sulphur, fixing nitrogen, chelating iron and copper. Phosphorus (P) frequently limits crop growth in organic production. Nitrogen fixing bacteria are miniature of urea factories, turning N_2 gas from the atmosphere into plant available amines and ammonium via a specific and unique enzyme they possess called **nitrogenase**. Although there are many bacteria in the soil that 'cycle' nitrogen from organic material, it is only this small group of specialized nitrogen fixing bacteria that can 'fix' atmospheric nitrogen in the soil. **Arbuscular mycorrhizal fungi** (AMF) are root symbiotic fungi improving plant stress resistance to abiotic factors such as phosphorus deficiency or deshydratation.

The fourth major plant nutrient after N, P and K is sulphur (S). Although elemental sulphur, gypsum and other sulphur bearing mined minerals are approved for organic production, the sulphur must be transformed (or oxidized) by bacteria into sulphate before it is available for plants. Special groups of microorganisms can make sulphur more available, and do occur naturally in most soils.

One of the most common ways that PGPR improve nutrient uptake for plants is by altering plant hormone levels. This changes root growth and shape by increasing root branching, root mass, root length, and/or the amount of root hairs. This leads to greater root surface area, which in turn, helps it to absorb more nutrients.

How PGPR Promote Plant Growth

- Increasing nitrogen fixation in legumes.
- Promoting free-living nitrogen-fixing bacteria.
- Increasing supply of other nutrients, such as phosphorus, sulphur, iron and copper.
- Producing plant hormones.
- Enhancing other beneficial bacteria or fungi.
- Controlling fungal and bacterial diseases.
- Controlling diseases.

Disease control

PGPR have attracted much attention in their role in reducing plant diseases. Although the full potential has not been reached yet, the work to date is very promising and may offer organic growers some of their first effective control of serious plant diseases. Some PGPR, especially if they are inoculated on the seed before planting, are able to establish themselves on the crop roots. They use scarce resources, and thereby prevent or limit the growth of pathogenic microorganisms. Even if nutrients are not limiting, the establishment of benign or beneficial organisms on the roots limits the chance that a pathogenic organism that arrives later will find space to become established. Numerous rhizosphere organisms are capable of producing compounds that are toxic to pathogens like HCN.

Challenges with PGPR

One of the challenges of using PGPR is **natural variation**. It is difficult to predict how an organism may respond when placed in the field (compared to the controlled environment of a laboratory). Another challenge is that PGPR are **living organisms**. They must be able to be propagated artificially and produced in a manner to optimize their viability and biological activity until field application. Like Rhizobia, PGPR bacteria will not live forever in a soil, and over time growers will need to **re-inoculate seeds** to bring back populations.

Application of PGPRs

Effectiveness of PGPRs does not depend only on suitable PGPRs strains but also on suitable methods and strategies for introducing and maintaining the organisms in crops.Most of the PGPRs strains arre usually applied as:

- Soil application
- Seed coating
- Foliar spray

Soil application: The granule formulation of the PGPR strain has been developed specially for the soil application. Sometimes it can be placed near the root zone along the seedlings during transplanting.

Seed coating: Seed coating /bacterization is recommended to those PGPR strain, which have sufficient rhizosphere competence so that they may proliferate easily in rhizosphere , increased to sufficient number to express the biocontrol and growth promoting potentiality. In general the agents like *Pseudomonas* or *Bacillus* are applied through **seed bacterization**. Seed treatment may be given as dry seed treatment, wet seed treatment and slurry seed treatement.

Foliar application: The foliar application of PGPR strain is comparatively less common as compared to seed or soil application. However, for the biocontrol of certain aerial plant pathogens the wet formulation is suspended and applied through sprayng in case of bocontrol of bacterial blight of rice the spray method of Pseudomonas was found to reduce the disease intensity.

Precaution

- Formulation of biocontrol should be purchased from an authorized/ recommended company shop or retailer. The date of manufacturing and expiry of utilization must be verified before delivery.
- During storage packets should not be exposed to direct sunlight and should also not be stored with chemical fertilizers and pesticides.
- Formulation should be stored in cool, and dry place.
- The entire contents of the pack should be used at one time.

Mass Multiplication of Biocontrol Agents

a) Mass multiplication of Trichoderma viride

Preparation of mother culture

Molasses yeast medium is prepared as detailed below.

Molasses : 30 g

Yeast : 5 g

Distiller water : 1000 ml

The medium is prepared and dispensed into conical flasks and sterilized at 15 lb pressure for 15 minutes in an autoclave. After the medium is cooled it is inoculated with 10 days old fungal disc of *T. viride* and then incubated for 10 days for fungal growth. This serves as mother culture.

Mass multiplication

Molasses yeast medium is prepared in fermentor and sterilized as described earlier. Then after the medium is cooled, the mother culture is added to the fermentor @ 1.5 lit / 50 lit of the medium and incubated at room temperature for 10 days.Then the incubated broth containing the fungal culture is used for commercial formulation preparation using talc powder.

b) Mass production of Pseudomonas fluorescens

Preparation of mother culture

Mother culture is prepared by using the king's B medium

Peptone : 20.0 g

K_2HPO_4 : 1.5 g

Mg SO_4 : 1.5 g

Glycerol : 10 ml

Distilled water : 1000 ml

The above broth is dispersed into conical flasks and autoclaved at 15 lb pressure for 15 minutes and cooled and inoculated with a loop of *P.fluorescens* and incubated for 2 days.

Mass multiplication

The kings B medium is prepared and poured into the fermentor and sterilized at 15 lb pressure for 15 minutes. After the broth has cooled below the mother culture of *P.fluorescens* is added to the king's B medium in the fermentor at the rate of 3 lit for 40 lit of the broth. Then it is incubated in the fermentor for 2 days with frequent mixing of the broth by operating the stirrer. Then the broth containing the bacterial growth is collected in plastic buckets and used for mixing with talc powder for commercial formulation.

c) Mass multiplication of Bacillus subtilis

Preparation of mother culture

The nutrient broth medium is prepared as detailed below

Glucose	: 5.0 g
Peptone	: 5.0 g
Beef extract	: 3.0 g
Sodium chloride	: 3.0 g
Distilled water	: 1000 ml

The above medium is dispensed in conical flasks and autoclaved at 15 lb pressure for 15 mts. A loop of *B.subtilis* is inoculated into the medium and incubated for 2 days. This serve as the mother culture.

Mass multiplication

The nutrient broth is prepared in fermentor and sterilized at 15 lb pressure for 15 mts. Then the mother culture is added @ 1 lit / 100 lit of the medium and incubated at room temperature for 2 days. The medium containing the bacterial growth of *B.subtilis* is used for mixing with talc powder.

Preparation of Products

a) Trichoderma viride

The fungal biomass collected from fermentor is mixed with talc powder at 1:2 ratio. The mixture is air dried in shade and mixed with carboxy methyl cellulose (CMC) @ 5 g / kg of the product. It is packed in polythene bags and should be used within 4 months.

Quality Control Parameters

1. Fresh product should contain not less than 28 x 10^6 cfu / g
2. After 4 months of storage at room temperature, the population should be 20 x 10^6 cfu / g.
3. Maximum storage period in talc is 4 months.
4. The talc size should be 500 microns
5. The product should be packed in polythene bags
6. Moisture content of the final product should not be more than 20%.

a. Pseudomones fluorescens

The broth containing the bacterial growth is collected from fermentor and added @ 400 ml / kg of talc powder. Then CMC is added @ 5 g /kg mixed well air dried to 20% moisture level and packed in polythene bags.

b) *Bacillus subtilis*

The broth containing the bacteria is collected from fermentors and mixed with 250 kgs of sterilized neat soil for 100 lit of broth. Then 37 kgs if calcium carbonate is added thoroughly mixed, dried is shade and packed in polythene bags. This can be stored upto 6 months.

Quality control parameters

1. Fresh produce should contain 2.5 x 10^8 cfu/g.
2. After 3 months of storage at room temperature the population should be 8-9 x 10^7 cfu/g.
3. Storage period is 3-4 months.
4. Minimum population load should be 1.0 x10^8 cfu /g.
5. Moisture content should not exceed 20% in the final product.
6. Population per ml of the broth should be 2 x 108 cfu /g.

Commercialization of biological control products

Growers are interested in reducing dependence on chemical inputs, so biological controls (defined in the narrow sense) can be expected to play an important role in **Integrated Pest Management** (IPM) systems. A model describing the several steps required for a successful IPM has been developed . In this model, good cultural practices, including appropriate site selection, crop rotations, tillage, fertility and water management, provide the foundation for successful pest management by providing a fertile growing environment for the crop. The use of pest- and disease-resistant cultivars, developed through conventional breeding or genetic engineering, provides the next line of defense. However, such measures are not always sufficient to be productive or economically sustainable. In such cases, the next step would be to deploy biorational controls of insect pests and diseases These include BCAs, introduced as inoculants or amendments, as well as active ingredients directly derived from natural origins and having a low impact on the environment and non-target organisms. If these foundational options are not sufficient to ensure plant health and/or economically sustainable production, then less specific and more harmful synthetic chemical toxins can be used to ensure productivity and profitability. With the growing interest in reducing chemical inputs, companies involved in the manufacturing and marketing of BCAs should experience continued growth.

However, **stringent quality control** measures must be adopted so that farmers get quality products. New, more effective and stable formulations also will need to be developed.

Most pathogens will be susceptible to one or more biocontrol strategies, but practical implementation on a commercial scale has been constrained by a number of factors. **Cost**, **convenience**, **efficacy**, and **reliability** of biological controls are important considerations, but only in relation to the alternative disease control strategies. **Cultural practices** (e.g. good sanitation, soil preparation, and water management) and **host resistance** can go a long way towards controlling many diseases, so **biocontrol** should be applied only when such agronomic practices are **insufficient** for effective disease control. As long as petroleum is cheap and abundant, the cost and convenience of chemical pesticides will be difficult to surpass. However, if the infection court or target pathogen can be effectively colonized using inoculation, the ability of the living organism to reproduce could greatly reduce application costs. In general, though, regulatory and cultural concerns about the health and safety of specific classes of pesticides are the primary economic drivers promoting the adoption of biological control strategies in urban and rural landscapes. **Self-perpetuating biological controls** (e.g. **hypovirulence** of the chestnut blight pathogen) are also needed for control of diseases in forested and rangeland ecosystems where high application rates over larger land areas are not economically-feasible. In terms of efficacy and reliability, the greatest successes in biological control have been achieved in situations where environmental conditions are most controlled or predictable and where biocontrol agents can preemptively colonize the infection court. Monocyclic, soilborne and postharvest diseases have been controlled effectively by biological control agents that act as bioprotectants (i.e. preventing infections). Specific applications for high value crops targeting specific diseases (e.g. fire blight, downy mildew, and several nematode diseases) have also been adopted. As research unravels the various conditions needed for successful biocontrol of different diseases, the adoption of **BCAs** in **IPM** systems is **bound** to **increase** in the years ahead.

BIOPESTICIDES

Defnition

Many biologically based products are currently available, and these products are often referred to as **"biorationals"** or **"biopesticides"**. Biorational is an undefined term used in broad reference to **any biologically based product used in agriculture** that includes fertilizers, pesticides, herbicides, plant growth regulators, and various other products. **A biopesticides** is defined by the U.S. Environmental Protection Agency (EPA) **as a pesticide derived from natural materials**.

FAO Definition

"A compound that kills organisms by virtue of specific biological effects rather than as a broader chemical poison. Differ from biocontrol agents in being passive agents, where as biocontrol agents actively seek the pest. The rationale behind replacing conventional pesticides with biopesticides is that the latter are more likely to be **selective** and **biodegradable**."

Classification of Biopesticides

Biopesticides fall into three major classes:

- **Microbial pesticides:** contains microorganism as the main active ingredients that function as biological control agents, affecting the pathogen directly or indirectly through the compounds they produce or by stimulating specific plant responses. It consist of bacteria, entomopathogenic fungi or viruses (and sometimes includes the metabolites that bacteria or fungi produce). Entomopathogenic nematodes are also often classed as microbial pesticides, even though they are multi-cellular.
- **Biochemical pesticides** are naturally occurring substances that control pests by non toxic mechanisms. Substances that control diseases in this category include potassium bicarbonate, hydrogen dioxide, phosphorus acids, plant extracts, and botanicals
- **Plant incorporated protectants (PIPs):** are least common type of biopesticide. These are pesticidal substances produced by plants that contains genetic material added to the plant of tenthrough genetic engineering.(e.g GM crops)

Difference between biopesticde and chemical pesticide.

Biopesticides	Chemical pesticides
These do not harm non target species	Nontarget species are also harmed
They do not pollute the environment	Cause pollution; sometimes serious
No harmful residues remain in food, fodder and fibers	Harmful residues may often remain in food, fodder and fibers
Relatively cheaper	Relatively costlier
Insects are expected not to develop resistance to biopesticides	Insects may become resistant, e.g., **Heliothis** has become resistant to most insecticides
Since they are highly specific, correct identification of the pest is essential	It is often not critical
High specificity may often make the use of two or more biopesticides necessary	Often not required
Performance may be variable due to the influence of biotic and abiotic factors of the environment	This is not often the case

Benefits of Biopesticides

Some of the unique features and benefits of biopesticides include:

- The ability to provide alternative modes of action to traditional products which makes them a critical component in most IPM programs.
- Registration in less time than conventional chemical products because biopesticides exhibit minimal impact on the environment and humans.
- The ability to extend the life of conventional chemicals by providing resistance management benefits in agricultural programs.
- Exemption from tolerances, such as reduced preharvest restrictions and application in environmentally sensitive areas, which permits biopesticides that have no Maximum Residue Levels (MRLs) to be used on crops intended for export and in urban settings.
- A high degree of worker safety and the shortest reentry intervals allowed by law.
- Value-added benefits, such as improved plant health, yields and quality and an increase in beneficials, in both traditional and organic cultivation programs.

Biopesticides can be used in almost any crop production program because of they offer unique modes of action and have low impact on the environment and human health. They are especially suited for use in:

- Rotation with chemicals in traditional programs to manage for pesticide resistance.
- Certified organic production systems.
- Grower programs where pesticide residue management is important for harvest management and/or export markets.
- Crops with intensive labor demands to gain maximum flexibility in managing work crews.

Disadvantages

- High specificity, which will require an exact identification of the pest/ pathogen and may require multiple pesticides to be used.
- Often slow speed of action (thus making them unsuitable if a pest outbreak is an immediate threat to a crop).
- Often variable efficacy due to the influences of various biotic and abiotic factors (Since biopesticides are usually living organisms, which

bring about pest/pathogen control by multiplying within the target insect pest/pathogen.)

- Living organisms evolve and increases their resistance to biological, chemical, physical or any other form of control. Unless the target population is completely exterminated or is rendered incapable of reproduction, the surviving population will inevitably acquire a tolerance of whatever pressures are brought to bear- this result in an evolutionary arms race

Effective use of Biopesticides

Even though many biopesticides are formulated, packaged and applied in a very similar fashion to conventional pest control products, the active ingredients on which they are based are quite different. These products, many of which are based on living organisms, are much more susceptible to slight changes in conditions which would have little to no impact on the performance of conventional products. Handling, storage and expectations around efficacy therefore need to be adjusted accordingly. Considerations include:

- Biopesticides are not generally intended to be **"silver bullets"**, and should always be used in conjunction with other pest control tactics. Some of these products are labelled for **suppression** rather than control, meaning that a smaller portion of the pest population is controlled.
- One of the most crucial factors influencing efficacy of biopesticides is **right timing** of applications. Many of these products are designed to be **preventative** and won't work once diseases or pests are present in large numbers. This is particularly true for many biofungicides, which are based on beneficial microbes that colonize the surfaces of plant roots and act as a barrier to invading plant pathogens. If the pathogen has already invaded the roots prior to application, the biopesticide will not have any impact on it. Timing can also be influenced by the life stage or activity of the pest.
- Biopesticides can be extremely sensitive to environmental conditions such as sunlight, temperature, rain or humidity. There are quite a few products which are intended for suppression of various plant pathogens in soil. These contain live spores of beneficial microbes which suspend activity at lower soil temperatures and their efficacy will be greatly reduced if they are applied to cool soils.
- Because the mode of action of a biopesticide is different from that of a conventional pesticide, the way to determine the product's

effectiveness is also different. The best way to measure the effectiveness of a biopesticide product is not only through field performance trials that measure number of pests or amount of leaf spots, but through marketable yield and quality of the edible or final product.

- Thorough coverage of plant surfaces is also vital to the efficacy of most biopesticides. Because most of these products require direct contact with the pest to be effective, **all affected plant parts must be thoroughly covered**.
- Because of their environmental sensitivity, many biopesticides have limited residual activity. Biopesticides which work by forming barriers on exposed plant surfaces are often dislodged by wind or rain. Others are quickly degraded and don't provided long term control. For these products, **repeat applications** may be **compulsory**.
- Biopesticides can also be impacted by conditions in the spray tank. Factors to consider include temperature, pH and other compounds in the spray water, compatibility with other products and life of the spray mix. For instance, some biofungicides which contain beneficial fungi should not be tank mixed with fungicides. Other products break down or otherwise change when left in spray tanks for extended periods, so pay careful attention if product labels specify that the product should be sprayed within a certain period of mixing with water.
- Because biopesticides often contain live organisms, they may have **specialized storage** instructions. It is not uncommon for labels to specify that a product can be stored for a several months if refrigerated but only a few weeks if stored at room temperature. This is in contrast to many conventional products, which can often be stored for much longer periods.

In conclusion, biopesticides can be a useful tool for harder-to-control diseases and pests. Though it is imperative to ensure the products are registered and acceptable to our certifying body. Additionally, awareness to specific application and storage instructions on product labels is particularly important to make sure optimum efficacy of biopesticides. Failure to closely follow instructions related to timing and environmental conditions can consequence in disappointing results with these products. At the same time, it is essential to balance the level of pest suppression with any costs associated with applying the product. To do this, it can be helpful to leave untreated portions of the field as a check when trying biopesticides.

Table 24 : Some commercially available biocontrol products/biopesticdes to control plant diseases

Product/Trade name	Species/strain of *Trichoderma*	Agency/Company
Ecofit	*Trichoderma viride*	*Fusarium, Rhizoctonia, Pythium, Phytophthora, Nectria*
Trichogourd	*Trichoderma viride*	*Fusarium, Rhizoctonia, Pythium, Phytophthora, Nectria*
Defense SF	*Trichoderma viride*	*Fusarium, Rhizoctonia, Pythium, Phytophthora, Nectria*
Tricho-X	*Trichoderma viride*	*Fusarium, Rhizoctonia, Pythium, Phytophthora, Nectria*
Biogourd	*Trichoderma viride*	*Fusarium, Rhizoctonia, Pythium, Phytophthora, Nectria*
Top shield, Root shield	*Trichoderma harzianum T-22*	*Fusarium, Rhizoctonia, Pythium*
F-Stop	*Trichoderma harzianum*	*Rhizoctonia, Pythium*
Trichodex	*Trichoderma harzianum strain T-39*	*Colletotrichum, Monilinia, Plamopara, Rhizopus, Sclerotinia*
Bioderma	*Trichoderma viride+* *Trichoderma harzianum*	*Fusarium, Botryosphaeria, Fusarium*
Ecoderma	*Trichoderma viride+ Trichoderma harzianum*	*Rhizoctonia, Pythium, Phytophthora*
Binap- T&W	*Trichoderma harzianum+ T. polysporum*	Wood decay fungi
Gilogard and Soil guard	*Trichoderma virens*	*Rhizoctonia, Pythium*
AQ 10 biofungicide	*Ampelomyces quisqualis*	Powdery mildew
Biotrox C	*Fusarium oxysporum* (non pathogenic)	*Fusarium oxysporum*
Fusaclean	*Fusarium oxysporum* (non pathogenic)	*Fusarium oxysporum*
Contans WG, Intercept WG	*Coniothyrium minitans*	*Sclerotinia scelrotiorum S. minor*
Diptera Biocontrol	*Myrothecium verrucaria*	Parasitic nematode
Polygandron	*Pythium oligandrum*	*Pythium ultimum*
Galltrol	*Agrobacterium radiobactor* strain 84	*A tumefaciens*
Companion	*Bacillus subtilis strain GB03*	*Pythium, Phytophthora, Fusarium, Rhizoctonia*
Histick N/T	*B subtilis Str.MB 1600*	*Fusarium, Rhizoctonia, and Aspergillus*

Contd...

Kodiak	*Bacillus subtilis strain GB03*	*Fusarium, Rhizoctonia,* and *Alternaria*
Deny	*Burkholderia cepacia*	*Fusarium, Rhizoctonia,* and several nematode
Intercept	*A. cepacia*	*Fusarium, Pythium, Rhizoctonia*
Biosave 10LP, 110	*P.syringae*	*Botrytis, Mucor, Penicillium*
Dagger G	*P.fluorescens*	*Rhizoctonia, pythium*
Actino-Iron	*Streptomy-ces lydicus WYEC 108 plus iron*	*Soilborne fungal species of Pythium, Rhizoctonia, Phytophthora, Verticillium, and Fusarium* spp.
Actinovate	*Streptomy-ces lydicus WYEC 108 plus iron*	Soilborne fungal species of *Pythium, Rhizoctonia, Phytophthora, Verticillium,* and *Fusarium* spp.
Bio-Save 10 LP Bio-Save 110Bio-Save 1000	*Pseudomo-nas syringae strain ESC-10*	*Postharvest decay: blue mold, gray mold, mucor rot,* and *potato dry rot and silver scurf*
Cease	*Bacillus subtilis*	*Broad spectrum*

CHAPTER - 35

Host Plant Resistance

INTRODUCTION

Plant pathogens can spread rapidly over great distances, vectored by water, wind, insects, and humans. Across large regions and many crop species, it is estimated that diseases typically reduce plant yields by 10% every year in more developed nations or agricultural systems, but yield loss to diseases often exceeds 20% in less developed settings, an estimated 15% of global crop production.

Disease control is reasonably successful for most crops. Disease control is achieved by use of plants that have been bred for good resistance to many diseases, and by plant cultivation approaches such as crop rotation, pathogen-free seed, appropriate planting date and plant density, control of field moisture and pesticide use. However, the most attractive form of control is provided by **disease resistance**, for as long as it remains effective, it provides protection at **no cost** to the farmers or the community. So plant resistance is a highly useful strategy that can be applied in the control of diseases. It does not require any special action from growers and constitute **cheap** and **practical** input in the integrated disease management system. The use of resistant varieties cannot only ensure protection against diseases but also save the **time**, **energy** and **money** spent on other measures of control. In addition to these advantages, resistant varieties, if evolved, can be the only practical method of control of such diseases as viruses, phytoplasmas wilts, and rusts etc. in which chemical control is very **expensive** and **impractical**. In crops of low cash value, chemical and other methods of control are often too expensive to be applied. In such crops development of varieties resistant to important diseases can be an acceptable recommendation for the farmer.

Definition of Host Plant Resistance (HPR)

Those characters that enable a plant to avoid, tolerate or recover from attacks of pathogens under conditions that would cause greater injury to other plants of the same species.

or

Those heritable characteristics possessed by the plant which influence the ultimate degree of loss done by the disease.

or

The inherent ability of an organism (i.e., the crop plant) to resist or withstand the pathogen is called resistance

Classification of Resistance

Each plant species is affected by hundreds of kinds of pathogen. Frequently a single plant is attacked by hundreds of individuals of a pathogen. Yet, those plants survive which are resistant, adapting a number of mechanisms classified variously.

1. Based on existence

a. Preformed

When the resistance is already present in the plant even in the absence of the pathogen, it is known as **preformed**, **axenic** or **passive** resistance. For instance, mildew resistance in barley variety Nigrete

b. Induced

When the resistance is not present in the plant in the absence of the pathogen, but with its contact the resistance is induced, it is known as **active**, **apergic** or **induced** resistance. For instance, seedlings of cotton are susceptible to many pests due to absence of gossypol but once infected by *Verticillium,* gossypol is synthesized by induction and seedlings become resistant.

2. Based on type of host response

a. Immune

Immunity is exempt from infection or hundred per cent freedom from disease. No symptom develop. For instance, potato is resistance to karnal bunt.

b. Resistance

Resistance characterizes those situations in which some degree of host pathogen interaction is evoked. Therefore, resistance is **partial**, that is ,always some symptoms appear contrary to immunity, where no symptoms appear.

c. Tolerance

Tolerance is defined as the inherent or acquired capacity of the host to endure disease. **Tolerance** means disease tolerance where yield losses are minimum even in the presence of disease. Therefore, tolerance is the capacity of the host genotype to compensate yield losses even when diseases.

3. Based on growth stage of host plant

Various terms such as seedling resistance, post seedling resistance, adult resistance, etc. have regularly been used to reveal the precise stage of the host growth when it shows resistance. For instance, resistance of wheat to leaf rust (*Puccinia recondita*) may be articulated at the "first leaf stage". The term adult plant resistance is used in the logic that a cultivar is susceptible at first leaf stage but at later stages of development it becomes resistant. For instance, adult plant resistance has been reported in wheat varieties having Sr 2 gene for resistance to stem rust.

4. Based on number of genes

a. *Monogenic resistance*: Controlled by single gene.
    - Easy to incorporate into plants by breeding.
    - Easy to break also.
b. *Oligogenic resistance*: Controlled by few genes.
c. *Polygenic resistance*: Controlled by many genes.
d. *Major gene resistance* : Controlled by one or few major genes (**vertical resistance**).
e. *Minor gene resistance*: Controlled by many minor genes. The cumulative effect of minor genes is called adult resistance or mature resistance or field resistance. Also called **horizontal resistance**.

5. Based on mode of inheritance

a. Monogenic (controlled by a single gene)

Monogenic resistance is frequently sufficiently effective to qualify as immunity. It is stable under a broad array of environmental fluctuations, but is generally specific for certain race virulence gene of the pathogen.

b. Polygenic (controlled by several genes).

Polygenic resistance is more sensitive to environmental fluctuations, does not result in immunity, but is more evenly effective against variants of the pathogen.

c. Cytoplasmic

Such resistance is governed by cytoplasmic factors. For instance, all Tms cytoplasm of miaze used in hybrid seed production is susceptible to T race of Southern Corn Blight. Contrary to it , C or S cytoplasm are also male sterile but are resistant to T race of the pathogen.

6. Based on epidemiological terms

a. Vertical resistance

When a plant variety is more resistant to a few races of pathogen than to others, the resistance is called **'vertical'** or **'perpendicular'**. Vertical resistance reduces the effective amount of initial inoculums from which the epidemic starts. A characteristic of vertical resistance is that the infection rate is as fast in the vertically resistant as the completely susceptible variety after the initial infection has occurred. In other words, the pathogen may mutate and cause severe diseases in the vertically resistant variety. The vertical resistance may break rapidly whenever new races are formed. Vertical resistance is generally controlled by one or few genes thereby the name **monogenic** or **oligogenic**.

b. Horizontal resistance

When host resistance is equally effective against all races of a pathogen- it is termed **horizontal** or **'lateral'**. It may operates before or after infection through defense mechanisms which delay or reduce infection, colonization of the plant and/or production of spores by the pathogen. Horizontal resistance is controlled by many genes, there by the name **polygenic** or multigenic resistance. Each of these genes alone may be rather ineffective against the pathogen and may play a minor role in the total horizontal resistance.

Horizontal resistance is recommended for **subsistence agriculture while vertical** resistance is for **intensive agriculture**.

Diverse complementary terms have been in use to illustrate the genetic concept of resistance. They are summarized in Table-25.

Table 25 : Terms often used to convey genetic concept of resistance

General Resistance	Specific Resistance
Horizontal	Vertical
Minor	Major
Polygenic	Monogenic
Race nonspecific	Race specific
Quantitative	Qualitative
Multiple gene	Multiple allele
Durable	Nondurable
Non hypersensitive	Hypersensitive
Low to moderate	High

7. *Based on mechanism of resistance*

The various mechanisms of disease resistance are as follows

1. Mechanical

Mechanical or structural resistances are due to external or internal peculiarities of the host plant. The first line of defense is the **surface**. Thick hairs, cuticle, wax and hairs on plant parts and foliage check the germination and entry of pathogen in the host tissue. The epidermal cells of rice varieties resistant to blast are lignified. Formation of cork layer beyond the infection point of *R solani* in potato , or abscission layer around diseased spot in peach against *Xanthomonas pruni* are the few examples to further check the spread of pathogen.

2. Hypersensitivity

In the large number of cases, immune reaction is due to the **hypersensitive** reaction of the host. The mechanism is found in case of **biotrophic** organisms or obligate parasites. Immediately after infection, several host cells surrounding the point of infection die. This leads to death of the pathogen or at least prevents its spore production.

3. Nutritional

The reduction in growth and in spore production is generally supposed to be due to an unfavorable physiological conditions within the host. Most likely, a resistant host does not fulfill the nutritional requirements of the pathogen and thereby limits its growth and reproduction.

8. Based on population/Line concept

Pureline resistance: Exhibited by lines which are phenotypically and genetically similar

Multiline resistance: Exhibited by lines which are phenotypically similar but genotypically dissimilar

9. Miscellaneous categories

Cross resistance: Variety with resistance incorporated against a major disease, confers resistance to minor disease.

Multiple resistance: Resistance incorporated in a variety against different environmental stresses like insects, diseases, nematodes, heat, drought, cold, etc.

10. Based on evolutionary concept

Sympatric resistance: Acquired by coevolution of plant and disease (gene for gene) Governed by major genes

Allopatric resistance: Not by co-evolution of plant and disease. Governed by many genes

11. Based on cological Resistance or Pseudo resistance

Apparent resistance resulting from transitory characters in potentially susceptible host plants due to environmental conditions.

Pseudo resistance may be classified into 3 categories:

a. Host evasion

Host may pass through the most susceptible stage quickly or at a time when insects are less or evade injury by early maturing. This pertains to the whole population of host plant.

b. Induced Resistance

Increase in resistance temporarily as a result of some changed conditions of plants or environment such as change in the amount of water or nutrient status of soil

c. Escape

Absence of infestation or injury to host plant due to transitory process like incomplete infestation. This pertains to few individuals of host.

Following situations may explain the disease escape

- Early maturing or short duration variety may escape serious disease attack (wheat rust and potato late blight)
- Rapid germination of seed and growth of seedling may escape attack by damping off pathogens.
- Perceptive growth stage of host may not coincide with conducive condition for disease development(*Botrytis* and *Alternaria* are more severe on old senescing plants)
- Plant may escape owing to patchy distribution of soil inoculums.
- Environmental conditions (temperature, humidity, wind and rain) play crucial role in escape of disease. Good planning and adjustment of cultural practices may help to lessen.

Difference between vertical and horizontal resistance

Factor	Complete Resistance	Partial resistance
Synonyms	Monogenic inheritance Race specific resistance Major gene resistance Juvenile plant resistance Vertical resistance	Polygenic inheritance Non-race specific Minor gene resistance Adult plant resistance Field resistance Rate-reducing resistance Horizontal resistance
Genetic control	One or few genes	Few to many genes
Expression by host	Usually all growth stages	Increases with plant development; lower expression by seedlings
Mechanism	Limits initial infection; none to low symptom development and pathogen reproduction	Slow progress of infection, colonization, lesion development and pathogen reproduction – resulting in slowed disease progress
Efficiency	Highly efficient to avirulent races; high degree of failure against virulent races	Some degree of symptom severity and pathogen reproduction, but similar reaction to all races of pathogen
Primary inoculum	Primary inoculum has little effect	Effectiveness declines as primary inoculum increases; most true for monocyclic diseases
Secondary inoculum	Not a factor because primary inoculum failed to form	Slowed pathogen reproduction; plus fewer successful infections
Environment	Usually stable across range of environments	Effectiveness declines as environment favors pathogen or predisposes host

Contd...

Pathogen virulence	Exerts strong selection pressure on pathogen population; emergence of new races	Exerts weak selection pressure on pathogen population; slows emergence of new races
Other control tactics	Limited response to additional control tactics	Enhance effectiveness of other control tactics

Resistance Breeding

Resistance breeding differs from breeding for any other traits (quantitative or qualitative), in that one will have to consider the biology of the pest over and above the breeding system of crop plants and the types and genetics of resistance. The use of disease resistant crop plants is an environmentally favourable method of controlling disease but the process of breeding for disease resistance is subject to several constraints among them **is the variability of pathogens** in relation to host resistance race specific and race non specific resistance. The use of specific resistance demands the identification and use of strong genes against which the stabilizing selection operates.

There are various ways in which strong gene can be used.

- Singly
- Deployment
- In combination
- Multiline

a. Use of single resistance gene

Here the **single gene** is used one at a time. This strategy results in homogeneity of the crop, which imposes strong selectional forces on pathogen population. As a consequence there is a development of a race which can over come this resistance and thus there starts a **boom –bust** cycle. The use of **single R-gene** is thus **risky** and its use has been questioned on the ground of its failure to provide permanent resistance.

b. Gene Deployment

This involves distribution of varieties with different resistance genes in **space** (spatial gene deployment) and in **time** (temporal gene deployment).The geographical or temporal deployment of varieties with different R. gene causes disruptive selection. Different R gene can be used in different seasons where more than one crop is taken per year. Gene deployment in space would be most effective against pathogens/ parasite that migrate over long distance and cycling against those that do not. Thus, by adopting such strategy, the stabilizing could be switched on and off and directional selection is thus under human control.

Here R- gene could be stored and used again at later date i.e. **recycling of R-gene** can be done. This sequential pattern involves regular control of disease through changes from R-gene to another. The gene deployment strategy has been used for controlling many plant diseases such as bacterial blight of rice, rusts of wheat, crown rust of oat, leaf rust of barley, rust of bean etc.

c. Pyramiding of genes

When two or more known resistance genes are introduced into a single variety it is called **pyramiding** or **stacking** of gene. The aim here is to increase the strength of vertical resistance by way of combining to such a point that the matching pathogen genotype lacks ability to overcome the combined resistance. It increases the longevity of resistance due to low probability of mutation to multiple virulence. Considering mutation rates, 4 or 5 genes for resistance might provide stable resistance for centuries. This has been successfully attempted in a number of crops against different diseases *viz,* rusts of wheat, bacterial leaf blight of rice, blast of rice, rust of bean, powdery mildew of pea etc.Pyramiding of genes for susceptible resistance may act in **complementary** or **additive** fashion and thus enhance the level of resistance shown by one particular gene separately.

Thus this approach is **superior** to **gene deployment** or **multilines**. However, the problems in developing a variety with combined resistances are as follows:

- Many of the desired resistance genes are **allelic** or closely linked and so cannot be easily **combined**.
- As the sources of different resistance, genes will be different host plants, which may create breeding problems, or the isolated advanced line may have undesirable characters linked with resistance gene.
- The development and cultivation of varieties with multi genes for resistances may lead to the development of **super race** sooner.

d. Multilines

The introduction of genetic variability in host population through development of multiline can reduce the **fitness of the pathogens** and thus can break the **boom and bust cycle. Multiline varieties** are mixtures of **several purelines** of similar height , flowering and maturity dates, seed color and agronomic characteristic, each of which has a different gene for resistance to the given disease. The idea of multiline varieties was put forward by **Jenson in 1952** for use in **cereals**. Disease control in multilines can be due to the following reasons:

- Interception of spore by resistant plant called **barrier effect**.
- Reduction in density of susceptible host variety and the consequent spore production and transmission.
- Induced resistance (due to the non virulent pathogen biotype or cross protection)
- Competitive inhibition
- Modification of micro climate due to different plant types.

Multiline variety appears to be useful approach to control diseases like **rusts** where **new races** are continuously produced. In India, three multiline varieties viz., KSML3, MLKS 11 and KML 7406 have been released in wheat

Boom and Burst Cycle

In varietial improvement programmes, it is easy to incorporate the monogenic vertical resistance genes. But the success of exploiting the monogenic host resistance invariably does not last long. Whenever a single gene-based resistant variety is widely adopted, the impact would be the arrival of new matching pathotypes. These pathotypes soon build up in population to create epidemics and eventually the variety is withdrawn. This phenomenon is generally called **"boom and burst"**. The boom burst cycle can be broken by

- Localized usage of R- gene
- Cycling of R- gene
- Use of polygenic resistance
- Combination of above
- Multigenic resistance
- Multiline variety

Durable Resistance

To avoid boom- bust, use of durable resistance is advocated. When a pathogen is not able to overcome the host resistance easily due to fitness reasons, the burst stage is delayed and resistance is noted as durable. This type of resistance remains effective, though the variety is grown over a long period of time. For example, oat variety, Red Rust Proof is still resistant against crown rust even after a hundred years. Wheat varieties, Thatcher and Lee have withstood stem rust for 55 and 30 years, respectively. Cappelle Desprez expresses at adult stage, a moderate resistance to yellow rust and this has been maintained for the last 20 years. Two of the genes like Lr34 for resistance of leaf rust and

Sr2 for resistance to stem rust have been recognized for durability. Wheat cultivars such as HD2189, HP1102, DL153-2, DL803-3 and DL802-2, which possess Lr34 with other gene combinations have a good degree of resistance and had become popular with growers.

Vertifolia Effect

In the **boom and bust cycle**, there is a special kind of **host erosion of horizontal resistance** when **Vander plank** (1963) has named the **vertifolia effect**, after the potato cultivar vertifolia which was bred for vertical resistance to blight and which proved exceptionally susceptible when the vertical resistance breakdown. The process of neglecting of losing horizontal resistance in the course of breeding for vertical resistance has been termed as **'vertifolia effect'**. This failure occurs because of two reasons:

- The level of horizontal resistance in the varieties carrying oligogenes for resistance is usually low.
- The pathogen is able to evolve the virulent pathotype.

Pre-emptive breeding

Pre-emptive or **anticipatory** breeding for resistance is breeding for resistance to **future patho types**. Its success depends on the ability of the breeder to predict the likely pathogen phenotypes (pathopypes) that will be important at some future time. Because durability of resistance can not be assumed, resistance breeding strategies are usually supported with the maintenance of genetic diversity to provide buffering against extreme crop losses in the event of significant pathogenic changes.

BREEDING METHODS FOR DISEASE RESISTANCE

The methods of breeding varieties resistant to diseases do not differ greatly from those adopted for other characters. The following methods are used:

1. Introduction
2. Selection
3. Hybridization followed by selection
4. Back cross method
5. Induced mutagenesis
6. Development of multilines and
7. Tissue culture techniques

1. Introduction

It is a very simple, quick and inexpensive method of obtaining resistant varieties. Varieties resistant to a particular disease somewhere else may be thoroughly tested in the regions in which they are proposed to be introduced. Their yield performance and disease resistance should be confirmed by large scale cultivation. Introductions have served as a useful method of disease control.

Table 26 : Resistance variety introduced in India from other countries

Name of Crop	Name of Variety	Introduced from	Introduced in	Remarks
Wheat	Ridley	Australia	India	Rust resistance
wheat	Kalyan Sona and Sonalika	CIMMYT, Mexico	India	Rust resistance
Rice	Manila	Philippines	Karnataka	Tolerance to blast, bacterial leaf blight and sheath blight.
Rice	Intan,	Indonesia	Karnataka	Resistant to blast
Rice	Munal	U.S.A.	West Bengal	Tolerant to blast, bacterial leaf blight and leaf folder
Sugarcane	Co.475		Mumbai	Conquered red rot but brought in leaf rust and whip smut

2. Selection

Selection of resistant plants from a commercial variety is the **cheapest** and **quickest** method of developing a resistant variety. This is better method than introduction and has more chances of success in obtaining disease-resistant plants. The work of selection is carried out either in the naturally infected fields under field conditions or under artificially inoculated conditions. The resistance in such individuals will occur in nature by **mutation**. To ensure the resistant character of a plant, large population of crop plant may be exposed to the attack of pathogen under artificial conditions and the non-infected plants may be chosen. Sugandh of Bihar is a selection from Basmati rice of Orissa tolerant to bacterial leaf blight. Rice varieties Sudha (Bihar), Patel 85 (Madhya Pradesh), Janaki (Bihar), Sabita, Nalini (West Bengal), Improved White Ponni (Tamil Nadu), Ambika (Maharashtra), are some of rice selections resistant to one or more diseases. Kufri Red, a potato selection from Darjeeling Red Round is a disease resistant variety.

3. Hybridization

Hybridization is the most common method of breeding for disease resistance, Hybridization serves the following two chief purposes: (1) transfer of disease resistance from an agronomic ally undesirable variety to a susceptible but otherwise desirable variety (by back crossing). and (2) combining disease resistance and some other desirable characters of one variety with the superior characteristics of another variety (by pedigree method).In the **back cross** method, the new variety is agronomically the same as the susceptible variety, but is disease resistant. In the **pedigree method**, on the other hand, the new variety is expected to be superior to both the parents in agronomic characteristics and at the same time would be disease resistant.

In both the cases, one parent is selected for disease resistance; it should have a high intensity of resistance to as many races of the pathogen as possible, and the resistance whould be governed by few oligogenes. When the resistant varicty is updatcd and agronomically undcsirablc, **backcross** method is the obvious choice. But when the resistant variety is well adapted and has some other desirable features as well, the **pedigree** method of breeding is preferred. This method is **suited** for **small grains** and beans but unsuited to fruits and vegetables.

4. Back Cross Method

The back cross method is useful in transferring genes for resistance from variety that is undesirable in agronomic characteristics to a susceptible variety, which is widely adapted and is agronomically highly desirable. is widely used to transfer disease resistance from wild species. Interspecific hybridization is made to transfer the gene or genes for resistance to the cultivated species. Resistance to grassy stunt virus from *Oryza nivara* to *O.sativa*, late blight resistance from *Solanum demissum* to cultivated potato, rust resistance from *durum* to *aestivum* wheat are some of the examples involving interspecific hybridization. Depending upon the number of genes governing resistance and the nature of the gene, whether dominant or recessive, the procedure varies. The number of back crosses to the cultivated species may be **five to six**. Once the back cross progeny resemble the cultivated parent, then they are selfed and segregating progeny screened for disease resistance.

5. Induced Mutagenesis

While following mutation breeding for disease resistance, a large number of mutation progeny should be produced and screened under artificial epiphytotic condition to select resistant plants. **MCU10** cotton, a resistant variety to bacterial blight was evolved in Tamil Nadu by subjecting seeds of a susceptible variety CO4 to **gamma rays** followed by rigorous screening and selection. Resistance to Victoria blight (caused by *Helminthosporium victoriae*) in oats was induced by irradiation with X-rays or thermal neutrons; resistant mutants were also isolated spontaneously in low frequencies. Some other cases in induced mutations for disease resistance are as follow; resistance to stripe rust in wheat, crown rust in oats, mildew in barley and leaf spot (tikka).

6. Somaclonal Variation

Disease resistant somaclonal variants can be obtained in the following ways. First, plants regenerated from cultured cells or their progeny are subjected to disease test and resistant plants are isolated (screening). Secondly, cultured cells are selected for resistance to the toxin or culture filtrate produced by the pathogen and plants are regenerated from the selected cells (Cell selection). In most cases, these plants are also resistant to the disease in question. Cell selection strategy is most likely to be successful in cases where the toxin is involved in disease development. Somaclonal variations for disease resistance are reported in *Zea mays* for *Drechslera maydis* race T-toxin resistance, in *Brassica napus* for resistance/tolerance to *Phoma lingam*, early and late blight resistance in potato, *Pseudomonas* and *Alternaria* resistance in tobacco, besides smut and rust disease resistance in sugarcane.

TESTING OF DISEASE RESISTANCE

Disease resistance tests may be carried out in the **field** or in the **glass house. Glass house tests** are more **reliable** since the favourable environment for disease development can be provided more readily in a glass house than in a field. An optimum humidity and temperature are necessary, though the optimum conditions for one disease may vary significantly from that for another. The common inoculation techniques used for different categories of pathogens are briefly outline below.

1. Soil Borne Pathogens

Diseases *viz.,* damping off, root rot, wilt etc., are produced by fungi present in the soil. Commonly, **sick plots** are created for testing resistance to such diseases. **Sick plots** are fields that have a sufficient inoculums load of the pathogen to infect all the susceptible plants of the host population. Sick plot may be produced by adding the remains of diseased plant, or by adding inoculums produced in a laboratory on host seeds, seedlings or on a nutrient medium or by mixing the soil from other sick plots. The pathogen inoculums may be increased by growing a susceptible variety for one or more years. Glass house tests may be carried out using the soil from a sick plot.

2. Air Borne Diseases

Diseases like smuts, rusts, blight, mildews, leaf spots etc., are produced by air borne fungal pathogens. Inoculation of such a disease may be done by dusting spores from infected plants onto test plants, spraying a suspension of spores or mycelium , injecting a spore suspension into individual plants or leaves, or, in some cases, by planting rows of a highly susceptible variety, normally called **infectior**, to produce a large inoculums, which is spread by natural factors, e.g., wind. In the case of wheat rust, infectors are commonly used. **Agra Local wheat** is the common **infector** for all the three **rusts**. In the case of air borne fungi infecting ovary e.g., loose smut of wheat and barley, spores are introduced in the flowers at the time of anthesis with the help of a forecep or a hypodermic needle.

3. Seed Borne Diseases

Some diseases are seed borne, e.g., some smuts, bunt etc. Mostly the smut spores are present on the surface of the seed or under the hull. In artificial inoculation of seeds with smut spores, the seeds and spores are thoroughly mixed before planting. In hill bunt of wheat and grain smut of jowar dusting of spores on the seed is enough for inoculation. In smut diseases of barley, oats, etc. usually the seeds are treated with spore suspension under vacuum to facilitate deposition of spores on the seed. In diseases where the pathogen is both soil as well as seed borne mostly soil inoculation is preferred.

4. Insect Transmitted Diseases

Most of the viral diseases are transmitted either by **insects** or **mechanically**. The following procedures are adopted in testing varieties.

a. **Transmission by insect vectors**; Insects which fed on diseased plants are collected and left on healthy plants to continue feeding. Mostly these insects **aphids** or **white fly**. The healthy plants are grown in insect proof cages so that unwanted insects do not visit them and the vectors being used do not move out. Obviously, such tests cannot be conducted on a large number of plants under field conditions. The insect vectors must feed on the diseased and healthy plants for the minimum period requirement for becoming infective.

b. Mechanical transmission: The juice from infected plants rubbed on healthy leaves. To facilitate contact with healthy cell sap artificial wounds or scratches are created by rubbing **carborundum powder** separately or with the infected juice.

CHAPTER - 36

Regulatory Methods - Plant Quarantine

INTRODUCTION

The current food crisis has put the agriculture production on a tight leash, not allowing the producers any lassitude whatsoever. Even though we have outgrown from our 'ship to mouth existence'; our least negligence can torpedo our efforts to maintain the steady state of progress achieved in food grain production. Around 35% of what is produced is lost due to pest and diseases. In this situation, plant protection assumes significance. Unfortunately our plant protection regime begins and ends with pesticides. It is the default option in the plant protection menu and all the other options more or less remain defunct and unused. Even though, our major thrust areas of plant protection are promotion of Integrated Pest Management: ensuring availability of safe and quality pesticides for sustaining food production from the ravages of pests and diseases, streamlining the quarantine measures for accelerating the introduction of new high yielding crop varieties, besides eliminating the chances of entry of exotic pests; we remain largely insulated from these aspects in IPM.

With the Globolization and liberalization in International trade of plants and plant material in the wake of Sanitary and Phytosanitory (SPS) Agreement under WTO, the plant quarantine measures have become more imperative. Liberalization of trade policies have helped the world agriculture trade to prosper which is key sector for many countries like India whose economies are dependent on agrarian industry. But the likehood of the presence of disease/pest inherent in the import material can very well geopardize the trade. Activities are meant to help agricultural development and **Plant quarantine service** are charged with the responsibility of preventing the entry of hazardous **pests, pathogens** and **weeds**, but to deny entry of valuable genetic re-sources would be against national interest. These activities are meant to help agricultural development and they are complementary to each other and therefore are necessary, and we on our parts need to be fairly vigilant. As has been very truly said-**An ounce of prevention is worth a pound of cure.**

PLANT QUARANTINE

The term **'Quarantine'** is derived from the Latin word ***quarantum,*** meaning **40**. It refers to the 40 days period of detention of ships from countries with **bubonic plague** and **cholera** in the Middle Ages. The first such quarantine was imposed in **Venice in 1374**. Present quarantine laws now include **plants**. Plant quarantine, restrict entry of plants, plant products, soil, cultures of living organisms, packing materials, and commodities, as well as their containers and means of conveyance to protect agriculture and the environment from avoidable damage by hazardous organisms.They exclude dangerous organisms while permitting plants and plant products to enter. The term *exclusion* convey this objective more clearly than *plant quarantine.* **Exclusion** relates to keeping organisms out; **plant quarantine** relates to keeping plants out.

In strict sense 'Plant Quarantine' refers to the holding of plants in isolation until they are believed to be healthy. Now, broader meaning of the plant quarantine covers all aspects of the regulation of the movement of living plants, living plant parts/plant products between politically defined territories or ecologically distinct parts of them. Intermediate quarantine and post entry quarantine are used respectively to denote the detention of plants in isolation for inspection during or after arrival at their final destination.

The term frequently used in plant quarantine are *hazard, risk*, and *safeguards*.

- **Hazard**: is the danger that a specified pathogen is known or perceived to present to the agriculture of the importing country should the pathogen gain entry on imported items and subsequently become established.
- **Risks**: is the chance that a hazardous organism will enter and become established.
- **Safeguards**: are action taken to reduce the risk of introducing hazardous organisms.

Importance

The importance of plant quarantine has increased because of the increase in exchange of seeds or grains for consumption along with better means of transportation. The international exchange of plants or their parts is practiced widely to improve crops of a country and their genetic base. In addition, shiploads of grains for consumption or large quantities of seeds for direct sowing are imported in many countries. Even minute quantities of soil and plant debris contaminating true seeds can disseminate pathogens.

The entry of a single exotic insect or disease and its establishment in the new environment continues to cause great, national loss (Table-27) till such time it is brought under effective control. In certain cases a country has to spend a few million rupees before success in controlling the introduced insect pest or disease is achieved.

Table 27 : Losses caused by introduced plant diseases

Disease	Host	Country	Introduced From	Losses Caused
Bunchy top	Banana	India	Sri Lanka	Rs.4 crores
Wart	Potato	India	Netherlands	2500 acres infected
Canker	Citrus	U.S.A	Japan	$ 13 million; 19.5 million trees destroyed
Dutch elm	Elm	U.S.A.	Holland	$ 25 million -$ 50,000 million
Powdery mildew	Grapevine	France	U.S.A	80% in wine production
Downy mildew	Grapevine	France	U.S.A	$ 50,000 million
Blue mould	Tobacco	Europe	U.K	$ 50 million

Goal of Plant Quarantine

The goal of regulatory actions are

- To delay or prevent entry of the pathogen along manmade pathways.
- If entry succeeds, to prevent infection.
- If infection succeeds, to prevent establishment of pathogens entering on manmade and natural pathways.
- If established, to minimize or retard spread.

Basic Principles of Plant Quarantine

- The basic principles of plant quarantine is to check the entry and spread of potentially dangerous plant pathogens and insects imported along with the germplasm.

Prerequisites of Plant Quarantine Regulations

In spite of quarantine regulations, plant pathogens have been introduced in different countries. Plant quarantine regulations have certain prerequisites. They must be

- Only pathogens and pest that pose a threat to major crops or forest.

- Formulated to control or prevent the pests and not to hinder trade or attainment of other objectives.
- Derived from adequate legislation and operated solely under the law.
- Modified as conditions change or further facts become available.
- Those responsible for quarantine measures should be properly trained and experienced.
- Professional workers and the public must co-operate on an international scale for effective operation of quarantine regulations.

Component of Plant Quarantine

The plant health or quarantine services in most countries, usually have three components.

1. Exclusion of pathogens and pests of quarantine and economic significance that might unintentionally be moved along manmade pathways.
2. Containment, suppression and eradication of exotic pathogens and pests recently introduced along natural and manmade pathways.
3. Assistance to exporters of plant products, such as fruits, vegetables, plants, cut flowers, commodities, etc., in meeting the quarantine or exclusion requirements of importing countries and , therefore, based on plant health, biologically facilitating the acceptance of imports.

1. Pest Risk Analysis

Pest risk defines the chances that a pathogen or pest of quarantine significance will enter along a manmade pathway. Risk often is expressed as low, medium or intermediate, and high.

- **Low risk:** means that there is little chance that the pathogen or pest will enter.
- **High risk:** means that chances are high that the pathogen or pest could enter.
- **Acceptable risk:** Means that the benefits derived after taking risk are high enough to justify taking the risk, with safe guards , in the first place.

The rules and regulations governing seed entry should be based on a matching of risk with entry decisions. If the risk is low, the entry should be liberal; if risk is high, the entry atus should be conservative: and when the risk is unknown, quarantine officer need to be policy of an importing countries might prohibit all plants of high risk and by doing so take no risk, but at the cost of receiving no benefits from crop improvement.

2. Movement of pathogens

Plant pests of quarantine importance can move along with natural and man made pathways, depending upon the life cycle of the organism, the environment through which it moves, and human activities. At the end of the pathway, the establishment of a pathogen or pest in a new area depend on the level of inoculums or pest carried by seeds, the susceptibility of host crop(s), and the environment. Exchange of germplasm creates the risk of introducing pathogens or pests of quarantine importance. The considerations are two fold; that exotic organisms or more virulent strains of existing ones might be introduced. Quarantine regulations to prevent movement of feces derived products as a potential source of introduction should be considered . Viable teliospores of *T.caries*, *T. indica* and *T. controversa* are present in feces of chickens, grasshoppers and cow. Hence quarantine established to prevent movement of spore contaminated seeds may miss an important avenue of potential introduction by animal and animal product movements.

3. Legal basis of plant quarantine

Quarantines are regulations promulgated by governments to reduce the risk of introducing hazardous pathogens and pests on articles, including seeds from foreign countries. The legal basis of quarantine comprises.

- Legislation enacted by national and sometimes state or provincial governments.
- Enabling legislation that directs the Minister of Agriculture to issue necessary rules, orders or directives.
- Legislation by a regional parliament representing groups of countries such as the EEC or Andean Pact Nations.
- The legal umbrella that covers international plant quarantine matters is the **International Plant Protection Covention of 1951** (Rome Certificate). Most countries either are signitories of the Rome Convention or follow its mandates.

4. Requirement for a Quarantine program

- A **phytosanitory certificate** that attests to the inspection, origin and identification of the seeds.

- A permit requirement for added declaration on the phytosanitory certificate that the mother plants were inspected during the growing season.
- A requirement for treatment at origin.
- The acceptance of a special certification or safe guarding program at origin, such as may be practiced at International Agricultural Research Centers (IARC)
- Inspection and treatment , if necessary ,upon arrival at port of entry.
- Isolation, special testing, or additional quarantine after entry.

National and International Regulations

- The first plant quarantine law was passed in **1873 in Germany to** prohibit importation of plants and plant products from the United States to prevent the introduction of the **Colorado potato beetle**.
- In 1875, France imposed measures against the American pest.
- In 1877, United Kingdom Destructive Insects Act prevented the introduction and spread of this beetle.
- In 1891, first plant quarantine measure was initiated in the United States by setting up a seaport inspection station at San Pedro, CA.
- **In 1912, first U.S. quarantine** law was passed.
- In 1909, Federal Plant Quarantine Service was established in Australia.
- In **1914, Destructive Insects and pest Act** was passed in **India**.
- In 1971, Government of Greece prohibited introduction of rice seeds for sowing infected with *P. oryzae*.
- In 1980, Phillipine government introduced seed health testing plants of rice for *P. oryzae*.in addition to field inspections for breeder and foundation seeds.

On a global basis, the **first International Plant Protection Convention** (the Phyllozera Convention) was signed in **1881** with the objective of **preventing the spread of severe pests**. This convention was amended in 1889,1929 and 1951. The International Plant Protection Convention (IPPC or Rome Convention) under the Food and Agriculture Organization was established to prevent the introduction and spread of diseases and pests through legislation and organizations across international boundaries. This convention provided a model phytosanitary certificate (Rome certificate) to be adopted by member countries. Within this convention, ten regional plant protection organizations have been established on the basis of biogeographical areas.

- The European and Mediterranean Plant Protection Organization (EPPO)
- The Inter-African Phytosanitary Council (IAPSC)
- Organismo International Regional de Sanidad Agropecnario (OIRSA)
- The Plant Protection Committee for, the South East Asia and Pacific region (SEAPPC)
- Near East Plant Protection Commission (NEPPC)
- Comit'e Interamericano de Protection Agricola. (CIPA)
- The Caribbean Plant Protection Commission (CPPC)
- The North American Plant Protection Organization (NAPPO).
- Organismo Bolivariano de Sanidad Agropecuria (OBSA)
- Association of South East Asian Countries (ASEAN)

The regional organizations are concerned with the co ordination of legislation and regulations within their area, agreement on the quarantine objects, inspection procedures, etc.

Criteria for Determining Organisms for Quarantine Significance

1. General criteria

- The organism does not occur in the country but is known to cause economic damage elsewhere.
- The organism occurs in the country but is not extensively spread in the ecological range of its host in that country; is under a national domestic suppression or eradication programme; has exotic strains of quarantine importance that do not occur in the country; and/or causes economic damage or has a potential to cause such damage on economically important crops.
- The organism is a general pathogens established in the importing country. But government regulations require that commercial growers use pathogen-tested seed stocks so that imported stocks meet domestic standards.

2. Criteria based primarily on Pathogen Characteristics

The criteria are based on the general characteristics of a pathogen.

- Able to survive and move easily in international trade.
- Capable of developing a high population in a short time.

- Difficult to detect by general inspection or field survey.
- Capable of damaging and / or reproducing on many hosts.
- Has a potential for rapid dispersal , especially along manmade pathways.
- Has a potential for significant reduction in the quality and quantity of crop yields.
- Capable of adversely affecting the environment.

Problems in Plant Quarantines

Quarantine serves as a filter against the introduction of dangerous pathogens, however pathogens are still introduced. Probable reasons are that

- Difficult to detect all types of infectious pathogens by conventional methods.
- Methods may not be sensitive enough to detect traces of infection.
- Latent infections may pass undetected under post entry quarantine.
- Destruction of all infected or suspected material and
- Sensitive methods for testing fungicide treated seeds may be lacking.

Organisms of Quarantine Significance

Organisms of quarantine significance may include any pathogen or pest that a government (or intergovernmental organization) considers to pose a threat to the agriculture and environment of the country or region. Such organism generally are exotic to that country or region but may include exotic strains or races of domestic strains.

Plant Quarantine Methods

There are number of plant quarantine methods which are used individually or jointly to retard or prevent the introduction and establishment of exotic pests and pathogens. The components of plant quarantine activities are:

1. Complete embargoes

This is the most effective measure to exclude specified plants and plant products completely from a country infected or infested with highly destructive diseases or pests or that could be transmitted by the plant or plant products under consideration and against which no effective plant quarantine treatment can be applied or is not available for application. However, in practice it is difficult to achieve because of more and more exchange of diverse genetic material among countries.

2. Partial embargoes

Partial embargoes, applying when a pest or disease of quarantine importance to an importing country is known to occur only in well defined area of the exporting country and an effectively operating internal plant quarantine service exists that is able to contain the pest or disease within this area.

3. Inspection and treatment at point of origin

It involves the inspection and treatment of a given commodity when it originates from a country where pest/disease of quarantine importance to importing country is known to occur.

4. Inspection and certification at point of origin

It involves pre-shipment inspection by the importing country in cooperation with exporting country and certification in accordance with quarantine requirements of importing country.

5. Inspection at the point of entry

It involves inspection of plant material immediately upon arrival at the prescribed port of entry and if necessary subject to treatment before the same related.

6. Utilization of post entry plant quarantine facilities

It involves growing of introduced plant propagating material under isolated or confined conditions.

Plant Quarantine Organizations in India

The first plant quarantine measure in India dates **to 1906**, when the danger of introducing the **Mexican boll weevil** had the Government of India directed that all cotton imported from the New World should only be admitted after **fumigation** with **carbon disulphide**. Two categories of regulatory measures are in operation for controlling pests, diseases and weeds:

- **Destructive Insects and Pests (DIP) Act of 1414 of Central Government**, which regulates the introduction of exotic diseases and pests into the country or their spread from one state or Union Territory to another.
- The **Agricultural Pests and Diseases Acts** of various states, which suppress or prevent the spread of diseases and pests in areas within a State or Union Territory.

DIP Act

The legislative measures against crop pests and diseases were initiated under the DIP Act of 1914 which was passed by the then Governor General of India in Council on 3 February 1914. The quarantine regulations are operative through The Destructive Insects and Pests Act, 1914 (which has been revised 8 times from 1930 to 1956 and amended in 1967 and 1992). The provisions of the DIP Act are

- It authorizes the Central Government to prohibit or regulate the import into India or any part.
- It authorizes the officers of the Customs at every port to operate, as if the rules under DIP Act are made under the Sea Customs Act.
- It authorizes the Central Government to prohibit or regulate the export from a State or the transport from one State to another State in India of any plants and plant material, diseases or insects, likely to cause infection or infestation. It also authorizes the control of transport and carriage and gives power to prescribe the nature of documents to accompany such plants and plant materials and articles.
- It authorizes the State Governments to make rules for the detention, inspection, disinfection or destruction of any insect or class of insects or any article or class of articles, in respect of which the Central Government has issued notification.
- It also authorizes the State Governments for regulating the powers and duties of the officers whom it may appoint on its behalf.
- It provides penalty for persons who knowingly contravene the rules and regulations issued under the Act.
- It also protects the personnel from any suit or prosecution or other legal proceedings for anything done in good faith as intended to be done under this Act.

The plant quarantine service is centrally organized and administered through the **Directorate of Plant Protection, Quarantine and Storage** established under the **Ministry of Agriculture** (Department of Agriculture and Co-operation) which is headed by the **Plant Protection Adviser** to the Government of India and having its headquarters at N.H. IV, **Faridabad, Haryana State**.

Import Regulations

When plants are imported there are certain principles which, if followed ensure that as few risks as possible are taken.

- Import from a country where, for the crop in question, pathogens which are mainly to be guarded against are absent.

- Import from a country with an competent plant quarantine service, so that inspection and treatment of planting material before dispatch will be thorough, so reducing the likelihood of contaminated plants being received.
- Take planting material from the safest known source within the chosen country.
- Take an official certificate of freedom from pests and diseases from the exporting country.
- The smaller the amount the less the chance of its carrying infection, and inspection as well as post-entry quarantine.
- Check material watchfully on arrival and treat (dust, spray, fumigate, heat treat) as necessary.
- Import the safest type of planting material, For instance, seeds are usually safer than vegetative material, unrooted cuttings than rooted. axenic cultures of meristem tip tissues (micropropagation).
- If other precautions are not thought to be adequate, the consignment for import should be subject to intermediate or post-entry quarantine. Such quarantine must be carried out at properly equipped station with suitably trained staff.

Seed was not originally included in the DIP Act, but because of the changing circumstances and to meet up the present necessities, the Government of India passed the Plants, Fruits, Seeds (Regulation of Import into India) Order 1984 which came into effect in June 1985. The conditions for the import of 17 crops are stipulated in this order. The main features of the order are:

1. **Seed** has been brought under the purview of the DIP Act.
2. No consignment can be imported into the country without valid import permit issued by the Plant Protection Adviser to the Government of India.
3. No consignment can be imported without an official phytosanitary certificate issued by the plant quarantine agency of the exporting country.
4. Post-entry growth of the particular crops at approved locations.

1) Conditions for import

- No consignement of seeds/planting materials shall be imported into India without a vilid **'Import permit'**, which is to be issued by a competent authority, to be notified by the Central Government from time to time in the Official Gazate.

- No consignment of seeds/ planting materials shall be imported into **India** unless accompanied by a **Phytosanitory Certificate**, issued by the official Plant Quarantine Service of the source country.
- All plants on arrival at port, shall be inspected and if required **fumigated**, **disinfested** or **disinfected** by Plant Protection Adviser to the Government of India or any other officer authorized by him on his behalf.
- Seeds and plants which call for post-entry quarantine inspection shall be grown in post-entry quarantine facilities approved by the Plant Protection Adviser to the Government of India.
- Import of **hay** or **straw** or **any material of plant origin** used for packing is **prohibited**.
- Import of **soil**, **earth**, **compost**, **sand**, **plant debris** accompanying **seeds/planting materials** shall not be **permitted**. However, soil can be imported for research purposes under a special permit issued by the Plant Protection Adviser to the Govt, of India.

Note: Cut flowers, garlands, bouquets, fruits and vegetables weighing less than 2 kg for personal use may be imported without a permit or phytosanitary certificate, but are subject to inspection.

Special conditions In addition to the general conditions, there are special conditions for certain notified plants as follows.

Prohibition from certain areas

Name of the plant	Countries from where prohibited
Sugarcane	Australia, Fiji, Papua New Guinea
Sunflower	Argentina, Peru
Rubber	South America,West Indies
Coffee beans	Africa, South America, Sri Lanka
Cocoa and all species of Sterculiaceae and Bombaceae	Africa, Sri Lanka, West Indies

1. **Prohibited for general public**: Coffee plants and seeds, coconut plants and seeds, cotton seeds and unginned cotton, forest tree seed (*Pinus, Ulmus Castanea,*), groundnut seeds and cuttings, potato, sugarcane, tobacco seeds and wheat seeds.
2. **Plants/seeds which require post entry quarantine**: Potato, sugarcane, sunflower, tobacco and wheat, cocoa, citrus, coconut, groundnut. Additional declarations necessary for notified plants (see Table below)

Plant/seed additional declarations for freedom of pests

All species of *Solanum* (Potato)	• Wart (*Synchytrium endobioticum*) • Freedom of parent crop from virus diseases
All species of *Hevea* (Rubber)	• South American leaf blight (*Microcyclus ulei, Sphaerostilbe repens*)
All species of *Saccharum* (Sugarcane)	• Leaf scald (*Xanthomonas albineans*) • Gummosis (*Xanthomonas vasculorum*) • Sereh downy mildew • Chlorotic streak • Fiji disease.
All species of *Medicago* (Lucerne)	• Bacterial wilt (*Corynebacterium incidiosum*)
All species of *Arachis* (Groundnut seeds)	• Production of seeds in areas free of *Puccinia arachidis* and *Sphaceloma arachidis*. • Inspection of parent crops in active growing seasons and certification for freedom from peanut mottle peanut stunt, marginal chlorosis and peanut stripe viruses
All species *Cronartium ribicola, Endothea* of *Pinus, Ulmus, Castanea* (Forest tree seeds)	• *Ceratocystis ulmi,* • *Dothiostroma pini.*
Cotton seeds	• Bacterial blight (*Xanthomonas axonopodis* pv.*malvacearum* and *Glomerella gossypii*)
Coffee – plants, seeds	• American leaf spot (*Omphali flavida*)· Virus diseases
Coconut seeds and all species of *Cocos*	• Lethal yellowing • Cadang· • Bronze leaf wilt • Guam • Coconut disease • Leaf scorch
All species of *Citrus* (lemon, lime, orange etc.,)	• Mal Secco (*Deuterophoma tracheiphila*)
Cocoa and all species of the family Sterculiaceae and Bombaceae	• Pod rot (*Monilia rorei*), • Mealy pod (*Trachysphaeria* and *fructigena*),

Contd...

	• Witches' broom (*Crinipellia perniciosus*) • Swollen shoot virus
All species of *Allium* (onion, garlic, leek, chive, shallot, etc.)	• Smut (*Urocystis cepulae*)

2. Agencies involved in plant quarantine

The authority to implement the quarantine rules and regulations framed under DIP Act rests basically with the Directorate of plant Protection, Quarantine & Storage, under the Ministry of Agriculture. This organization handles bulk import and export of seed and planting material for commerical purpose. Under this organization **9 seaports, 10 airports** and **7 land frontiers** are functioning. These are the recognized ports for entries for import of plant and plant material.

The names and places of the ports and stations are as follows.

A. Airports

i. Amritsar - Punjab
ii. Calcutta - West Bengal
iii. Chennai - Tamil Nadu
iv. Hyderabad - Andhra Pradesh
v. Tiruchirappalli - Tamil Nadu
vi. Trivandrum - Kerala
vii. Varanasi - Uttar Pradesh
viii. Mumbai - Maharashtra
ix. New Delhi - New Delhi
x. Patna - Bihar

B. Seaports - Place State / Union territory

i. Bhavnagar - Gujarat
ii. Nagapattinam - Tamil Nadu
iii. Rameswaram - Tamil Nadu
iv. Tuticorin - Tamil Nadu
v. Visakhapatnam - Andhra Pradesh
vi. Calcutta - West Bengal

vii. Chennai - Tamil Nadu

viii. Cochin - Kerala

ix. Mumbai - Maharashtra

C. Land frontiers

i. Bangaon Benapol Border - West Bengal

ii. Gede Road Railway Station - West Bengal

iii. Kalimpong - West Bengal

iv. Sukhia Pokhri - West Bengal

v. Amritsar Railway Station - Punjab

vi. Attari Railway Station - Punjab

vii. Attari-Wagah Border- Punjab

The Government of India has also approved three other national institutions to act as official quarantine agencies, especially for research material.

- *National Bureau of Plant Genetic Resources (NBPGR)*

  The NBPGR in New Delhi and its regional station at Hyderabad is the agency involved in processing of germplasm, seed, plant material of agricultural, horticultural, and silvicultural crops of all the institutions of Indian Council of Agricultural Research (ICAR) functioning in the country

- *Forest Research Institute (FRI), Dehra Dun* : for forestry plants
- *Botanical Survey of India (BSI)* : for other plants.

3. Domestic Quarantine

Under the DIP Act, the Directorate of Plant Protection, Quarantine and storage has the accountability to take the essential steps and regulate the inter-state movement of plants and plant material in order to prevent the further spread of destructive pest and diseases that have already entered the country. The solitary object of enforcing domestic quarantine is to prevent the spread of these diseases from infected to non-infected areas. Presently, domestic plant quarantine exists in four diseases, **wart** (*Synchytrium endobioticum*) of potato from 1959, **bunchy top** (virus) of banana from 1959, **mosaic** (virus) of banana from 1961 and **apple scab** (*Venturia inaequalis*) from 1979. Most of the states in India have plant quarantine laws to avoid entry of plant pests and diseases.

Export Regulations

- In India, the plant quarantine measures for exporting plants and material including seeds have been streamlined and strict inspections are imposed before the material is permitted to be landed into the country.
- Currently plant quarantine regulations differ with different countries for major agricultural commodities that are being exported out of India.
- The Central Government has authorized officers of the Directorate of Plant Protection, Quarantine & Storage, ICAR Research Institutes, Botanical Survey of India, National Institutes like Forest Research Institute, and the Directorates of Agriculture of all States.
- The quarantine authorities have also framed terms and conditions pertaining to inspection, fumigation or disinfection of the exportable plants and plant material in India including the following schedule/or fee for inspection and issue of phytosanitary certificate, and/or fumigation or disinfection in respect of plants, plant material, seeds, and plant products to issue phytosanitary certificate.
- All the plants and plant material are subjected to inspection by officials issuing certificate.
- Infested materials are given necessary treatment with chemicals and fumigated if required.

The list of plant quarantine and fumigation stations in India is given below.

Maharashtra

I. Plant Quarantine and Fumigation Station, Haji Bunder Road, Sewri, Mumbai

New Delhi

I. Plant Quarantine and Fumigation Station, Palam Airport, New Delhi-10.

II. Plant Quarantine and Fumigation Station, Garden Reach Road, Calcutta-24.

III. Plant Quarantine and Fumigation Station Sukhiapokri, Darjeeling District.

Gujarat

i. Plant Quarantine and Fumigation Station, Haryana Plot No.75, Behind Yusuf Bagh, Bhavnagar

Andhra Pradesh

i. Plant Quarantine and Fumigation Station, The Harbour, Visakhapatnam-1.

Punjab

i. Plant Quarantine and Fumigation Station, Hussainiwala, Ferozepur District.
ii. Plant Quarantine and Fumigation Station, Attari – Wagah Border, near Attari Bus Stand, Attari, Ferozepur District.
iii. Plant Quarantine and Fumigation Station, Civil Aerodrome, Rajasansi, Amritsar.

Tamil Nadu

i. Plant Quarantine and Fumigation Station, 6, Clive Battery, Chennai-1.
ii. Plant Quarantine and Fumigation Station, 335, Beach Road, Tuticorin-1.
iii. Plant Quarantine and Fumigation Station, 110, Railway Feeder Road, Rameswaram.
iv. Plant Quarantine and Fumigation Station, Tiruchirappalli Airport, Tiruchirappalli.

Kerala

Plant Quarantine and Fumigation Station, Willingdon Island, Cochin-3.

CHAPTER - 37

Chemical in Plant Disease Management

INTRODUCTION

The use of chemical for protecting plants from the ravages of the pathogens is not an innovation of the 20th century. Chemicals have been used for over 200 years to protect plants against fungal diseases. At present about 150 chemicals belonging to different classes are used as fungicides in world agriculture. Most of the recommended treatments generally provide 90% or greater control of target diseses. Even when a crop has been grown from pathogen free soil and the crop seems superficially healthy, the use of fungicides in some circumstances become unavoidable. Resistant varieties of potato are attacked by late blight if rain occurs during tuber formation. To control this disease use of fungicides become vital to avoid any loss of the crop. Thus, even in the case of resistant varieties, judicious use of chemical protection will extend the life of resistance in the variety. For killing different groups of pathogens, different types of chemicals are required. The chemicals mainly used for controlling diseases are: fungicides for killing fungus, bactericide for killing barteria, nematicides for killing nematodes, and viricides for killing viruses.

ANTI-PATHOGEN CHEMICALS

The chemical substances that help to retard the activity of pathogens like fungus, bacteria and nematodes are said to be **anti-pathogen** chemicals.

Types of Anti-Pathogen Chemicals

Pesticide type	Target pest
Fungicide	Fungi
Insecticide	Insect
Herbicide	Weeds
Acaricide	Mites, spiders, ticks
Nematicide	Nematodes
Rodenticide	Rodents

Aim of Use of Chemicals in Plant Disease Control

The aim and of use of chemicals in plant disease control are

- To create a toxic barrier between the host surface or tissue and the pathogen .
- To eradicate the pathogen present at a particular site on the host, such as seed, foliage, roots etc.

Functions of Chemicals in Plant Disease Control

- Reduction in inoculum density or eradication of inoculum from source of growth, multiplication and survival.
- Inactivaion or destruction of the pathogen when it lands on the treated surface, and
- Cure of the diseased plant.

Characters of anti-pathogen chemicals or pesticides

In general, the anti-infection chemicals or fungicides having following characters are supposed to be ideal.

- High field performance
- Easy availability of the active constituents.
- Absence of toxicity for the host, man and animals.
- High toxicity for the pathogen at low concentration.
- Retention of toxicity on dilution.
- Stability in storage.
- Slow or no loss of toxicity in storage.
- Good spreading quality on host surface.
- High tenacity on the host surface i.e. it should be retained on the surface.
- Compatibility with pesticides, nematicides, herbicides, vermicides and fertilizers

Advantages of using Pesticides

- **Cost effectiveness**: Pesticides are an economical way of controlling pests. They require low labour input and allow large areas to be treated quickly and effectively. It has been estimated that there is a four-fold return on every dollar a farmer spends on pesticides.

- **Quality, quantity and price of produce**: Using pesticides means there is a plentiful supply and variety of high quality products at reasonable prices. Modern society demands nutritious food free from damage caused by pests and diseases which look untouched. This would be very difficult without pesticides.
- **Prevention of problem**: Pesticides are often used to stop the spread of pests in imports and exports, preventing weeds in gardens and protecting house and furniture from destruction.
- **Protection of pets and humans**: Under the blanket use of pesticides is pet flea products, fly and insect spray and other household products which make life bearable.
- **Flexibility**: A suitable pesticide is available for almost all pest problems with variation in type, activity and persistence.
- **Protection of the environment**: Currently, weeds are controlled by herbicides, but without them, land would need to be cultivated, increasing land degradation.

Disadvantages of Pesticides

- **Drift of sprays and vapour**: Pesticides can affect other areas during application and can cause severe problems in different crops, livestock, waterways and the general environment. Wildlife and fish are the most affected.
- **Reduction of beneficial species**: Animals which interact with the targeted pest can also be affected by he chemical application. The reduction in these other organisms can result in changes in the biodiversity of an area and affect natural biological balances.
- **Residues in food**: There is the possibility of pesticides in human food, either by direct application onto the food, or by bio-magnification along the food line. Not all levels are undesirable but unnecessary and dangerous levels must be avoided through good agricultural practice.
- **Contamination of ground water**: Chemicals can reach underground aquifers if there is persistent product use in agricultural areas.
- **Resistance**: Overuse of the same pesticide can encourage resistance in the target pest.
- **Poisoning hazards**: Pesticide operators can risk poisoning through

excessive exposure if safe handling procedure are not followed and protective clothing is not worn. Poisoning risks depend on dose, toxicity, duration of exposure and sensitivity.

- **Other possible health effects**: As pesticides used now have been through rigorous testing, most health problems stem from misuse, abuse or overuse.

CLASSIFICATION OF CHEMICALS

There are many chemicals which are available for plant disease control but all are not equally safe, effective and popular. The success of any chemical depends on the **selection of suitable chemical** and **its use at appropriate time** and **place** and **its proper application**. The chemicals can be broadly classified on the basis of their mode of action against pathogen and type of pathogen.

A. According to Mode of Action

Depending upon their mode of action the chemicals can be grouped as protectants, eradicants and therapeutants. They are briefly discussed as under.

1. Protectants

Protectants are **prophylactic** in their behaviour. These may be applied to seeds, plant surfaces or the soil but cannot penetrate deep into plant tissues. Therefore, they **act outside** the plant parts as a cover to check the invasion by the pathogen. They include thiram, captan, agallol, zineb, sulphur, ceresan and streptocyclin.

2. Eradicants

Eradicants help to **eradicate** the dormant or active pathogen from the host completely. They are effective in checking the entry (by covering surfaces) and penetrating in the tissue killing pathogen in the host plant. These chemicals can be used as **protectant** as well as **eradicant**. Examples are lime, sulphur, organo mercurials, such as phenyl mercury acetate, methoxy ethyl mercury chloride.

3. Therapeutants

Therapeutants is an agent that inhibits the growth and development of a disease **already entered** in a plant, when applied appropriately. This therapy can be achieved by physical means, such as solar energy treatment or hot water treat- ment, but quite often by chemical means and is called **chemo- therapy**. Usually the chemo-therapeutants are **systemic** in their action, i.e. they enter the plants and affect deep-seated infection. e.g. plantvax, vitavax, brassicol, dithane M-45, dithane Z- 78, bordeaux mixture, streptocyclin and agromycin.

B. According to Type of Pathogen

Based on the type of pathogens, the chemicals can be grouped as

(1) fungicides

(2) bactericides and

(3) nematicides

1. Fungicides

The chemicals which kill **fungus** are called fungicides. Most of the plant diseases are caused by fungus only. Some diseases remain on the surface of the plant while others are deeply seated. These fungicides can again be classified as **non systemic** and **systemic** based upon their action in plant.

I. Non- Systemic or Contact Fungicides

Non-systemic or contact fungicides are the chemicals which do not enter inside the plant tissue, but kill the pathogen by **surface contact**. Some of the important categories of chemicals used for disease control are given here.

A. Sulphur Fungicides

Sulphur fungicides are the **oldest method** of disease control. Inorganic sulphur is used in the form of elemental sulphur or as lime sulphur mixture. Elemental sulphur can be in dust form or. as wettable powder, the latter is used more commonly. However, the most popular fungicides in sulphur groups are the organic compounds known as **dithio-carbamates**. Some of the important chemicals under dithiocarbamates are thiram, ferbam, ziram, nabam, zineb and maneb.

1. Thiram

The trade name for thiram is arasan, tundas, terson, tulisan, etc. It is a leading chemical for **seed treatment**. It is also used in the control of foliage disease *Pythium, Rhizoctonia, Fusarium* and *Protomyces*.

2. Zineb

Zineb is also known as dithane Z- 78, parzate or lonacol. It is effective as foliar spray against late blight of potatoes and tomatoes, blast of rice, ripe rot of chillies and downy mildew of maize.

3. Maneb

Maneb is called as dithane M-22, manzate or **dithane M-45**. It is effective against bean anthracnose, downy mildew and anthracnose of cucurbits, fruit rot of chillies, citrus greasy spot, maize leaf blight and blights caused by **Alternaria**, **Phytophthora** and **Cercospora** on crops.

B. Copper Fungicides

Bordeaux and **Burgundy** mixtures are the dispersible forms of cuprous oxide and basic carbonates are among the important copper fungicides.

1. Bordeaux mixture

Bordeaux mixture (5: 5 : 50) is prepared as

Ingredient	Quantity
Copper sulphate (Blue stone)	5lb (2.26 kg)
Stone or hydrated lime	5 lb (2.26 kg)
Water	50 gallons

It is specific against dowy mildew, late blight of potato, coffee rust, various leaf spots diseases, blights, anthracnoses etc.

2. Burgundy mixture

Burgundy mixture is also known as **"Soda bordeaux"** It is prepared as.

Ingredient	Quantity
Copper sulphate (Blue stone)	10 lb (4.5 kg)
Stone or hydrated lime	12.21b (5.6 kg)
Water	50 gallons.

3. Chestnut compound

Chestnut compound contains **two parts of copper sulphate** and **11 parts of ammonium carbonate**. The two substances are well powdered and thoroughly mixed and the dry mixture stored in an airtight receptacle for 24 hours before being used. It is used against damping -off disease.

4. Chaubattia paste

Chaubattia paste is prepared by mixing **copper carbonate -800 g**, **red lead -800 g** and **raw linseed oil or lanolin -1littre**. This paste was developed as a **wound dressing** fungicide to be applied to pruned parts of pears, apples and peaches for the control of disease, such as stem black, stem-brown, pink disease, stem canker and collar rot of apples, peaches, apricots and plums.

C. Meceury Fungicides

Many mercury compounds are highly effective as fungicides and bactericides. Mercuric chloride ($Hg\,CI_2$) and mercurous chloride (Hg_2C1_2) are used as 1 : 1000 dilutions for soaking the seeds, rhizomes and corms of vegetables and flowers to mainly control certain bacterial and fungal diseases. It is used against club root disease of brassica seedlings.

D. Quinone Fungicides

Some common quinone fungicides are mentioned here.

1. Chloranil

Chloranil is mainly used in seed treatment. It is sold as spergon and is used in seed and bulb treatment of legume flowers and vegetables. It is also used as soil drench.

2. Dichlone

Dichlone is used as seed treatment as well as foliar spray also. It is 4-8 times more effective than chloranil in the protection of legume and cotton seed.

E. Benzene Fungicides

Benzene is used as a dormant spray for the control of many diseases of fruit trees and ornamental plants and for the treatment of wounds in trees.

1. Dinocap (Karathane)

Dinocap is an excellent substitute **for sulphur** for the control of **powdery mildew** and is highly specific against them. It is also effective against **mites**.

2. Chloronil

Chloronil is active against *Rhizoctonia solan; Sclerotium rolfsii* and *Phytophthora cinnamoni*. This fungicide has been used for the most part as a seed or in-furrow treatment of cotton.

3. Penta chloronitrobenzene (PCNB)

Penta chloronitrobenzene is sold as quintozene, PCNB terrachlor brassicol etc. They control many soil-borne diseases caused by *Rhizoctonia, Sclerotium* etc.

F. Hetero-Cyclic Nitrogen Compound

Hetero-cyclic nitrogen compound are used as foliage protectants and eradicants of fruits and vegetables. **Glyodin** and **captan** are the two important fungicides of this group.

1. Captan

Captan is sold under different names like capton 50W, 75W, orthocide dust etc. It is effective for seed treatment for seedling diseases of vegetables, cotton etc, smuts, and bunt of wheat. It is also used as spray fungicide against, downy mildew and powdery mildew of grapevines, apple scab, brown rot of stone fruits and mango anthracnose.

2. Difoltan

Difoltan has properties similar to captan. It is a good fungicide for the control of early and late blight of potatoes and tomatoes.

3. Folpet

It is sold under the trade names of phaltan, orthophaltan etc. Wettable powder and dust are applied for foliage diseases of fruits and ornamentals. Folpet is eftective against *Sphaerotheca pannosa*

G. Organo-Phosphorus Fungicides

1. Ediphenphos

It is the common name to the fungicide sold under the trade name **Hinosan**. It is an effective against **blast** of rice.

H. Organo-tin Compounds

1. Brestan

Brestan is effective against *Cercospora, Alternaria*, *Spetoria* and many other fungi.

2. Du- Ter,

Du-Ter is used effectively against diseases caused by *Cercospora, Helminthosporium, Alternaria*, *Pythium, Phytophthora* and *Rhizoctonia.*

I. Soil Fumigants

The most promising method of controlling nematodes in the field has been through the use of chemicals called **nematicides**. Some of these, including chloropicrin, methyl bromide, vapam and vorlex, give off gases after being applied ; to the soil. Some of the soil fumigants are mentioned here.

1. Formalin

Formalin is used to control damping-off and seedling blights. A solution of 37-40% in water is used.

2. Chloropicrin

Chloropicrin is useful both as a fungicide and a larvicide. It is injected into the soil at a depth of 3-6" in holes 9-12" apart. The soil is then covered with impervious cloth or sheet for 48 hours.

3. Vapam

Vapam is a colourless liquid which decomposes rapidly in moist soil to release a fumigating gas. It has been used as nematicide and also as selective weedicide. It is also quite effective in the control of wilt of cotton, damping-off of papaya and root rot of beet.

4. DD Mixture (Dichloropropene and Dichloropropane)

DD Mixture is extensively used as nematode control. Also used as control of soil borne diseases in pineapple.

II. Systemic Fungicides

Sysyemics fungicides are the fungicitoxic compounds which when applied on different parts of the plant are absorbed by the plant tissues and then translocated upwards, downwards and both ways and act on the pathogen either directly or through its metabolite products and control plant diseases away from the point of application.

An ideal systemic fungicide should have the following characteristics.

1. The substance may either be toxic to the pathogen concerned or be converted in the host plant to such a fungitoxicant.
2. Alternatively, the substance may alter the metabolism of the host so that biochemical or physical resistance to pathogen may be induced or enhanced.

3. It must not adversely affect the host plant to such an extent that the quantity or quality of the crop is reduced.
4. Systemic fungicides are highly selective i.e. toxic to the pathogen but not to the host.
5. In systemicity the substance must be absorbed sufficiently the translocated from the point of application to the site of the pathogen and should have a considerable degree of stability within the host plant.
6. Most systemic fungicides are translocated in the **apoplast**, though some mainly compound related to the **benzimidazoles**, appear to move in the **symplast** also.
7. Systemic fungicides are advantageous over non systemic fungicides because of more coverage, systemic and mobile nature.so that concealed pathogens are also targeted, more specific in mode of action and thus less quantity is required against fast growing fungi.
8. However, there are some disadvantages also like narrow spectrum of activity, development of resistance of pathogen, higher cost and residual toxicity if it is not metabolized in the system.
9. If it is applied to an edible portion of the plant the mammalian toxicity must be low enough to avoid residue problems at the consumer stage.

On the basis of chemical structure, systemic fungicides can be classified as follows.

1. Oxathins and Related Compounds

These were the **first systemic fungicides** to be discovered in 1966. They selectively concentrate in cells of fungi and inhibit succinic hydrogenase (enzyme involved in mitochondrial respiration). Oxathins are systemic fungicides which are effective only against *Basidiomycetous fungi*, such as rusts, smuts, Rhizoctonia etc. Two types of oxathins are there.

a. Vita vax or carboxin

Vitavax or carboxin has become the most popular fungicide for seed treatment to control loose smut in wheat and barley. It gives satisfactory control of bunt and flag smut also.

b. Plant vax or Oxycarboxin

Plant vax or Oxycarboxin is toxic to *Helminthosporium sativum, Curvularia, Aspergillus, Cladosporium, Botrytis, Monilinia* etc.

2. Benzimidazoles

Benzimidazole fungicides were introduced for disease control in the 1960s and 1970s as foliar fungicides, seed treatments and for use in post harvest applications.They possessed unique properties not seen before in the protectants. These includes low use rates, broad spectrum and systemicity with post infection action that allowed for extended spray interval. All these qualities made them very popular with growers. These fungicide show broad spectrum activity against fungi but are **not effective** against **lower fungi** and **bacteria**.

a. Benomyl

This is also marketed as benlate. It is effective against *cercospora* leaf spot of sugarbeet, rice blast, apple scab, powdery mildew of curubits, cereals and legumes. Dipping of fruits and roots has controlled banana fruit rots, root rot of sweet potato, corn rot of gladiolus etc

b. Carbendazim

It is sold as Bavisitin, Derosol, MBC, Tagstin, Agrozim or Jkenstin.Carbendazim is effective against a wide range of fungal pathogens of field crops, fruits, ornamentals and vegetables as spray, seedling dip, seed treatment, soil drench and as post harvest treatment.It is very effective against wilt diseases,, turmeric leaf spot and rust diseases.

c. Thiabendazole (TBZ)

It is sold as Thiabendazole, Mertect, Tecto, Storite. Thiabendazole is a broad spectrum systemic fungicide effective against species of *Botrytis, Ceratocystis, Coletotrichum, Fusarium, Cercospora, Rhizoctonia, Sclerotinia, Septoria* and *Verticillium.* it is also used to control post harvest storage diseases of fruits and vegetables.

3. Acylalanines

These are was introduced in 1977, brought a completely new level of control to **oomycetes** through their systemic properties by offering protection to the plants as seed treatments, and soil or foliar applications. These include metalaxyl, furalaxyl or banalaxyl. These fungicides are highly effective against downy mildews, *Pythium* and *Phytophthora* diseases including late blight.

4. Thiophanates

These compounds are the derivatives of thioallophanic acid representing a new group of systemic fungicides. The aromatic nucleus of these fungicides is converted into benzimidazole ring for their activity. Hence, thiophanates are often classified under benzimidazole group.Two compounds are developed under this group are Thiophanate and Thiophanate –methyl .The former has a broad range of action and is effective against *Venturia* spp. on apple and pear, powdery mildews, *Botrytis* and *Sclerotinia* spp.Thiophanate methyl is also recommended for use in the management of apple scab, powdery mildews and some leaf spots.

5. Morpholines

Morpholine fungicides are best known for their excellent control of cereal diseases, powdery mildew on vegetable and grapes, and sigatoka of banana. Tridemorph and Dodemorph are the common morpholine fungicides sold as Calixin ,Bradew and Beacon etc. Among the recently developed systemic fungicides, **Tridemorph** has excellent prophylactic and curative action against powdery mildew of cereals, sigatoka disease of banana and other ascomycetous pathogens. Dodemorph is widely used in the management of powdery mildew of roses.

6. Sterol biosynthesis inhibitor(SBIs) fungicides

SBIs have proved most successful fungicides for about three decades since their release in 1970's. Their mode of action is inhibition of **sterol (ergosterol)** biosynthesis, an important component of cell membranes of Asco- and Basidiomycotina.Sterol biosynthesis inhibitor fungicides include Pyrimidines, Piperidines, Imidazole and Piperazine. Among all SBIs, **triazoles** are the most commonly used. Triazoles are one of the most effective fungicides such as **triadimefon** (Bayleton,) and **triadimenol** (Baytan), both of which are effective against powdery mildews. Others in this group are hexaconazole (Contaf 5EC, Anvil 5 EC), triazbutyl (Indar or RH 124) , **propiconazole** (Tilt 25 EC) and terbuconazole (Folicur 25 EC) etc. In addition to powdery mildew , hexaconazole is effective against rusts, propiconazole against rust and leaf spots, terbuconazole as seed treatment fungicide against smuts, penconazole and difenoconazole and cyperocoanazole against leaf spots and rusts and porbenazole is specific against rice blast.

7. Strobilurins fungicides

Strobilurins are a group of chemical compounds used in agriculture as fungicides. They were extracted from the fungus **Strobilurus tenacellus** and hence the name strobilurin. These fungicides have become very important in the control of wide range of plant diseases caused by all major groups of fungi, Asco, Basidio, and the Oomycota. They have a suppressive effect on other fungi, reducing competition for nutrients; they inhibit electron transfer in mitochondria, disrupting energy metabolism and preventing growth of the target fungi. They are part of the larger group of **QoI inhibitors**, which act to inhibit the respiratory chain at the level of **Complex III**. Some common Strobilurins are azoxystrobin, kresoxim-methyl, picoxystrobin, fluoxastrobin, oryzastrobin, dimoxystrobin, pyraclostrobin and trifloxystrobin. Strobilurins represented a major development in fungus-based fungicides. Strobilurins are miracle fungicides ever developed.

This group of fungicides should be applied preventively or as early as possible in the disease cycle. They are effective against spore germination and early mycelium growth. Once the fungus is growing inside the leaf tissue, QoI fungicides have little or no effect. Most of the Q_0I fungicides exhibit **translaminar movement** (which means "across the lamina", or leaf blade). When these fungicides are applied, most of the active ingredient is initially held on or within the waxy cuticle of plant surfaces. Some of the active ingredient "leaks" into the underlying plant cells. For those fungicides with an affinity for the waxy cuticle (such as trifloxystrobin and kresoxim methyl), active ingredient that "leaks" all the way through the lamina quickly rebinds to the cuticle on the far side of the leaf blade. Thus, the fungicide can be found on both leaf surfaces even if only one leaf surface was treated. Translaminar movement can take one to several days to be fully effective. The fungicide **azoxystrobin** moves **translaminarly** as well as **systemically** (in the plant's vascular system, or "plumbing"). The fungicides kresoxim methyl and trifloxystrobin move translaminarly but not systemically. These latter fungicides, however, appear to move as a gas in the layer of still air adjacent to the leaf surface called the *boundary layer*. As they move in the vapor phase, they readily re-bind to the cuticle. Fungicides such as kresoxim methyl and trifloxystrobin—which are not true systemics but which redistribute by these other mechanisms—have been referred to as "mesostemics", "quasi-systemics", or "surface systemics". Most have a residual period of approximately 21 days. Since the mode of action of the Q_0I fungicides is highly specific. Of the millions of biochemical reactions that occur in the fungal cell, these fungicides interfere with just one, very specific biochemical site. It is a very important biochemical site for the fungus, to be sure, but it is just one site. Thus, these are called **site-specific fungicides**. This is important because, commonly, just one mutation at that biochemical site (the target site of the fungicide) can result in a fungicide-resistant strain. If such a fungicide-resistant strain occurs, repeated application of Q_0I fungicides can lead to buildup of a fungicide-resistant pathogen subpopulation. Experience with the Q_0I fungicides worldwide indicates there is a **high risk** of development of resistant pathogen subpopulations. Worldwide, resistance has been reported in an increasing number of pathogens of field crops, fruit, vegetable, and nut crops, ornamentals and turfgrass.

Recommendations for avoiding fungicide resistance:

- Tank mix QoI fungicides with fungicides that have a different mode of action.
- Apply a maximum of two QoI fungicide-containing sprays per season.
- Apply QoI fungicides according to manufacturers' recommendations for the target disease at the specific crop growth stage indicated.
- Apply the QoI fungicide preventively or as early as possible in the disease cycle. Do not rely on management of diseases when QoI fungicides are applied during early infection.
- Reduced rate programs accelerate the development of resistant populations and therefore must not be used.

FUNGICIDE MIXTURES

Fungicide mixtures

Containing two or more fungicides with different mode of action, have been developed with the twin objectives of broadening the activity spectrum against diverse plant diseases and to check the development of resistance in the target pathogens. In recent years several prepacked mixtures of specific site and contact fungicides have been introduced by different manufacturers. Theoretically the use of pre packed mixtures offer several advantages: (a) the protectant component should control the resistant isolates, (b) the dose of the systemic component may be reduced to additive or synergistic levels (c) reduced concentration of systemic component should reduce the selection pressure for resistance, (d) multiple disease control and most importantly and (e) the use of pre packed mixtures is an enforceable strategy. Some of the recently developed and commonly used fungicide mixtures are depicted in Table 28.

Table 28 : Some of the recently developed fungicide mixtures

Common name	Name of Fungicide mixtures'	Effective against
Ridomil Gold	Mefenoxam + Ancozeb	Downy mildew, *Pythium* and *Phytophthora* diseases.
Input	Prothioconazole + Spiroxamine	Powdery mildew, *Fusarium*, *Septoria*, rusts in cereals.
Twinline	Yraclostrobin + Metaconzole	Cereal rusts
Amistar Top	Azoxystrobin + Difenoconazole	Various diseases on diverse crops.
Prosaro	Prothioconazole + Tebuconazole)	*Fusarium* head scab in cereals
Sensation	Fluopyram + Trifloxystrobin	Gray mold, powdery mildew, *Sclerotinia* and *Monilia* in fruits.

2. Antibiotics

Antibiotics are substances which are produced by micro- organisms and which act against micro-organisms. It is also defined as secondary metabolites produced by microorganism, which inhibits the growth of another microorganism, Most antibiotics known uptill now are products of **actinomycetes** and some are from fungi and bacteria. The use of the antibiotics in managing plant diseases, particlulaty the disease caused by bacteria, mycoplasma and ricketsia, is well demonstrated and are thought to be effective means because of their selective action directed towards causal agents not to the infected host. The mode of action of the antibiotics varies depending on site of action which in turn determines their specificity towards given target host, (Table-29). Some time mixture of antibiotics are in practice in managing the diseases to reduce, delay the chances of resistance development against a particular antibiotic by the causal agent. The most useful antibiotic mixture is **streptocycline**, which contains streptomycin and tetracycline.

Table 29 : Important antibiotics and their mode of action

Name	**Source**	**Effective against**	**Mode of action**
Penicillins	*Penicillium* spp.	Prokaryotes	Inhibits murein synthesis
Cephalosporins	*Cephalosporium* spp.	Prokaryotes	Inhibits murein synthesis
Streptomycin	*Streptomyces griseus*	Prokaryotes	Binds to protein S12 of 30S causing aberrant inhibiton complex
Kanamycin	*S. kanamyceticus*	Prokaryotes	Affect 30S risbosomal aubunits and prevents the translation.
Neomycin	*S. fradiae*	Prokaryotes	Affect 30S risbosomal aubunits and prevents the translation.
Erythromycin	*Streptomyces erythraeus*	Prokaryotes	Inhibits translation by binding to the 50S ribosome
Carbomycin	*S.halstedii*	Prokaryotes	Inhibits translation by binding to the 50S ribosome
Chlorotetracyclin	*S. aureofaciens*	Prokaryotes	Inhibits binding of aminoacyl- t- RNA to A site of 30S ribosomes; specifically binds to the protein S & near A site, resulting change in topology
Oxytetracycline	*S. riomosus*	Prokaryotes	Inhibits binding of aminoacyl- t- RNA to A site of 30S ribossomes; specificallybinds to the protein S & near A site,

			resulting change in topology
Rifampin	*Amycolatopsis rifamycinica*	Prokaryotes	Inhibits DNA dependent RNA polymerase in bacterial cells by binding its betasubunit, thus preventing transcription to RNA and subsequent translation to proteins.
Bacitracin	*B. subtilis*	Prokaryotes	Destroys murein biosynthesis
Polymixin-G	*Bacilus polymyxa*	Prokaryotes	Destroys cytoplasmic membrane.
Chloramphenicol	*Streptomyces venezuelae*	Prokaryotes	Inhibits peptidyl transferase activity of 50S ribosome and affects translation.
Nystacin	*S. nouresii*	Eukaryotes (Fungi)	Inactivates membrane containing sterols by making pore through which kions, small molecules.
Amphotericin	*S. nodosus*	Eukaryotes (Fungi)	Inactivates membrane containing sterols by making pore through which kions , small molecules.
Aureofungin	*Streptoverticillium cinnamoneus var terricola*	Eukaryotes (Fungi)	Inactivates membrane containing sterols by making pore through which kions , small molecules.
Natamycin/ Pimaricin	*Streptomyces natalensis*	Eukaryotes (Fungi)	Inactivates membrane containing sterols by making pore through which kions , small molecules.

3. Nematicides

The chemicals which kill the nematodes are called nematicides. The nematicides commonly used are, nemaphos, D.D, DBCP, carbofuran, phorate, telone, terracur, terracur-P, methon M-sodium and vapam.

MODES OF ACTION FOR PLANT DISEASE MANAGEMENT CHEMICALS

Application of chemicals to plants in order to prevent or inhibit disease development is a fundamental means of managing diseases caused by fungi. Knowledge of the effectiveness of particular compounds is important for achieving effective disease control. Equally important is an understanding of the underlying physiological mode of action of plant disease management materials. Fungicides are metabolic inhibitors and their modes of action can be classified into four broad groups.

1. Inhibitors of electron transport chain.
2. Inhibitors of enzymes.
3. Inhibitors of nucleic acid metabolism and protein synthesis.
4. Inhibitors of sterol synthesis.

1. Inhibition of electron transport chain (Respiration in mitochondria)

- **Sulfur**

  Disrupts electron transport along the cytochromes

- **Strobilurins** (azoxystrobin, kresoxim-methyl, pyraclostrobin, trifloxystrobin)

  Inhibit mitochondrial respiration, blocking the cytochrome bc1 complex.

2. Inhibition of enzymes

- **Copper**

  Nonspecific denaturation of proteins and enzymes.

- **Dithiocarbamates** (Maneb, Zineb, Mancozeb, etc)

  Inactivate –SH groups in amino acids, proteins and enzymes.

- **Substituted aromatics** (Chlorothalonil, PCNB)

  Inactivate amino acids, proteins and enzymes by combining with amino and thiol groups.

- **Organophosphonate (fosetyl-Al)**

  Disrupts amino acid metabolism.

3. Inhibition of nucleic acid metabolism and protein synthesis

- **Benzimidazoles** (Thiophanate-methyl, Carbendazim, Benolmyl)

  Inhibit DNA synthesis (nuclear division).

- **Phenylamides** (metalaxyl, Mefenoxam)

  Inhibits RNA synthesis.

- **Dicarboximides** (Iprodione, Vinclozolin)

  Inhibits DNA and RNA synthesis, cell division and cellular metabolism.

4. Inhibition of sterol synthesis

- Imidazoles (imazalil)
- Triazoles (propiconazole, myclobutanil, tebuconazole, triflumazole)
- Morpholines (dimethomorph)
- Inhibits sterol production at different site than imidazoles and triazoles. Affects cell wall production.

Table 30 : Classification of fungicides based on their mode of action

Mode of action	Chemical family(group)	Active ingredients
Mitosis and cell division	Benzimidazoles	Thiabendazole, carbendazim, Benomyl
	Thiophanates	Tthiophanate-methyl
Multi-site contact activity	Iinorganic	Sulphur
	Inorganic	Copper
	Dithiocarbamates and relatives	Ferbam, mancozeb, maeb,metiram thiram, ziram
	Phthalimides	Captan
	Chloronitriles	Chlorothalonil
	Guanidines	Dodine
Respiration		Iprodione
		Vinclozolin
Sterol synethesis	Imidazoles	Imazilil
	Piperazines	Triforine
	Pyrimidines	Fenarimol
	Ttriazoles	Bitertanol, cyproconazole, difenoconazole Fenbuconazole. flusilazole, ipconazole, metconazole, myclobutanil, propiconazole, prothioconazole, tebuconazole, tetraconazole, triadimefon triadimenol, triticonazole
Nucleic acid synethesis	Acylalanines	Metalaxyl, metalaxyl-M
Protein synthesis		Cyprodinil
Respiration	Oxathins	Carboxin
Respiration	Methoxyacrylates	Azoxystrobin, picoxystrobin

	Methoxy-carbamates	Pyraclostrobin
	Oximino acetates	Trifloxystrobin, kresoxim-methyl
	Oxazolidine-dionenes	Famoxadone
	Dihydro dioxazines	Fluoxastrobin
	Imidazolinones	Fenamidone
	2,6-dinitro-anilines	Fluazinam
Lipids and membranes		Chloroneb, dicloran, quintozene (PCNB)
Cell wall synthesis	Peptidyl pyrimidinenucleoside	Polyoxin
	Cinnamic acid amides	Dimethomorph
	Mandelic acid amidesh	Mandipropamid
Protein synthesis		Kasugamycin, streptomycin, oxytetracycline
Host plant defense induction	Benzo thiadiazole, BTH	Acibenzolar-S-methyl

PESTICIDE FORMULATIONS

Defnition of Pesticide Formulation

Pesticide formulation is the process by which the pesticide is put into a form which can be easily produced, stored, transported and applied by practical methods in order to achieve a safe, convenient economic and effective method of pest control.

When a pesticide active ingredient (a.i) is manufactured, it is not in a usable form as it may not mix well with water or may be unstable. Therefore, it is mixed with other compounds to improve its effectiveness, safety, handling and storage. These other compounds can include solvents, mineral clays, stickers, wetting agents, or other adjuvant. **The mixture of a.i. and inert (inactive) ingredients is called a pesticide formulation**. Some formulations are premixed while others must be mixed before use. A single a.i. is often made into several formulations.

Objectives of Pesticide Formulations

The objective of formulating pesticide active ingredients for crop protection is:

- To uniformly spread a small amount of the active ingredient over a large area.
- To ensure safety in handling and application

- To optimize pesticide doses for better efficacy.

How to Choose a Formulation?

Selection of the most appropriate formulation for a given application includes an analysis of the following factors:

Application safety: Different formulations create varied degrees of hazards for the applicator. Some products are easily inhaled, while others may readily penetrate skin, or cause injury when splashed in the eyes.

Pest biology: The growth habits and survival strategies of pests are also key factors in determining which type of formulation provides optimum contact between the active ingredients and the pest.

Environmental concern: Special precautions need to be taken with formulations that are prone to drift in the air or move off target into water. Wildlife may also be affected in varying degrees by different formulations.

Available application equipment: Some pesticide formulations require specialized application equipment. This includes safety equipment and, in special cases, containment structures.

Surface to be protected: Applicators must be aware that certain formulations can stain fabrics, discolor linoleum, dissolve plastic, or burn foliage. These surfaces require protection.

Cost: Product prices may vary substantially, based on the ingredients used and the complexity of delivering active ingredients in specific formulations.

Conventional Pesticide Formulations

Solid formulations: These are divided into two types: Ready to use, and concentrates which must be mixed with water in order to be applied as spray able suspensions. Of the six solid formulations dust, granules, and pellets are ready to use, while other three wettable powders, dry flowable powders, and soluble powders are intended to be mixed with water before applying in the field.

Dusts: These are manufactured by the sorption of an active ingredient onto a finely ground, solid inert such as clay, chalk or talc. Usually the concentration of active ingredients in these formulations is **less than 10%**.

A granule is defined by size. Granule sized products should pass through a 4 mesh sieve and be retained on an 80 mesh sieve.

Granules: The manufacture of granular formulations is similar to that of dusts except that the active ingredient is sorbed onto a larger particle. The inert solid may be clay, sand or ground plant materials. Granules are applied in the dry state and are usually intended for soil applications where they have the advantage of weight to carry them through foliage to the ground below.

Pellets: The active ingredient is combined with inert materials to form slurry (a thick liquid mixture) and the slurry is then extruded under pressure through a die and cut at desired lengths to produce particles that are relatively uniform in size and shape. These pellets are typically used in **spot** applications.

Wettable powders: These powders are finely divided solids made of mineral clays to which an active ingredient is mixed and sorbed. These formulations are diluted with water and applied as a liquid spray. Under dilution, a suspension is formed in the spray tank. Apart from the active ingredient, wettable powders contain wetting and dispersing agents as an inert part of the formulation.

Dry flowable or water dispersible granules: They are diluted with water and applied as a spray suspension exactly in the same manner as wettable powders and dry flowables are expected to form a stable suspension with high susceptibility and they are also considered more environment and user friendly in comparison with wettable powders.

Soluble powders: Soluble powders provide most of the same benefits as wettable powders, without they need for agitation once they are dissolved in the spray tank.

Liquid powder: There are four types of liquid formulations available in the market. Prior to application these are diluted with water, but in some instances labels may permit the use of crop, oil, diesel fuel, kerosene, or some other light fuel oil as carrier. The four different types are:

Emulsifiable Concentrates: These are non aqueous solutions of pesticide along with emulsifiers, which, on dilution with water, produce a stable emulsion. **Emulsifiable concentrates** are mixed with **water** and applied as a **spray**. The emulsifing agents are long chain chemicals that roeint themselves around the droplets of oil and bind the oil water surfaces together to prevent the oil and water from separating. Emulsifiable concentrates allow oil soluble active ingredients to be sprayed in the field using water as a carrier.

Liquid Flowables: The manufacture of liquid flowable mirrors that of wattable powders with the additional step of mixing the powder, dispersing agents, wetting agents, etc., with water followed by wet grinding for making a stable suspension before packaging.

Microencapsulators: Microencapsulates consist of a solid and liquid inert, containing an active ingredient surrounded by a plastic, starch or polymers coating. The resulting capsules can be aggregated to form dispersible granules, or they may be suspended in water to form a **capsulated suspension**. Encapsulation enhances applicator safety along with minimization of residues, while at the same time providing timed release of the active ingredient. Liquid forms of microencapsulates are further diluted with water and applied as sprays. They form suspensions in the spray tank and have several properties similar to those of the liquid flowable.

Solutions: (Water soluble concentrates) These consists of water soluble active and inert ingredients to be used for further dilutions prior to field applications. They form a true solution in the spray tank and require no agitation after they are thoroughly dissolved. Solutions are not abrasive to equipment and donot plug strainers and screens. They include products containing paraquat, glyphosate and 2,4-D.

Aerosols and Fumigants: **Aerosols** really refers to a delivery system that moves the active ingredient to the target site in the form of **a mist** of very small particles. Solid or liquid drops. The particles can be released under pressure or produced by fog or smoke generators. **Fumigants** deliver the active ingredient to the target site in the form of **a gas**. Some fumigants are solids that sublime (turn into gas) in the presence of atmospheric moisture. Others are liquid under pressure that vaporizes when the pressure is released.

Disadvantages of Conventional Formulations	**Advantages of New Generation Formulations**
Bulky, dusty and inconvenient	Improved residual activity
Hazardous during manufacturing, packing and application	Longer application intervals
Highly flammable due to use of organic solvents	Reduction in application dosage
Can cause phytotoxicity	Reduction in spray drift
More impact on non target organism	Less impact on non target organisms
Poor rain fastness	Better rain fastness
Corrosive to metal and plastic	Less phytotoxicity
Expensive to pack and transport	Constant and delayed biological effect
Dermal hazards	Reduced environmental pollution
Extreme inhalation danger	Reduced volatilization and leaching
	Safe storage due to reduced flammability

FUNGICIDE RESISTANCE

Fungicides have been used for over 200 years to protect plants against fungal diseases. At present about 150 chemicals belonging to different classes are used as fungicides in world agriculture. Most of the recommended treatments generally provide 90% or greater control of the target disease, and give the farmer a benefit: cost ratio of at least 3:1. However, under certain circumstances, a fungicide might fail to control disease development. Poor disease control with fungicides can result from numerous causes, including inherently low fungicide effectiveness, inappropriate timing of application, inadequate dose, faulty method of application, longer interval between applications, expired product or exceedingly heavy disease pressure. Development of resistance to fungicides can also be the reason of poor disease control. *Resistance refers to a situation where a given fungicide once controlled a particular fungal population but, after one or more applications that fungicide no longer controls that population. Resistance to fungicides has become a challenging problem in the management of crop diseases and has threatened the performance of some highly potent commercial fungicides.* Worldwide, resistance in pathogen populations to more than 100 different active ingredient has been reported(Table-31). The first case of resistance to benzimidazoles occurred in powdery mildew in greenhouses in 1969 in New York, one year after introduction . Resistance to benzimidazioles has been reported to occur in about 126 fungal species including member of the Basidiomycetes, Ascomycetes and Deuteromycetes. Prior to the introduction of benzimidazoles (benomyl), farmers normally applied protectant fungicides *viz* dithiocarbamates without experiencing resistance problems and these are still used extensively and efficiently against several diseases. Superior disease control was frequently achieved with benomyl compared to the protective dithiocarbamates owing to its systemic activity. However within the few years wherever these fungicide was used intensively, sudden failures in control of disease were experienced with apple scab, powdery mildews, Botrytis grey mould and Peanut leaf spot. Majority of the fungicides developed and registered since the introduction of benzimidazoles have site specific mode of actions and carry risk of resistance. Therefore, strategies to manage the resistance risk need to be developed and implemented to avoid unexpected control failures and sustain the usefulness of new products.

Table 31 : Instances of resistance development to compounds of major classes of fungicides used in plant disease control.

Fungicide group/compound	Main Pathogens affected	Crops
Benomyl	*Botrytis cinerea*	Grape
Carbendazim	*Venturia inaequalis*	Apple
Metalaxyl	*Pseudoperonospora cubensis*	Cucurbits
	Plasmopara viticola	Grapes
	Phytophthora infestans	Potato
	Bremia lactucae	Lettuce
	Botrytis cinerea	Strawberry
	Corynespora cassiicola	Cucumber
	Botrytis cinerea	Grapes
	Alternaria alternata	Oil seeds
	Venturia inaequalis	Apple
	S. fuliginea	Cucurbit and Barley
	Mycosphaerella graminicola.	Cereal
Edifenphos	Magnoporthe grisea	Rice
Ethirimol	*Erysiphe graminis*	Barley
	Alternaria solani	Potato
	Colletotrichum graminicola	Barley
	Cercospora sojina	Soybean

Types of Fungicide Resistance

There are two types of fungicide resistance:

Qualitative resistance (discreate resistance): develops **suddenly** against fungicides that have a **single site of action**. A mutation in the gene of the target site alters the site of action of the fungicide that makes the fungicide totally ineffective the pathogen. The resistance is stable and persists even after the fungicide is withdrawn. This type of resistance is seen with the use of **benzimidazoles** and **QoI (Strobilurin)** fungicides. *Mycospharella musicola* , causing the Sigatoka disease of banana, become resistant to QoI fungicides due to a point mutation (single nucleotide change) in the gene encoding cytochrome b. The aminoacid glycine is replaced by aniline in the target protein (cytochrome b). The fungicide fails to bind to the protein and becomes ineffective.

Quantitative resistance (continuous resistance): develops **gradually** and is the result of accumulation of mutations in several genes (polygenic), each having a small additive effects.There is a continuous variation in sensitivity within the resistant population. The resistance is not present and the pathogens become sensitive again if the fungicide application is stopped. The **DMI** (demethylation inhibitor) fungicides induce quantitative resistance.

Preexisting resistance: Besides qualitative and quantitative resistance, caused by monogenic and polygenic mutations respectively, the resistance could be by built in mechanisms. The apple scab fungus, *Venturia inaequalis* develops resistance against DMI fungicides by upregulation of the target genes, resulting in hyperproduciton of the target proteins and making the fungicide less effective. Efflux of the fungicide out of the cell is reported in *Mycospharella*

Resistance Risk among Fungicides

The risk of resistance development depends greatly upon the chemical class to which a fungicide belongs and the mode of action of member fungicides. Over the past thirty years severe and wide spread problems of acquired resistance have affected the practical performance of most of the major groups of fungicides. Certain traditional major classes of fungicides such as those based on copper (cuprous oxide, copper oxychloride, Bordeaux mixture), phthalimides (e.g captan, captafol and folpet) and dithiocarbamates (e.g. mancozeb, maneb, zineb and thiram) have never been known to encounter practical resistance even after many years of use. These fungicides have a **multisite mode of action**, so that a number of simultaneous mutations would be needed in order to develop resistance. By contrast, all the compounds in some other classes, such as benzimidazoles e.g. benomyl, carbendazim, thiabendazole, pheylamides (e.g. metalaxyl and oxadixyl), dicarboximides (e.g. iprodione, peocymidoneand, vinclozolin) and the recently introduced strobilurins (e.g. azoxystrobin and kresoxim methyl) have met with serious resistance problems that arose in most of their target pathogens, within 2-10 years of their commercial introduction. Resistance to triazoles (e.g. triadimefon or flusilazole) has developed more gradually in stepwise process. Estimates of resistance risk in different chemical classes of fungicides are shown in Table-32.

Table 32 : Fungicides grouped by mode of action and relative risk for developing resistance problems.

Group name	Mode of action	Common Name	Mobility[1]	Uses[2]	Risk[3]
Phenylamide	Nucleic acid synthesis	Metalaxyl	S	ST, F, S	H
		Metalaxyl-M	S	ST, F, S	H
Benzimidazole	Mitosis and Cell divison	Thiophanate-methyl	S	ST, PH	H
		Thiabendazole	S	ST, F, S	H
Carboxamide	Respiration	Carboxin	S	ST	L
Strobilurin (Quinone outside inhibitor (QoI))	Respiration	Azoxystrobin	S	F, S, ST	H
Quinone insideInhibitor (QiI)	Respiration	Cyazofamid	S	F	M
Dicarboximide	Lipids andmembranes	Iprodione	P	F, S	M-H
		Vinclozolin	P	F, S	M-H
	Aromatic hydrocarbons	Chloroneb	P	ST	L
Demethylation Inhibitor (DMI)	Sterol synthesis	Cyproconazole	S	F	
		Difenconazole	S	ST, F	L-M
		Propiconazole	S	F, S	M
		Prothioconazole	S	F,S	M
		Tebuconazole	S	F, S, ST	M
		Triadimefon	S	F, S	M
		Triadimenol	S	ST	L
Cyanoaceta-mideoxime	Unknown	Cymoxanil	S	F	M
Phosphonate	Unknown	Fosetyl-AL	S	F	L
Inorganic	Multi-site	Copper salts, Sulphur	P	F	L
Dithiocar-bamate	Multi-site	Ferbam, ziram	P	F	L
		Mancozeb, Maneb, Thiram	P	F, ST	L
Phthalimide	Multi-site	Captan	P	F, ST	L
Chloronitrile	Multi-site	Chlorothalonil	P	F, S	L
Guanadin	Multi-site	Dodine	P	F	M

Source : http://osufacts.okstate.edu

1. P=protectant, S=systemic or penetrant.
2. S=soilborne diseases, F=foliar diseases, ST=seed treatment, PH=post-harvest treatment.
3. H-High Resistance, M-Moderate resistance, L-Low resistance

Mechanisms of Fungicide Resistance

There are several ways that populations of fungi can become resistant to fungicides, these include:

1. **Altered target site**: A fungicide has a specific target site where it acts to disrupt a particular biochemical process or function. If this target site is somewhat altered, the fungicide no longer binds to the site of action and is unable to exert its toxic effect. This is the most common mechanism that fungi use to become resistant

2. **Detoxification or metabolism**: Metabolism within the fungal cell is one mechanism a disease pathogen uses to detoxify a foreign compound such as a fungicide. A fungus with the ability to quickly degrade a fungicide can potentially inactivate it before it can reach its site of action.

3. **Removal:** A fungal cell may rapidly export the fungicide before it can reach the target site of action.

4. **Reduced uptake of fungicide**: The resistant pathogen simply absorbs the fungicide much more slowly than the susceptible.

Resistance Management

There are several ways to retard the development of resistance.These include:

1. **Tank mix with a fungicide with a different mode of action**. Mancozeb or chlorothalonil can be tank mixed effectively with benzimidazole or phenylamide fungicides.
2. **Apply a limited number of applications in a block at a critical period in the pathogen disease cycle**. A different mode of action should be used at other less critical times in the disease cycle, so as to minimize the exposure of the "at risk" fungicide. This has been recommended with some of the strobilurins.
3. **Alternate applications between or among two or more classes of fungicides with different modes of action**. This is a good strategy for resistance management of **triphenyltin** hydroxide, the sterol inhibitors, the dicarboximides and the strobilurins. Although the sterol

inhibitors and the phenylamides have some post-infection activity, they are best used in a preventive manner, which reduces the likelihood that resistance will develop.

4. **Limit the number of applications of an "at risk" fungicide per year**. This has been done with the phenylamide fungicides, the sterol inhibitors, and the strobilurins. Use of these fungicides may be restricted to the most critical parts of the season.
5. **Avoid reduced rates of fungicides.** These reduced rates may facilitate the development of resistance in fungi.
6. Do not use phenylamides as soil treatments against airborne pathogens.

CHAPTER - 38

Methods of Application of Fungicides

Proper selection of a fungicide and its application at the correct dose and the proper time are highly essential for the management of plant diseases. The basic requirement of an application method is that it delivers the fungicide to the site where the active compound will prevent the fungus damaging the plant. The fungicidal application varies according to the nature of the host part diseased and nature of survival and spread of the pathogen. The method which are commonly adopted in the application of the fungicides are discussed

1. Foliar or vegetative application
2. Soil application
3. Seed treatment

FOLIAR OR VEGETATIVE APPLICATION

Applying chemicals on the stem, leaves, flowers and fruits is called **foliar** or **vegetative** application. Foliar application is carried out in the form of **spray**, dust or paste.

a. Spraying

This is the most commonly followed method. Spraying of fungicides is done on leaves, stems and fruits. Formulations available in **wettable powder**, **solution** or **emulsified form** are used for spraying. The amount of spray solution required for a hectare will depend on the nature of crops to be treated. For trees and shrubs, more amount of spray solution is required than in the case of ground crops. Depending on the volume of fluid used for coverage, the sprays are categorized into high volume, medium volume, low volume, very high volume and ultra low volume. The different equipments used for spray application are: foot-operated sprayer, rocking sprayer, knapsack sprayer, motorised knapsack sprayer (Power sprayer), tractor mounted sprayer, mist blower and aircraft or helicopter (aerial spray). Generally, these chemicals are dissolved in water and sprayed using a pressure pump. Spraying of chemicals is more prevalent for controlling fungal diseases of foliage.

b. Dusting

Dusts are applied to leaves, stems and fruits of plants. It is used during **wet weather** which favours sticking of the chemical on the plant surface. Dry powders are used for covering host surface. The equipments employed for the dusting operation are: bellow duster, rotary duster, motorised knapsack duster and aircraft (aerial application).

c. Pasting and painting

Chemicals are occasionally mixed with water, alcohol, or other carriers and applied as a paint on injured surface or parts of the plant. When trees are pruned, application of paste or paint is necessary. For example, Bordeaux mixture can be made into a paint or slurry with linseed oil or water and can be applied to the cut portions of the trees.

SOIL TREATMENT

The aim of soil treatment with chemical is to eradicate or reduce plant pathogen population which is harboured in the soil. But the complete eradication of pathogen from soil is not feasible because of degradation of chemicals by physical, chemical and biological means. The soil treatment can be done by drenching of soil with solution or emulsion, and broadcasting of dusted granules.

a. Drenching

Chemicals mainly fungicides are mixed with water at the same concentration as for foliar spraying i.e. 0.01 to 0.03 per cent. The solution is applied to the soil surface either before or after planting. The sprinkled material should reach the depth of at least **10-15 cm**. This method is followed for controlling damping off, root rots, seedling blight or infection at the ground level.

b. Broadcasting of dusted granules

Sometimes non-volatile fungicides mixed with soil or fertilizer are scattered with hands as uniformly as possible over the field. They are mixed with the soil up to plough sole in depth. **i.e.** up to 6 inches by light ploughing or harrowing. This method is too expensive, since it requires a large quantity of chemicals.

c. Furrow application

The chemicals are applied in the furrows in the form of **dusts** and **granules**. This method is possible only in crop plants which are in furrows, such as, potato and sugarcane.

d. Fumigation

Application of certain chemicals to the soils can control fungi and nematodes. Such chemicals produce **a gas** that distributes itself through soil and are called **volatile** chemicals. By the release of gas, they kill the larvae of nematodes and other pathogens present in the soil. Applications of these highly toxic volatile substances is recommended some weeks before actual planting of crops. Methyle bromide, ethylene dibromide (EDB) and ED/CT mixture are examples of fumigants. The depth of application is maintained at 15-20 cm. A thin polythene sheet is required to confine the gas to the soil. This method is usually restricted to small areas.

e. Chemigation

In this method, the fungicides are directly mixed in the irrigation water. It is normally adopted using sprinkler or drip irrigation system.

SEED TREATMENT

The concept of seed treatment is the use and application of biological and chemical agents that control or contain primary soil and seed borne infestation of insect pests and diseases which otherwise causes considerable economic loss to crop production or productivity. Seed treatment is definitely a more safe and judicious use of agrochemicals. Treatment of seed results in good establishment of healthy plants leading to better yield. There are various types of seed treatment and broadly they may be divided into three categories (a) Mechanical, (b) Chemical and (c) Physical.

A. Mechanical Method

Some pathogen when attack the seeds, there may be alteration in size, shape and weight of seeds by which it is possible to detect the infected seeds and separate them from the healthy ones. In the case of ergot diseases of bajra, rye, sorghum, the fungal sclerotia are usually larger in size and lighter than healthy grains. So by sieving or flotation, the infected grains may be easily separated. Such mechanical separation eliminates the infected materials to a larger extent. Eg. Removal of ergot in sorghum seeds. Dissolve 2kg of common salt in 10 litres of water (20% solution). Drop the seeds into the salt solution and stir well. Remove the ergot affected seeds and sclerotia which float on the surface. Wash the seeds in fresh water 2 or 3 times to remove the salts on the seeds. Dry the seeds in shade and use for sowing. This method is also highly useful to separate infected grains in the case of 'tundu' disease of wheat.

B. Chemical methods

Using fungicides on seed is one of the most efficient and economical methods of chemical disease control. On the basis of their tenacity and action, the seed dressing chemicals may be grouped as (i) **Seed disinfectant**, are those which destroy the pathogen that has already infected the seed and established itself in the tissues. (ii) **Seed disinfestants**, which kill or inactivate the fungus or bacterium present on the seed but do not remain active for long after the seed has been planted and (iii) **Seed protectants**, which disinfect the seed surface and stick to the seed surface for sometime after the seed has been sown, thus giving temporary protection to the young seedlings against soil borne fungi. Now, the systemic fungicides are impregnated into the seeds to eliminate the deep seated infection in the seeds. The seed dressing chemicals may be applied by (i) Dry treatment (ii) Wet treatment and (iii) Slurry.

(i) Dry seed treatment

In this method, the fungicide adheres in a fine from on the surface of the seeds. A calculated quantity of fungicide is applied and mixed with seed using machinery specially designed for the purpose. The fungicides may be treated with the seeds of small lots using simple Seed treating drum or of large seed lots at seed processing plants using Grain treating machines. Normally in field level, dry seed treatment is carried out in dry rotary seed treating drums which ensure proper coating of the chemical on the surface of seeds. Eg. Dry seed treatment in paddy. Mix a required amount of fungicide with required quantity of seeds in a seed treating drum or polythene lined gunny bags, so as to provide uniform coating of the fungicide over the seeds. Treat the seeds atleast 24 hours prior to soaking for sprouting. Any one of the following chemical may be used for treatment at the rate of 2g/kg : Thiram or Captan or Carboxin or Tricyclazole. In addition, the dry dressing method is also used in pulses, cotton and oil seeds with the antagonistic fungus like *Trichoderma viride* by mixing the formulation at the rate of 4g/kg of the seed.

(ii) Wet seed treatment

This method involves preparing fungicide suspension in water, often at field rates and then dipping the seeds or seedlings or propagative materials for a specified time. The seeds cannot be stored and the treatment has to be done before sowing. This treatment is usually applied for treating vegetatively propagative materials like cuttings, corms, tubers, setts, rhizomes, bulbs etc., which are not amenable to dry or slurry treatment.

a. Seed Soaking

Seed soaking is essential for certain crops. Seeds treated by these methods have to be properly dried after treatment. The fungicide adheres as a thin film over the seed surface which gives protection against invasion by soil-borne pathogens. Eg. Seed dip treatment in Wheat. Prepare 0.2% of carboxin solution (2g/litre of water) and soak the seeds for 6 hours. Drain the solution and dry the seeds properly before sowing. This effectively eliminates the loose smut pathogen, *Ustilago tritici*. Eg. Seed dip treatment in paddy. Prepare the fungicidal solution by mixing any of the fungicides viz., carbendazim or tricyclazole at the rate of 2g/litre of water and soak the seeds in the solution for 2 hrs. Drain the solution and keep the seeds for sprouting.

b. Seedling Dip / Root Dip

The seedlings of vegetables and fruits are normally dipped in 0.1% carbendazin or 0.25% copper oxychloride solution for 5 minutes to protect against seedling blight and rots.

c. Rhizome Dip

The rhizomes of ginger, cardamom, and turmeric are treated with 0.1% emisan solution for 20 minutes to eliminate rot causing pathogen present in the soil.

d. Sett Dip / Sucker Dip

The sets of sugarcane and tapioca are dipped in 0.1% emisan solution for 30 minutes. The suckers of pine apple may also be treated by this method to protect from soil borne diseases.

(iii) Slurry treatment (Seed peletting)

In this method, chemical is applied in the form of a thin paste (active material is dissolved in small quantity of water). The required quantity of the fungicide slurry is mixed with the specified quantity of the seed so that during the process of treatment slurry gets deposited on the surface of seeds in the form of a thin paste which later dries up. Almost all the seed processing units have slurry treaters. In these, slurry treaters, the requisite quantity of fungicides slurry is mixed with specified quantity of seed before the seed lot is bagged. The slurry treatment is more efficient than the rotary seed dressers. Eg. Seed pelleting in ragi. Mix 2.5g of carbendazim in 40 ml of water and add 0.5g of gum to the fungicidal solution. Add 2 kg of seeds to this solution and mix thoroughly to ensure a uniform coating of the fungicide over the seed. Dry the seeds under the shade. Treat the seeds 24 hrs prior to sowing.

(iv) Special method of seed treatment

Seed biopriming: Treating of seeds with biocontrol agents and then incubating under warm and moist conditions until just prior to emergence of radical is reffered as **bioprimming**. This technique has potential advantages over simple coating of seeds as it results in rapid and uniform seedling emergence. *Trichoderma* conidia germinate on the seed surface and form a layer around bioprimed seeds. Such seeds tolerate adverse various soil conditions better. Biopriming could also reduce the amount of biocontrol agents that is applied to the seed.

Procedure of Seed Biopriming

- Pre soak the seeds in water for 28h.
- Mix the formulated product of *Trichoderma* with the pre-soaked seeds at the rate of 10 g/kg of seed.
- Put the treated seeds as heap.
- Cover the heap with moist jute sac to maintain high humidity.
- Incubate the seeds under high humidity for about 24 h at approximately 25-32^{0}C.
- Bioagents adhered to the seeds grows on the seed surface under moist conditions to form a protective layer all around the seed coat.
- Sow the seeds in nursery beds
- The seeds that bio-primed with bioagents provide protection against seed and soil borne plant pathogens, improving germination and seedling growth.

CHAPTER - 39

Application of Biotechnology in Plant Disease Management

Plant diseases are a threat to world agriculture. Significant yield losses due to the attack of pathogen occur in most of the agricultural and horticultural crop species. More than 70% of all major crop diseases are caused by fungi . Plant diseases are usually handled with applications of chemicals. For some diseases, chemical control is very effective; but it is often non-specific in its effects, killing beneficial organisms as well as pathogens. Chemical control may have undesirable effects on health, safety and cause environmental risks. A promising method for protecting plants against diseases is constructing and employing pathogen-resistant cultivars. Although a number of resistant cultivars have been developed through breeding programs, these cultivars become obsolete in a short time due to the rapid evolution of the phytopathogens and the emergence of virulent forms capable to overcome the plant resistance. Breeders are often confronted with the issue of using a limited number of plants in their breeding programs, undesirable traits transferred together with the valuable resistance genes, and, in recent years, also with the depletion of potential gene sources. Control of diseases is a subject of great interest for biotechnologists. The most significant development in the area of varietal development for disease resistance is the use of the techniques of gene isolation and genetic transformation to develop transgenic resistance to fungal, bacterial and viral diseases. Improvements in genetic transformation technology have allowed the genetic modification of almost all important food crops like rice, wheat, maize, mustard, pulses and fruits. Genetic engineering technology has proved to be beneficial in managing viral and bacterial diseases in plants. The advances in gene engineering technologies and the understanding of the molecular nature of plant protection mechanisms have provided means for developing principally new strategies of plant disease control, in addition to the traditional approaches based on employing chemicals or classical breeding schemes. Biotechnology will enhance our understanding of the mechanisms that control plant's ability to recognize and defend itself against disease caused by fungi. The integration of biotechnology with traditional agricultural practices will be the backbone for sustainable agriculture.

DEFINITION

Biotechnology - Bio means life and technology means the application of knowledge for practical use *i.e.*, the use of living organisms to make or improve a product.

Other Definitions for the Term Biotechnology

- The use of living organisms to solve problems or make useful products.
- The use of cells and biological molecules to solve problems or make useful products. Biological molecules include DNA, RNA and proteins.
- The commercial application of living organisms or their products, which involves the deliberate manipulation of their DNA molecules.
- Make a living cell to perform a specific task in a predictable and controllable way.

In modern terms "**biotechnology** is defined as the manipulation, genetic modification and multiplication of living organisms through novel technologies, such as **tissue culture** and **genetic engineering**, resulting in the production of improved or new organisms and products that can be used in a variety of ways.

Plant Biotechnology /Agricultural Biotechnology

Plant biotechnology is a precise process in which special techniques are used to develop molecular- and cellular-based technologies to improve plant productivity, quality and health; to improve the quality of plant products; or to prevent, reduce or eliminate constraints to plant productivity caused by biotic and abiotic stresses . In Nutshell it's the manipulation of plants for the benefit of mankind

Technologies Applied in Plant Biotechnology

Various technologies applied in plant biotechnology include

- Genetic engineering/ recombinant DNA technology
- Tissue culture
- Molecular pathology – MAS

GENETIC ENGINEERING

Genetic engineering allows the genetic modification of a plant by adding new traits through recombinant DNA technology. Genetic engineering makes possible the incorporation a single gene or a combination of genes into the plant genome in order to confer traits such as disease resistance, herbicide tolerance, tolerance to salt, drought and cold, increased productivity and increased nutritional value. The technology combines molecular biology, microbiology, tissue culture, cell transformation, plant selection and breeding techniques. Genetic engineering allow the development of genetically altered plants with defined traits and valuable properties without altering other desirable characteristics of the recipients. For instance genetic engineering is of special interest for the stable insertion of disease resistance genes into the genome of susceptible commercial varieties as method to protect such plants from phytopathogenic pathogens.

Methods for Gene Transfer

The uptake of foreign DNA or the recombinant DNA by cells is called **gene transfer** or transformation. Conventionally, the gene transfer necessary for crop improvement is obtained through sexual and vegetative propagation. However, biotechnological approaches like somaclonal variation, protoplast fusion etc. has successfully speeded up the process of generating genetic variation and introgression of foreign genes. The most potential biotechnological approach for transferring recombinant DNA is based on genetic engineering which involves various techniques for gene transfer. The transferred gene is called **transgene** and the plants that carry these stably integrated transgenes are called **transgenic plants**.

Various gene transfer techniques used are grouped into two broad categories:

- Direct gene transfer
- Indirect gene transfer (Agrobacterium mediated)

(i) Direct Gene Transfer

It is a process where no vector is involved and can be applied to any species or genotype. The methods for direct gene transfer are further classified into two classes:-Physical where usually naked DNA is directly transferred. Therefore, also referred to as DNA mediated gene transfer. The various physical methods for gene transfer are -

1. Electroporation: is a process where the cells are exposed to electrical impulses of high voltage to reversibly make cell membranes permeable for uptake of DNA. Electroporation has been used extensively for transformation of protoplasts. Recently, transformation of intact plant cells of sugarbeet and rice has been successfully reported. This method is convenient, simple and quick. However, electroporation cannot be applied to all the tissues, cell viability drops due to electric shock. Also, regeneration of plants from protoplasts is still difficult.

2. Particle bombardment: This is a relatively recent development but is widely used and is effective in introduction of DNA into plant cells. The technique involves coating 1μm diameter particles of tungsten or gold known as **microprojectiles** with DNA, which are then accelerated to high speed using a pulse of high pressure helium into an evacuated chamber containing the target tissues. These DNA coated particles penetrate through the cell wall releasing DNA from particles which can express transiently or get integrated into nuclear genome of that cell. With appropriate tissue culture and selection, transgenic plants can be regenerated. Particle bombardment has been used for transformation of monocotyledonous crop plants such as maize, rice, wheat etc.

3. Micro Injection: The plasmid DNA can also be delivered into host cells by mechanical means i.e. by microscopic needles also called **micro-injections**. This method does not have host range limitations. This method can be effectively used with different crop plants. However, in this method also regeneration from protoplasts is a basic requirement. Unfortunately, all crops do not regenerated from protoplasts. Hence, this method also has limited applications. Direct DNA transfer method does not require specialized equipment and is therefore, relatively inexpensive. However, it is more tedious than ballistic approach, as it requires efficient protoplast isolation and culture procedures which restrict its application.

4. Chemical mediated gene transfer : Direct DNA uptake by protoplasts can be stimulated by chemicals like polyethylene glycol (PEG). The technique is so efficient that virtually every protoplast system has proven transformable. PEG is also used to stimulate the uptake of liposomes and to improve the efficiency of electroporation. PEG at high concentration (15-25%) will precipitate ionic macromolecules such as DNA and stimulate their uptake by endocytosis without any gross damage to protoplasts. This is followed by cell wall formation and initiation of cell division. These cells can now be plated at low density on selection medium. Initial studies using the above method were restricted to *Petunia* and *Nicotiana*. However, other plant systems (rice, maize, etc.) were also successfully used later.

(ii) Indirect gene transfer (Vector-mediated)

The most commonly used vectors for gene transfer in higher plants are based on tumour inducing mechanism of the soil bacterium *Agrobacterium tumefaciens*, which is the causal organism for crown gall disease, A closely related species A. *rhizogenes* causes hairy root disease. Among the various vectors used in plant transformation, the Ti plasmid of *Agrobacterium tumefaciens* has been widely used. This bacterium is known as **"natural genetic engineer"** of plants because these bacteria have natural ability to transfer T-DNA of their plasmids into plant genome upon infection of cells at the wound site and cause an unorganized growth of a cell mass known as crown gall. Ti-plasmids are used as gene vectors for delivering useful foreign genes into target plant cells and tissues. The foreign gene is cloned in the T-DNA region of Ti-plasmid in place of unwanted sequences. To transform plants, leaf discs (in case of dicots) or embryogenic callus (in case of monocots) are collected and infected with *Agrobacterium* carrying recombinant disarmed Ti-plasmid vector. The infected tissue is then cultured (co-cultivation) on shoot regeneration medium for 2-3 days during which time the transfer of T-DNA along with foreign genes takes place. After this, the transformed tissues (leaf discs/calli) are transferred onto selection cum plant regeneration medium supplemented with usually lethal concentration of an antibiotic to selectively eliminate non-transformed tissues. After 3-5 weeks, the regenerated shoots (from leaf discs) are transferred to root-inducing medium, and after another 3-4 weeks, complete plants are transferred to soil following the hardening (acclimatization) of regenerated plants. The molecular techniques like PCR and southern hybridization are used to detect the presence of foreign genes in the transgenic plants.

Agrobacterium infection (utilizing its plasmids as vectors) has been extensively utilized for transfer of foreign DNA into a number of **dicotyledonous species**. The only important species that have not responded well, are major seed legumes, even though transgenic soybean (Glycine max) plants have been obtained. The success in this approach for gene transfer has **resulted** from improvement in tissue culture technology. However, **monocotyledons** could not be successfully utilized for **Agrobacterium** mediated gene transfer except a solitary example of Asparagus. The reasons for this are not fully understood, because T -DNA transfer does occur at the cellular level. It is possible that the failure in monocots lies in the lack of wound response of monocotyledonous cells.

Development of Genetically Modified Plants to Control Fungi, Bacteria and Viruses

The development of genetically modified plants that are resistant to disease caused by fungi, bacteria and nematodes has lagged behind that of virus resistant crop plants. However, examples of transgenic plants with high levels of resistance to fungi, bacteria and nematodes have been recently reported. To develop crop varieties that are resistant to bacteria, fungi and nematodes, genetically modified plants have been engineered to express proteins that are either toxic to the pathogen, degrade cell walls, or are involved in the plant defense response to pathogen infection. Pathogen derived resistances has also been used an approach to develop transgenic plants resistant to bacteria and fungi. We will discuss some of the significant achievements made in the field of plant resistance against different plant pathogens.

Resistant against Viral Diseases

Among various pest and diseases , management of viral diseases is most problematic. Because here is no direct control for the viruses. Generally cultural management are adopted and pesticides are applied to manage the insect vectors, if any, so that the spread of the disease is checked. Number of virus resistant varieties developed through conventional breeding are few. Therefore, effort are on to develop more and more transgenic crops to give protection against viruses.Several approaches have been used to engineer plants for virus resistance which are as follows:

- Coat protein gene
- cDNA of satellite RNA
- Antisense RNA approach
- Ribozyme mediated protection

Coat protein gene

Coat protein (CP) mediated resistance is most popular method, which involves transfer of coat protein gene of a virus into the genome of its host plant. Thus, the presence of viral coat protein within plant confers resistance against the challenging virus. Generally, the nucleic acid confined by coat protein is infectious part of the virus. Initially it was thought that when the nucleic acid of a virus enters into a CP mediated transgenic plants, the already present viral coat proteins immediately encircle the challenging nucleic acid and thus the infection is checked. But at the present level of knowledge , it is understood that coat protein present in transgenic plants inhibits the uncoating of the challenging virus provided that at least 60 percent homology exist between amino acid sequence of transgenic coat protein and that of challenging virus. However, the actual mechanism is not well understood.Powell-Able et al. for the first time in 1986 showed that transgenic tobacco plants expressing the coat proetein gene of tobacco mosaic virus. (TMV) were resistant against some strain of TMV. Subsequently, transgenic were developed against alfalfa mosaic virus (ALMV) in alfalfa, cucumber mosaic virus (CMV) in cucumber , papaya ring spot virus (PRSV) in papaya.

cDNA of Satellite RNA

Several RNA viruses have small RNA molecules, called **satellites**, which depend on the viral genomes for their replication, but not essential for viral infections. In several cases, satellite viruses increase or reduce the severity of disease produced by the virus carrying it. The cDNA copies of satellites that decrease disease severity have been integrated into host genomes; expression of the satellites has been shown to reduce disease symptoms as well as viral accumulation under both green house and field conditions. For instance, tobacco plants expressing the satellites of cucumber mosaic virus(CMV) showed reduced disease symptoms when infected with CMV. Likewise, transgenic tomato, potato and pepper plants expressing the CMV satellite and grown in the field showed reduced disease symptoms and less virus accumulation than control plants when inoculated with CMV.

Antisense RNA mediated resistance

Antisense RNA can be produced by inverting a cDNA copy of an mRNA with respect to the promoter in an expression vector; this yields a full length complementary copy of the mRNA sequence. Fragements smaller than full length can also be effective. Antisense RNA molecules are thought to interact with mRNA molecules by base pairing to form double stranded RNA. Transgenic tobacco plants expressing antisense RNA of the CMV coat protein gene showed reduced virus accumulation, and prevention of systemic spread at low concentrations of CMV inoculum.

Ribozyme mediated protection

Ribozymes are DNA molecules that exhibit enzyme activities. The ribozymes used to generate virus resistance gene, in fact, hybrid RNA molecules consisting of tobacco ring spot virus satellite RNA endoribonuclease catalytic sequences linked to the antisense RNA of specific genes against which they are targeted. The strategies consists of

- producing a ribozyme specific to the target virus genome
- to produce cDNA of plants ribozyme and
- to integrate it into the host plant genome

Transgenic tobacco plants expressing ribozymes against TMV showed some resistance to TMV infection. Ribozymes may be useful in producing resistance to several viruses within a group where conserved sequence exist.

Table 33 : Genetic engineered crops that show enhanced resistance to viral pathogens

Gene	Stage of infection cycle	Mode of action plant	Virus	Transgenic
Coat protein	Uncoating	Competition of RNA	TMV	Tobacco
Movement protein	Transport	Interfere with transport	TMV, PVY	Potato, Tobacco
Replicase protein	Replication	Competition for enzyme		Tobacco, Potato
Viral protease	Replication	Polyprotein processing	PVY	Potato
Antisense RNA	Translation	Blocks viral RNA and prevent translation	PLRV	Tomato
Satellite RNA	Assembly	Competes for capsids	CMV	Tobacco
Ribozyme	Translation	Cleaves viral RNA	CEVd	Tomato

Resistance against Fungal Diseases

Plants are continuously being challenged by innumerable aspiring pathogens, as compared that occurrence of disease is a rare phenomenon. It is because of the inherent defense mechanism of the plants. PR proteins, chitinase, glucanase, antifungal proteins , phytoalexins etc. play key role to provide protection against defense mechanisms. Through transgenic expression of these substances in host plant resistant varieties could be developed. Expression of **chitinases** and **glucanases** are induced in host plants in response to pathogen attack to degrade the fungal cell wall . Successful examples may be seen in Table-34.

Table 34 : Genetic engineered crops that show enhanced resistance to fungal pathogens

Gene/Protein product	Source	Target pathogen	Transgenic plant
Chitinase	Bean	*Rhizoctonia solani*	Tobacco
Chitinase	*Serratia marcescens*	*Alternaria longiceps*	Tobacco
Chitinase	Rice	*Rhizoctonia solani*	Rice
Chitinase	Tobacco	*Rhizoctonia solani*	Tobacco
Ribosome inactivation protein (RIP) from barley	Barley	*Rhizoctonia solani*	Tobacco
Stilbene synthase from grapevine	Grapevine	*Botrytis cinerea*	Tobacco
Chitinase +Glucanase		*Cercospora nicotianae*	Tobacco
Petete		*nicotiana.*	
Osmotin	Tobacco	*Phytophthora infestans*	Potato
Â-1.3-endoglucanase	Soybean	*Botrytis cinerea*	

Gene that induce artificial cell death			
Barnase and barstar		*Phytophthora infestans*	Potato
Glucose oxidase	*Aspergillus niger*	*Phytophthora infestans*	Potato
Cryptogein	*Phytophthora cryptogea*	*Erysiphe cichoracearum* *Botrytis cinerea*	Tobacco
Nettle agglutinin		*Botrytis cinerea*	Tobacco

Resistance against Bacterial Diseases

Strategies for developing transgenic plants resistant to bacteria are as follows

- Production of antibacterial protein of non plant origin.
- Inhibition of bacterial pathogenicity factors
- Enhancement of natural plant defenses

Antibacterial proteins of non plant origin include **lytic peptides**, lysozymes, **glycoproteins** etc. Lytic peptides are small protein which form pores in the bacterial membranes eg. cercopin, attacins etc. Cercopins have been expressed in transgenic potato and tobacco and attacins in apple plants. Lysozymes are ubiquitous enzymes with specific hydrolytic activities directed against the bacterial cell wall peptidoglycan. Lysozyme genes have been expressed in potato and tobacco. Inhibition of bacterial toxins by cloning and expression of a gene whose product either inactivates or is insensitive to bacterial toxin has been successfully employed to develop transgenic tobacco and bean plants.Recently, transgenic sugarcane was developed against leaf scald disease. The pathogen *Xanthomonas albilineans* produces a toxin albicidin which inhibits chloroplast development. It has been reported that a transgens from bacteria *Pantoca dispersa* detoxifies albicidin. In transgenic potato expression of a lectinolytic enzymes of *Erwinia carotovora* makes the plant less susceptible of bacterial rot caused by *E. carotovora.*

Table 35 : Genetic engineered crops that show enhanced resistance to bacterial pathogens

Gene/protein	Origin	Target	Transgenic plant
Lysozyme	T_4 bacteriophage	*Erwinia carotovora*	Potato
Tabtoxin acetyle transferase	*Pseudomonas syringae pv. tabaci*	*Pseudomonas syringae*	Tobacco
Horothionin	Barley seeds	*Pseudomonas syringae pv. tabaci*	Tobacco
Bacterio-opsin	*Halobacterium halobium*	*Pseudomonas syringae pv. tabaci*	Tobacco
Glucose oxidase	*Aspergillus niger*	*Erwinia amylovora*	Potato
Pectate lyase	*Erwinia carotovora*	*Erwinia carotovora*	Potato
Albicidin detoxi-fying gene	*Pantoea dispersa*	*Xanthomonas albilineans*	Sugarcane
Glucose oxidase	*Aspergillus niger*	*Erwinia carotovora*	Potato

TISSUE CULTURE

In crop improvement programs for desirable resistance, a number of strategies are used to acquire the desired trait. One source of plants with improved disease resistance can be material that is recovered from plant tissue culture. Plant tissue culture refers to the *in vitro* cultivation of all plant parts including single cells, tissues, and organ under aseptic conditions. The term plant tissue culture encompasses several different types of culture. Some specific types of culture include meristem culture, embryo culture, callus culture and protoplast culture.

Meristem Culture

Meristem culture involves the removal of the meristem with one to two leaf primodia and subsequent *in vitro* culturing of this explants. Many plant pathogens do not survive well in the actively dividing tissue of the apical parts, so this method is used to rid plant material of pathogens especially viruses. Meristem tip culture in combination with culture indexing can be used to establish stock material of ornamental plants that are free of fungi and bacteria. Meristem or shoot tips are removed from green house grown plants and established in tissue culture. Systemic pathogens, if present, will grow out into the tissue culture medium. Those explants that remain free of fungi or bacteria are grown up, transferred to a certification green house, and indexed an additional two times for systemic pathogens. Plant lines that remain free of the pathogens are used for propagation. Meristem culture has been applied to ornamental plants such as geraniums, New Gunea impatiens, and double flowered impatiens and seed potatoes. In seed potatoes, the bacterium *Erwinia carotovora var. atroseptica* was eliminated with 50% success using meristem tip culture.

The meritem tip culture has also been used to rid many plant species of viruses because it exploits the erratic distribution of viruses within plants. The viral diseases in plants transfer easily and lower the quality and yield of the plants. It is very difficult to treat and cure the virus infected plants therefore the plant breeders are always interested in developing and growing virus free plants. In some crops like ornamental plants, it has become possible to produce virus free plants through tissue culture at the commercial level. This is done by regenerating plants from cultured tissues derived from

- Virus free plants.
- Meristems that are generally free of infection.
- In the elimination of the virus, the size of the meristem used in cultures play a very critical role because most of the viruses exist by establishing a gradient in plant tissues.
- The regeneration of virus-free plants through cultures is inversely proportional to the size of the meristem used.
- Meristems treated with heat shock (34-36°C) to inactivate the virus
- Callus, which is usually virus free like meristems.
- Chemical treatment of the media- attempts have been made to eradicate the viruses.
- From infected plants by treating the culture medium with chemicals e.g. addition of cytokinins suppressed the multiplication of certain viruses.

Among the culture techniques, **meristem-tip culture** is the most reliable method for virus and other pathogen elimination. Viruses have been eliminated from a number of economically important plant species, which has resulted in a significant increase in the yield and production e.g. potato virus X from potato, mosaic virus from cassava etc. Even though meristem culture is not used regularly to produce disease resistance , it does give a source of pathogen free planting material. This is a vital element in the management of plant diseases where chemical control of a pathogen during growing season is either not available or too costly. One disadvantage to meristem culture is that because the explants is so minute the culture often takes a comparatively long time to grow. This predicament can be eliminated in the case of some virus diseases by adding up thermotherapy or antiviral compounds to meristem culturing.

Embryo Rescue

Embryo rescue is used to make sure the survival of immature embryos when wide crosses are made between distantly related plants. The incompatibility between distantly related plants often results in breakdown of the endosperm, embryos can be rescued by growing them on artificial medium until the plant can be transported to soil. Wide crosses are often attempted to transfer disease resistant traits from wild species to cultivated species. **Embryo rescue** is being used to introduce fungal, bacterial and virus resistance traits into plants. Potato leaf roll virus (PLRV) is a serious pathogen, reducing potato yields in developing countries. *Solanum etuberosum* is a wild non tuber bearing potato which is resistant to PLRV. Using embryo rescue, this trait was successfully introduced into a tuber bearing *Solanum*. *Oryza minuta*, a wild rice species, is resistant to the fungal diseases rice blast and bacterial blight, two devastating diseases of rice worldwide. Crosses made with the cultivated rice *Oryza sativa* and *O. minuta* resulted in progeny that were resistant to bacterial blight(*Xanthomonas oryzae pv oryzae*) or rice blast (*Pyricularia oryzae*). Embryo rescue was indispensable to recover hybrids and progeny from the backcross to *O. sativa.* Other crops where interspecific hybridization between cultivated species and wild species has been successful due to embryo rescue include lettuce (*Lactuca sativa* and *Lactuca* spp.) and tomato (*Lycopersicon esculentum* and *L. peruviianum*). These wild relatives are resistant to many diseases of these crops and could be used as a source of resistance in breeding programs. *Lactuca* sp. is a source for downy mildew resistance and wild *L. peruviianum* used is resistant to tomato spotted wilt. Embryo rescue has also been used to recover plants after intergeneric crosses. Hybrids from a cross between *Eruca sativa* and *Brassica campestris* were saved using embryo rescue. *Eruca sativa* is a source for resistance to white rust caused by the fungus *Albugo candida.*

Hence, pathogen and pest resistance can be transferred from wild species through embryo rescue, when desirable traits are not found in breeding material but are found in other species. **Embryo rescue** may allow recovery of plant between species where crossing barrier exists due to sexual incompatibility.

Somaclonal Variation

During the tissue culture process, genetic variability can occur. This variability is called **somaclonal variability**. based on the term somaclones which is used in reference to regenerated plants. The variability may arise from preexisting mutations in the cells of the explants, however, a large part of the variation is induced during tissue culture process. There have been numerous reports on somaclonal variation, some of which have been useful in crop improvement and some which have not. One application of somaclonal variants has been a source of disease resistant. The earliest report of somaclonal variation resulting in disease resistant material was in sugarcane. From the first report on disease resistant sugar cane until now, there are many examples of improved disease resistance in various crops via somaclonal variation. Table-36 contains some examples of disease resistant plants produced from somaclonal variation.

Table 36 : Disease resistant plants from somaclonal variation

Sl. No	Crop	Pathogen
1.	Potato	*Verticillium dahlia*
2.	Tomato	*Pseudomonas solanacearum Alternaria solani*
3.	Sugarcane	*Sugar cane mosaic virus*
4.	Apple	*Erwinia amylovora*
5.	Rice	*Xanthomonas oryzae*
6.	Poplar	*Septoria musiva*
7.	Straberry	*Fusarium oxysporum f sp.fragariae*

Somaclonal variation can be source of resistance in crops where genes of resistance are not available or are difficult to introgress in a breeding program. However, along with this improved resistance, other undesirable character may be introduced.

Protoplast Fusion

Protoplast means a plant cells lacking a cell wall. Proptoplasts are isolated by enzymatic degradation of the cell wall with cellulases, pectinases, and hemicellulases. The integrity of the protoplasts is maintained by inclusion of an osmoticum in the isolation method. If cultured in the appropriate medium, these protoplasts from new cell walls, then cell colonies, and possibly go on to regenerate plantlets. Beside from culturing the protoplasts for plant regeneration, the protoplasts can be fused, during which there is a mixing of cytoplasm. As a result of mixing , the nuclei may remain separate or they may fuse, resulting in what referred to as **somatic hybrids**. In some instances one nucleus completely disappears, but the cytoplasm remain mixed. This fusion product is referred to s **cybrid**.

The main advantage of protoplast fusion is that it provides a possible method of hybridization between two parents where crossing barrier may exist. These hybridization may be interspecific, intraspecific , or intergeneric. However, somatic hybrid that result need to be evaluated for morphological characteristic and fertility. Protoplast fusion is one of the methods that can be used to circumvent problems in introgressing disease resistance genes. Table-37 contains a list of some of the crops where protoplast fusion was used to transfer disease resistance.

Table 37 : Disease resistant plant from protoplast fusion

Sl.No	Species used for fusion	Disease
1.	*Brassica oleracea*	Club rot, Black rot
2.	*Brassica nigra*	Club root
3.	*Lactuca sativa*	Downy mildew
4.	*Solanum tuberosum*	Bacterial soft rot

All the tissue culture methods discussed can be used to alleviate the use of chemicals to control diseases. Tissue culture may help to reduce the amount of pesticides needed to control diseases by generating disease free plant through meristem culture, creating new sources of disease resistance as a result of somaclonal variation.

MOLECULAR PATHOLOGY

Marker : Easily identifiable traits are referred to as markers or marker traits. These markers are of three types.

Morphological markers: These are related to size, shape, color and surface of various plant parts.

Biochemical marker- Such markers are related to variations in proteins structure. for example, isozymes and storage proteins.

DNA-based and/or moleculars marker - refes to as unique sequence of nucleotides found on a strand of DNA.

Important Properties of Ideal Markers

- Abundant in number
- Polymorphic
- Easy recognition of all possible phenotypes (homo and heterozygotes) from all different alleles
- Demonstrates measurable differences in expression between trait types and/or gene of interest alleles, early in the development of the organism
- Has no effect on the trait of interest that varies depending on the allele at the marker loci
- Low or null interaction among the markers allowing the use of many at the same time in a segregating population.

Demerits of Morphological Markers

Morphological markers are associated with several general deficits that reduce their usefulness including:

- the delay of marker expression until late into the development of the organism
- dominance
- deleterious effects
- pleiotropy
- confounding effects of genes unrelated to the gene or trait of interest but which also affect the morphological marker (epistasis)
- rare polymorphism
- frequent confounding effects of environmental factors which affect the morphological characteristics of the organism.

To avoid problems specific to morphological markers, the DNA-based markers have been developed. They are highly polymorphic, simple inheritance (often codominant), abundantly occur throughout the genome, easy and fast to detect, minimum pleiotropic effect and detection is not dependent on the developmental stage of the organism. Numerous markers have been mapped to different chromosomes in several crops including rice, wheat, maize, soybean and several others. Those markers have been used in diversity analysis, parentage detection, DNA fingerprinting, and prediction of hybrid performance. Molecular markers are useful in indirect selection processes, enabling manual selection of individuals for further propagation.

Types of DNA Marker

There are several types of DNA markers . The DNA markers which are used in plant pathology is given below

1. **Hybridization based markers:**
   - Random Fragment Length Polymorphism (RFLP)
2. **PCB Based Markers:**
   - Random Amplified Polymorphic DNA (RAPD)
   - Microsatellites (SSR)
   - Amplified Fragemnt Length Polymorphism (AFLP)
3. **Sequencing –Based Markers**
   - Singlc Nuclcotide Polymorphism (SNPs)
   - Internal Transcribed Spacer (ITSs)

Table 38 : Comparison of the five most widely used DNA markers in plant pathology

Particulars	RFLP	RAPD	AFLP	SSR	SNP
DNA required (μg)	10	0.02	0.5-1.0	0.05	0.05
Quantity of DNA	High	High	Moderate	Moderate	High
PCR based	No	Yes	Yes	Yes	Yes
Number of polymorphism loci analysed	1-3	1.5-50	20-100	1-3	1.0
Prior information needed	Yes	No	No	Yes	Yes
Ease of use and development	Not easy	Easy	Easy	Easy	Easy
Reproducibility	High	Unreliable	High	High	High
Cost analysis	High	Low	Moderate	Low	Low
Automation	Low	Moderate	Moderate	High	High
Accuracy	Very High	Very low	Medium	High	Very High
Radioactive detection	Usually	Yes	No	No	Yes

Application of Molecular Markers in Plant Pathogens Genomic Analysis

1. Mapping and Tagging of genes
2. Plant pathogen species or strain identification.
3. Genetic structure
4. Polymorphism and genetic diversity.
5. Taxonomy and phylogeny.

Marker Assisted Selection (MAS)

Marker assisted selection (MAS) is **indirect selection process** where a trait of interest (i.e. productivity, disease resistance, abiotic stress tolerance, and/or quality) is selected not based on the trait itself but on a marker (morphological, biochemical or one based on DNA/RNA variation) linked to it. For example if MAS is being used to select individuals with a disease, the level of disease is not quantified but rather a marker allele which is linked with disease is used to determine disease presence. The assumption is that linked allele associates with the gene and/or quantitative trait locus (QTL) of interest. MAS can be useful for traits that are difficult to measure, exhibit low heritability, and/or are expressed late in development.

Steps in MAS

The marker aided selection consists of five important steps

1. Selection of parents

- Parents with contrasting characters or divergent origin should be chosen.
- For selection of parents, we have to screen germplasm and select parents with distinct DNA.
- The parents that are used for MAS should be pure (homozygous).
- In self pollinated species, plants are usually **homozygous**. In cross pollinated species, **inbred lines** are used as parents.

2. Development of breeding populations

- This is the second step for application of marker aided selection.
- The selected parents are crossed to obtain F_1 plants.
- F_1 plants between two purelines or inbreed lines are homogenous but are heterozygous for all the RFLPs of two parents involved in the F_1.
- The F_2 progeny is required for the study of segregation pattern of RFLPs.
- Generally 50-100 F_2 plants are sufficient for the study of segregation of RFLP markers.

3. Isolation of DNA

- The third step is isolation of DNA from breeding population.
- The DNA is isolated from each plant of F_2 population.
- The isolated DNA is digested with specific restriction enzyme to obtain fragments of DNA.
- The DNA fragments of different size are separated by subjecting the digested DNA to agarose gel electrophoresis.
- The gel is stained with ethilidium bromide and the variation in DNA fragments can be viewed in the ultraviolet light.
- The nuclear DNA of higher plants, when digested with specific restriction enzymes, produces millions of fragments in a continuous range of sizes.

- The DNA of chloroplasts, when digested with specific enzyme, produces about 40 fragments of different sizes.

4. Scoring RFLPs

- The polymorphism in RFLPs between the parents and their involvement in the recombinants in F_2 population is determined by using **DNA probes**.
- The labeled probes are used to find out the fragements having similarity.
- The probe will hybridize only with those segments which are complementary in nature.
- Generally ^{32}**P** is used for radioactive labeling of DNA probe.
- Now, non radioactive probe labeling techniques are alos available.
- In this way RFLPs are determined.

5. Correlation with morphological traits

- The DNA marker are correlated with morphological markers and the indirect selection through molecular markers is confirmed.
- Once the correlation of molecular markers is established with morphological markers, MAS can be effectively used for genetic improvement of various economic traits.

Practical Achievements

MAS has been mainly sued for developing disease resistant varieties in different crops (Table-39). In rice MAS has been successfully used for developing varieties resistant to bacterial blight and blast. For bacterial blight resistance four genes (Xa_4 Xa_5 Xa_{13} $Xa_{21)}$ have been pyramided using STS markers. The pyramided lines showed higher level of resistance to bacterial blight pathogen. In Indonesia, two bacterial blight resistant varieties of rice viz. Angke and Conde have been released through MAS. For blast resistance, three genes (Pi1, Piz 5 and Pita) have been pyramided in a susceptible rice variety Co39 using RFLP and PCR based markers. In soybean nematode resistant lines have been developed through SSR markers.

Table 39 : Disease resistant character being used for MAS in different crops

Crop	Disease Resistance
Rice	Bacterial blight, Blast, Rice tungro virus
Maize	Northern corn blight
Wheat	Leaf rust, Powdery mildew, Loose smut
Soybean	Mosaic virus, Cyst nematode
Pea	Powdery mildew, *Fusarium* wilt
Tomato	Bacterial wilt, Black mold, Yellow leaf curl virus
Potato	Late blight, Potato virus X
Barley	Powdery mildew, Stripe rust
Sunflower	Downy mildew

CHAPTER - 40

Integrated Disease Management

The over emphasis on the use of chemical pesticides and their improper use by the farmers has led to several complications such as residue in food, feed, fodder, development of resistance, resurgence, secondary outbreak, etc. and above all, environmental pollution, leading to a condition known as **Pesticide Treadmill** characterized by the need to spray ever greater quantities of chemical pesticides. In 1962, **Rachel Carson** in her book **'Silent Spring'** aroused worldwide concern about the excessive use of pesticides, which eventually led to the concept of Integrated Pest/Disease Management as an environmentally sound alternative to the sole use of chemicals.

The IDM Concept

In disease management, all the alternate control measures like cultural, biological, mechanical, resistant varieties, physical etc, are utilized in an integrated manner in order to maintain the disease below economic injury level. If the disease increases and reaches the economic threshold level, pesticides are used to bring the disease down. This is concept of an **Integrated Disease Management** in which minimum pesticides are used keeping in view of agro-ecosystem. Actually, we do not go for 100 percent control in disease management rather the disease is allowed below which can be tolerated i.e economic threshold. This also provides opportunity for bioagent to survive, managing upon the diseases keeping them at certain equilibrium level. Thus, the Integrated Disease Management concept aims at managing the disease through all the available tactics with favorable economic, social and ecological consequences.

What is IDM

IDM is a knowledge intensive and farmer based management approach that encourages natural control of disease problems and preventing pathogens from reaching economically damaging levels. IDM module is an appropriate technique, such as enhancing natural enemies, planting disease resistant crops, adopting cultural management and as a last resort, using pesticide judiciously to suppress rather than eliminate the population of target pathogens.

Important Features of IDM

The following are some of the important features of IDM

- IDM is an ecologically sound alternative to chemical disease management. It has also been shown to be economically viable and socially acceptable strategy for disease control for the farmers of our country.
- IDM is consistent with the needs of our agriculture. It provides food security by preventing and reducing crop losses; promotes self reliance by farmer participatory approach thereby, building on their understanding of local agro ecology; contributes to poverty alleviation by focusing on small and marginal farmers and protects environment and health by chemical inputs and conserving bio-diversity.
- The technologies developed have not yet exploited at the level to reach the small and marginal farmers of the country to make IDM as an effective alternative to use of chemical pesticides. Even though successful non chemical methods for the control of crop diseases have been developed, the transfer of this technology to the farmers and extension workers has been rather low. The coverage under IDM at present is estimated to be less than 10 percent of the total cultivable area in the country.
- The wide scale adoption of IDM faces a number of problems. These include the ready availability of appropriate technology and inputs, poor infrastructure and lack of adequate training and education.
- Availability of IDM technology alone is no guarantee that it will prove effective in the field. A top down technology driven approach is unlikely to succeed under Indian conditions .There is therefore, a need for farmers participation, including women, who play a dominant role in both seed selection and crop management

History

Benett(1956) coin the Phrase integrated control

Geier and Clark (1961) used the term Integrated pest management

Goals of IDM

The main goals of an integrated plant disease management programme are to:

- Eliminate or reduce the initial inoculums
- Reduce the effectiveness of initial inoculums
- Increase the resistance of the host
- Delay the onset of the disease
- Slow the secondary cycles.

Objective of IDM

Varied IDM objective are:

- It contributes significantly in the reduction in potential hazards to environment and people health.
- It provides improved control by conservation of natural enemies and employing traditional method.
- It helps in the production of improved quality produce.
- It help to reduce the cost of plant protection and thus render crop protection an economic venture.
- It helps in improvement on water and soil quality.
- It reduces farmers and consumer risk.
- It facilitates better pesticide management.

Why should we adopt IDM

- To avoid the collapse of control system based on single technology.
- To avoid disease control to enter exploitation, crisis and disaster phage.

1. **Explotation phage**: The disease control programme is dependent solely on chemical pesticides which are exploited to the maximum resulting in high yield.
2. **Crisis phage**: After many years of in exploitation phage and heavy use of pesticides, resistance, pathogen resurgence and out break of secondary diseases occur which increases the production cost.
3. **Disaster phage**: The use of pesticide increases the cost of production to the point where crop could no longer be grown profitably. High residue of pesticide in the food makes the produce unacceptable to consumers.

Framework of IDM strategy

IDM is an holistic guiding principle that encompasses all the activities from selection of crop to the harvest and storage. Broadly speaking, however , IDM strategies are based on thee main pillars.

1. Prevention.
2. Monitoring.
3. Intervention.

Most of the IDM activities emphasize heavily on the preventive measures. The first line of defense against disease is prevention through the use of agronomical practices or cultural practices which are unfavorable for the development of disease problems. Regular and sound monitoring of pathogen activity is essential for decisions in IDM. Selected control measures to check pathogens are to be taken at economic threshold level **(ETL)** or action threshold level **(ATL)**. IDM strives to **optimizes** rather than maximize pathogen control effects.

Economic injury level: It is the lowest disease index that will cause economic damage.

Economic Threshold level: It is the disease index at which control measures should be applied to prevent an increasing disease from reaching the economic injury level.

Tools of IDM

Monitoring of Pathogens: Monitoring is a vital component of an effective IPM program. Monitoring can be direct (looking for the pathogen or disease) or indirect (recording environmental conditions which affect disease development). Financial considerations weigh heavily in the choice of monitoring practice. Direct monitoring of diseases can be based on symptoms or signs of the pathogen. Identification of pathogens is commonly difficult, because pathogens generally are microscopic and can be detected typically after the disease process has begun. Most monitoring is actually for disease symptoms, with the control strategy aimed at reducing further spread. Even when visible symptoms are evident, levels of disease may be so low as to make detection very tricky. To optimize the chances of detection, one should concentrate on those areas where disease is most likely to occur, for example in low areas or areas of lush growth. If this is not possible, an array of sampling designs may be used, such as a diagonal across the field, a random walk, a stratified design where each subsection of the field is sampled, or a stratified random design where a random sample is taken in each subsection of the field . The appropriate sampling design will depend on the level of disease expected, the distribution of the disease and sampling schemes already in place for other pests. Disease distribution within a field is dependent, in large part, on the source of inoculum for the pathogen. If the disease is seed borne, in many cases the first diseased plants will be more uniformly distributed in the field. If the disease is soi lborne, it may often be found in clusters in the field. If it is transmitted by insects, the distribution may be more random, or a field edge effect may be apparent. Indirect monitoring of disease most often involves stand-alone, turn-key computer systems with probes or whole units in the field. Data commonly gathered include temperature, relative humidity, and leaf wetness. Data are typically recorded every 15 minutes, with data being used to update real time indices of the likelihood of disease at a given time. The Algorithms for the models are often developed from controlled environmental chamber experiments where the minimum, maximum, and optimum temperatures and relative humidity for fungal growth, germination, and/or disease development are identified. Leaf wetness, either monitored directly or by prediction of dew point based on the relative humidity and temperature conditions, is used if the pathogen requires free water for germination. The prediction of disease events through environmental monitoring has been very successful in a few cases and is used widely for those crops and diseases where sufficient research exists.

Genetic Host Resistance—The use of genetically resistant plants to minimize or avoid losses caused by insect pests and/or pathogens. The use of genetically resistant plants is often recommended by entomologists and plant pathologists as the first line of defense for avoiding or minimizing plant damage caused by insects and pathogens. In some cropping systems, such as large acreage field or row crop agriculture (corn, soybean, wheat, rice, cotton, etc.), the use of genetically resistant plants may be the only cost-effective means for managing a particular pest or disease. In some cases, the use of resistant cultivars or varieties might be the only means of effectively managing a disease or pest such as in the case of managing plant diseases caused by viruses. The development of resistant plant types may also reduce the need for using pesticides. Although genetic resistance should be considered when dealing annual cropping systems where new seed is sown each season thereby providing an opportunity to introduce new cultivars or varieties with insect or pathogen resistance. Although important in perennial cropping systems such as orchards, forests or home lawns, once the initial crop is planted, the introduction of resistant lines is limited due to the long-term nature of these crops.

Cultural Control

Cultural practices serve an important role in prevention and management of plant diseases. The benefits of cultural control begin with the establishment of a growing environment that favors the crop over the pathogen. Reducing plant stress through environmental modification promotes good plant health and aids in reducing damage from some plant diseases Sanitation practices aimed at excluding, reducing, or eliminating pathogen populations are critical for management of infectious plant diseases. It is important to use only pathogen-free transplants, especially for late blight, bacterial spot, viral diseases and early blight. In order to reduce dispersal of soilborne pathogens between fields, stakes and farm equipment should be decontaminated before moving from one field to the next. Reduction of pathogen survival from one season to another may be achieved by destruction of volunteer plants and crop rotation. Removal of cull piles and prompt destruction of crops should be applied as a general practice. Avoid movement of soil from one site to another to reduce the risk of moving pathogens. For example, sclerotia of *Sclerotinia sclerotiorum* and *Sclerotium rolfsii*, are transported primarily in contaminated soil. Minimizing wounds during harvest and packing will reduce post harvest disease problems. Depending on crops and other factors, sanitation of soil can be achieved to some degree by solarization. Crop rotation is a very important practice, especially for soilborne disease control. For many soilborne diseases, at least a 3-year-rotation using a non-host crop will greatly reduce pathogen populations. This practice is beneficial for Phytophthora blight of pepper and Fusarium wilt of watermelon, but longer rotation periods (up to 5-7 years) may be needed. Land previously cropped to alternate and reservoir hosts should be avoidedwhenever possible. Vegetable fields should be located as far as away as possible from inoculum and insect vector sources. Weed control is important for the management of viral diseases. Weeds may be alternate hosts for several important vegetable viruses and their vectors. Elimination of weeds might reduce primary inoculum. Cover crops help to reduce weed populations that may harbor pathogens between seasons. For this purpose use cover crops that grow fast and provide maximum biomass. Non-host cover crops will help to reduce weed populations and primary inoculum for soilborne pathogens. Excessive handling of plants such as in thinning, pruning and tying may be involved in spread of pathogens, particularly bacteria. It is advisable to handle plants in the field when plants are driest. Because some pathogens can only enter the host through wounds, situations which promote plant injury should be avoided. During pruning process and harvest, workers should periodically clean their hands and tools with a disinfectant, such as isopropyl alcohol. If applicable, plants can be staked and tied for improved air movement in the foliar canopy. A more open canopy results in less wetness discouraging growth of most pathogens. Soil aeration and drying can be enhanced through incorporation of composted organic amendments in the soil. Build up of inoculum can be reduced by removing all plant materials (infected and apparently healthy) after harvest. Between-row cover crops reduce plant injury from blowing sand. Polyethylene mulch can be used as a physical barrier between soil and above-ground parts of plants. This is an important practice for fruit rot control in the field. Highly UV-reflective (metalized) mulches repel some insects. It is beneficial to use metalized mulch during certain times of the year when insect vectors of some viral diseases are prevalent. *Tomato spotted wilt virus* (TSWV) incidence and associated vector thrips populations have been demonstrated to be effectively reduced by using metalized mulches on tomatoes.

Mechanical control: It involves use of mechanical or manual operation and mechanical barriers for the control of diseases. For example- pruning of diseased part of the plants, rouging of viral infected plants etc. This is especially very effective in high value crops where area under cultivation is less.

Physical control: It involves manipulation of temperature, humidity, lght and sound water etc for controlling diseases. Hot air treatment at 54^{0}C for 8h, effectively eliminates RSD pathogen without impairing the germination of buds. Similarly, grassy shoot disease of sugarcane has also been controlled by hot air at 54^{0}C for 8 h.

Biological Control—. Biological control is the use of one organism or a group of organisms to suppress, kill, or restrict the activity of a pest or pathogen. The use of biological control is considered advantageous and environmentally sound as it provides an eco-friendly alternative to the use of pesticides. Unfortunately, however, few biocontrol products are available that provide consistent and commercially acceptable levels of pest or disease control. Biocontrol organisms kill or suppress pathogens and pests by either (a) parasitizing the pest or pathogen, (b) out competing the pest or pathogen for space or nutrients, (c) producing toxins that kill or make the pest or pathogen sick, and/or (d) inducing a physiological or biochemical change in the host plant making it less susceptible to (more tolerant of) pest or pathogen attack. Biocontrol agents for use in plant disease management are increasing in use especially among organic growers. These products are considered safer for the environment and the applicator, than conventional chemicals and are mainly used against soilborne diseases. Examples of commercially available biocontrol agents include the fungi *Trichoderma harzianum* and *Trichoderma virens*, an actinomycete *Streptomyces griseoviridis*, and a bacterium *Bacillus subtilis*. Bacteriophages (phages) have been found as an effective biocontrol agent for the management of bacterial spot on tomato. Phages are viruses that infect bacteria. It is best to run small trials on one's own farm to fully evaluate the applicability of biocontrol to particular farming operations.

Regulatory Measures—the use of quarantines and pest eradication programs to limit the introduction or spread of deleterious plant pests and/ or pathogens. Strict government inspections and quarantines of imported plants, plant products, and soil can be an effective way to keep a pest or pathogen out of a region or area. However, given the global nature of modern society, the possibility of moving and introducing pests dangerous to people, plants, and animals is real. Government eradication programs are conducted when a serious insect or disease pest breaks out. Often the trouble is eliminated before it has a chance to spread. Such programs require highly trained personnel who know the potential insect and disease problems and are able to recognize the pathogens and the symptoms of their activities. On the grower level, many greenhouses and nurseries also use quarantine measures. They often keep the new material separated from the old. If a disease were to come in on the new material it would not impact the rest of the greenhouse or nursery.

Chemical control: Fungicides and bactericides are an important component of many disease management programs.It is important to remember that chemical use should be integrated with all other appropriate tactics mentioned in this chapter. Information regarding physical mode of action of a fungicide will help producers improve timing of fungicide applications. Physical modes of action of fungicides can be classified into four categories: protective, after infection, pre-symptom, and anti-sporulant (post-symptom). Protectant fungicides include the bulk of the foliar spray materials available to producers. In order to be effective, protectant fungicides, such as copper compounds, mancozeb etc., need to be on the leaf (or plant) surface prior to arrival of the pathogen. Systemic [(therapeutic) fungicides, based on their level of systemicity, true systemic (i.e. Aliette), translaminar (i.e. Quadris), meso-systemic (i.e. Flint)], are active inside of the leaf. Systemic fungicides may stop an infection after it starts and prevent further disease development. If necessary fungicides must be used based on recommended fungicide resistance management strategies. A new startegy to chemically manage plant diseases without direct interference with the pathogen is the triggering of plant defense reaction. Acibenzolar-S-methyl (Actigard), a chemical in this category, was registered for the control of bacterial spot and speck on tomatoes. Chemicals must be used at recommended rates and application frequencies. Besides selection of the most efficacious material, equipment must be properly calibrated and attention paid to the appropriate application technique. As always, the key to effective disease management is correct diagnosis of the problem. Always read the pesticide labels and follow the instructions carefully. Remember, the label is the law. Fumigants can be used to manage soilborne pathogens. Before applying, it is important to review the disease history of the specific site when choosing fumigant materials.

Key Components or Steps in the Implementation of IDM

1. **Correct disease Identification :** What diseases/pests and stages are causing the damage. This is foundation of all decision making.
2. **Understanding of disease and crop dynamics :** We must have enough information about the nature of the pathogens encountered to assess the potential risk that the disease poses and determine the best possible management strategy.
   - How much disease is tolerable?
   - What are the expected losses of the disease if controls are not used?
   - What is the most vulnerable stage for management?
3. **Planning preventive strategies** as the preferred management strategy in IDM; a careful examination of field history and all aspects of the crop production system should be made to determine if the crop can be grown or treated to prevent disease from exceeding economic levels.
   - Can any cropping practice, such as time of planting, crop rotation, or tillage, be manipulated to reduce disease attack?
   - Are the chances of economic disease losses great enough to justify a preventive pesticide strategy?
   - What are the benefits and risks of pesticides?
   - What are the existing natural control agents that can be augmented or conserved?
4. **Monitoring** : involves periodic assessment of diseases, natural control factors, crop characteristics, and environmental factors to the need for control and the effectiveness of any management action. Different methods and sampling frequencies are used, depending on the nature of diseases and monitoring objective.
5. **Decision making :** involves an evaluation of the monitoring information to assess the relevant economic benefits versus the risks of disease management actions. What will I lose if I do nothing? What will I gain?
   - Is there enough natural control agents present to reduce the disease incidence/severity below economic levels?
   - Is the incidence/severity potential of the disease more costly than the control?

- Estimates of incidence/severity size are compared to "economic thresholds" or "action thresholds" which serve as references for loss potential at particular crop growth stages or sets of crop conditions.

6. **Selection of optimal disease control tactics** to manage the problem while minimizing economic, health and environmental risks.

   - Are there opportunities to integrate nonchemical tactics?
   - How well will the control option fit into the total management system?
   - How well will the tactic control the disease? What effects will this action have on the user, society as a whole, and the environment?
   - Will this action impact, either positively or negatively, the other species or natural enemies present in my crop?

   For chemical controls, important questions at this step are: What is the best fungicide for the target disease? What is the optimal rate? Is it legal? What are the safety requirements and use restrictions?

7. **Implementation** Once the management options are selected, they should be deployed on a timely manner with precision and completeness.

   - What can be done to improve effectiveness of the management tactics?
   - Is the pesticide application equipment calibrated properly and in good working condition?
   - If pesticides are used, what is the appropriate chemical and rate for the target diseases?
   - Can the pesticide be applied in a manner that will be least disruptive on natural enemies while still provide effective control?
   - In certain situations, it may be desirable to leave small non treated areas to evaluate control effectiveness.

8. **Evaluation** Always take time to follow-up and evaluate disease control actions to determine if you got your money's worth. Review what went wrong but more importantly what went right.

   - Was the choice of control action appropriate?
   - Was the management action implemented on time and according to recommendations?

- What changes to the management tactics can be made to improve control if the same disease problem occurs in the future?
- What future changes in the production system can be made to achieve more permanent suppression of the disease problem?

Advantages of IDM

Some of the advantages of an integrated approach are as follows:

- Promotes sound structures and healthy plants.
- Promotes the sustainable bio based disease management alternatives.
- Reduces the environmental risk associated with management by encouraging the adoption of more ecologically benign control tactics.
- Reduces the potential for air and ground water contamination.
- Protects the non-target species through reduced impact of plant disease management activities.
- Reduces the need for pesticides and fungicides by using several management methods.
- Reduces or eliminates issues related to pesticide residue.
- Decreases workers, tenants and public exposure to chemicals.
- Alleviates concern of the public about pest & pesticide related practices.
- Maintains or increases the cost-effectiveness of disease management programs.

Constraints in the Implementation of IDM

A. Information and technological constraints

- Though IDM technology in rice, cotton, red gram, certain vegetable etc. is available, there is a lack of multiple resistant varieties.
- There is a need for a number of selective pesticides against diseases of crops which are safe against the natural enemies.
- One important prerequisite for a sound IDM package is information on economic threshold levels. These have not been worked out for most of the diseases.
- Precise disease surveillance and monitoring methods and forecasting models have not been standardized.

- The techniques of mass multiplication of several potential bio control agents are still not well developed.
- Identifying cropping sequence, plant based pesticides and biocides develop system analysis (SA) based plant protection package.

B. Institutional Constraints

- There is an immense need for multidisciplinary approaches inter institutional collaboration to develop sound IDM technology.
- Human resource development in IDM through training of trainers and farmers.
- Large scale demonstration of field tested IDM policies.
- Participatory approach among state extension functionaries scientists of SAV and research institutes, NGO and farmers group.
- Pesticide industry should also continue their effort to ensure the availability of safe, selective environment friendly and quality pesticides.

Chapter - 41

Glossary

A

Acervulus (pl. Acervuli)—A saucer-shaped, spore-producing body of a fungus embedded in host tissue.

Actinomycctcs Filamentous bacteria that produce several antibiotics and give soil its earthy smell.

Active ingredient: In pesticides, the chemical responsible for the desired effect.

Aggressiveness: Virulent forms of pathogen cause differing degrees of symptom severity.

Alternate Host—One of two kinds of plants on which a parasitic fungus (e.g., rust) must develop to complete its life cycle.

Anamorph—Asexual stage of a fungus.

Antagonism: The counteraction between organisms or groups of organisms.

Anthracnose—Disease caused by acervuli-forming fungi (order *Melanconiales)* and characterized by sunken lesions and necrosis.

Antibiotic—A complex chemical substance produced by one microorganism that inhibits or kills other microorganisms (e.g., streptomycin).

Antibody—A specific protein formed in the blood of warm-blooded animals in response to the injection of an antigen.

Antigen—Any foreign chemical (normally a protein) that induces antibody formation in animals.

Antiseptic—A substance that prevents, retards, or destroys microorganisms.

Apothecium—An open, cuplike, or saucer-shaped sexual fungal fruiting body containing asci.

Aquisition period: The period of time need for a virus vector to aquire a virus while feeding on an infected plant host.

Asci—Several saclike cells in which meiosis occurs and which generally contain eight spores each.

Ascomycetes—A group of fungi characterized by the production of sexual spores within an oval or tubular membranous sac called an ascus.

Asexual—Vegetative; without sex organs, sex cells, or sexual spores, as the anamorph of a fungus.

Atrophy - A lack of development of certain plant parts or tissues.

Autoecious—The need of only one host for completing the life cycle of a rust.

Avirulence: The inability of a pathogen to cause disease.

AVR gene: Avirulence gene, a pathogen gene whose product is recognized by a plant and leads to a resistant reaction in the plant.

B

Bactericide - A compound toxic to bacteria.

Bacterium (pl. Bacteria)—Microscopic one-celled organism. Cell type lacks a distinct nucleus, sexual recombination, and chlorophyll. It does have cell walls and DNA.

Basidiomycetes—A group of fungi characterized by the pro-duction of sexual spores on a club-shaped filament called the basidium.

Basidiospore—A haploid spore formed externally on a basidium.

Basidium—Short, club-shaped fungus cell on which basidiospores are produced.

Biotroph: A plant pathogenic fungus that requires living host cells i.e. an obligate parasite.

Biotype: The smallest morphological unit within a species, the members of which are usually genetically identical.

Blight—Any sudden, severe, and extensive spotting, discoloration, or destruction of leaves, flowers, stems, or entire plants, usually attacking young, growing tissues.

Blotch—A blot or spot, usually superficial and irregular in shape and size, on leaves, shoots and fruit.

Burn—The condition in which the cells of the host become reddish or dark brown and collapse.

C

Callus—Parenchyma tissue that grows over a wound or graft and protects it against drying or other injury.

Calyx—Outermost whorl of organs of a flower.

Canker - A diseased or dead area in the bark and wood of trees or shrubs characterized by a drying out of the tissues.

Carrier—A plant or animal that carries a virus or other infective agent without showing symptoms.

Chemotherapy—Treatment of disease by chemicals working internally. Chemical agent has toxic effect directly or indirectly on the pathogens without injury to the host plant.

Chimera—A plant with several tissue sectors or layers differing in genetic or chromosomal constitution from the original plant.

Chlamydospore—A thick-walled asexual resting spore formed by the modification of a fungus hypha.

Chlorosis—The abnormal plant color of yellowish-white or gray condition of plant parts resulting from the incomplete destruction of the chlorophyll.

Circulative transmission : refers to vector transmission of a virus where virus particles must circulate through the vectors hemolymph and enter the salivary glands to be tramsitted. In this case the vector aquisition and retention time is longer than with non or semi-persistant transmission.

Cirrus—A curllike tuft; a tendrillike mass or "spore horn" of forced-out spores.

Cleistothecium—Closed, usually spherical, ascus-containing structure of powdery mildew fungi. A sexual fruiting structure.

Collateral host: The wild host of same families of a pathogen is called as collateral host.

Conidiophore—The specialized fungal hyphal branch that bears the conidium.

Conidium—Asexual spore formed by abstriction and detachment of part of a hyphal cell at the end of a conidiophore and germinating by a germ tube.

Coremium—A cluster of erect fungus filaments (hyphae) that are joined together to form a column and that bear asexual spores (conidia).

Crop Damage: It is defined as any reduction in the quality or quantity of yield or loss of revenue resulting from crop injury.

Cultivar—A cultivated plant variety. Used synonymously with variety.

Curative: Chemical control method aimed at inhibiting the development of an established infection.

Curl—The distortion, fluting, and puffing of a leaf resulting from the unequal development of its two sides.

D

Damping-off—Decay of seeds in the soil or young seedlings before or after emergence.

Deficiency: Abnormality or disease.

Diagnostic—A distinguishing characteristic serving to identify or determine the presence of a disease or other condition.

Dieback—Progressive death of shoots, branches, and roots generally starting at the tips.

Differential hosts; Host range can be tested and compared to known pathogens for identification.

Diploid—Having a double set of chromosomes (2*n* chromosomes) per cell.

Disease cycle: The chain of events involved in disease development.

Disease incidence: The number or proportion of individuals that are diseased.

Disease progress curve: A graph that plots disease vs. time.

Disease severity:The amount or proportion of tissue that is diseased.

Disease syndrome: The set of varying symptoms characterizing a disease are collectively called a syndrome.

Disease: Any deviation in the general health, or physiology or function of plant or plant parts, is recognized as a disease.

Disease-gradient curve: A graph that plots disease vs. distance from an inoculum source.

Disinfectant—Any agent for destroying the causal agent of disease after infection.

Disinfestant—Any agent that removes, kills, or inactivates disease-causing organisms *before* they can cause infection.

Dissemination—The spread of infectious material (inoculum) from a diseased to a healthy plant by wind, water, humans, insects, animal, machinery, or other means.

DNA fingerprinting: Technique for pathogen identification where restirction enzymnes are used to cut genomic DNA, producing a pattern specific to a pathogen.

Dormancy—Nongrowing (inactive, quiescent) state of a plant.

Dwarfing—The underdevelopment of any organ of a plant.

E

Ecology - The study which deals with the effect of environmental factors, such as soil, climate, and culture on the occurrence, severity, and distribution of plant diseases.

Ectoparasite— A parasite that feeds from outside the host.

ED 50: Effective dose, the amount needed to have the desired effect in 50% of the population.

ELISA: Enzyme linked immunosorbent assay – a test used to detect antigens. Antibodies can be created to detect pathogen proteins.

Enation—Epidermal outgrowth.

Endogenous—Produced inside.

Endoparasite- A parasite that enter and feed from inside the host.

Endophytic—Living within another plant.

Enphytotic—Plant disease that causes about the same amount of injury each year.

Environment - The external conditions and influences that surround living organisms.

Epidemiology—The study of factors influencing the initiation, development, and spread of infectious disease.

Epiderm - The superficial layer of cells occurring on all plant parts.

Epinasty—An abnormal downward-curving growth or movement of a leaf, leaf part, or stem.

Epiphytotic—The widespread and destructive development of a disease on many plants in a community or communities.

Eradicant—Chemical used to eliminate a pathogen from a host or an environment.

Eradication—Control of disease by eliminating the pathogen after it is already established.

Escape—Plants in a given population that remain free of disease where it is prevalent, although they possess no natural inherent resistance to the disease.

Etiolation—Yellowing and long, spindly growth as a result of insufficient light.

Etiology—The description of the cause of disease.

Exclusion—Control of disease by preventing its introduction into disease-free areas.

Exogenous—Produced outside.

Exudate—A substance (usually liquid) formed inside a plant and discharged from diseased or injured tissue. The presence of an exudate often aids in diagnosis (e.g., fire blight bacteria).

F

Facultative Parasite—An organism that is ordinarily saprophytic but under proper conditions may be parasitic.

Facultative Saprophyte—An organism that is ordinarily parasitic but under proper conditions may be saprophytic.

Fasciation—A distortion of a plant caused by an injury or infection that results in thin, flattened, and sometimes curved shoots.

Fission: Bacterial reproduction by simple cell division.

Flagellum—A long hairlike or whiplike contractile filament protruding from certain bacterial cells and spores of fungi and that enable movement.

Flagging—The loss of turgor and the drooping of plant parts, usually following a water deficit.

Fleck—A small, white to translucent lesion (spot) visible through a leaf.

Frass—Excrement of an insect, usually mixed with plant debris.

Fruiting Body—Any of various complex, spore-bearing fungal structures.

Fumigant—Vapor-active chemical used in the gaseous phase to kill or inhibit the growth of microorganisms or other pests.

Fungi Imperfecti—A major group of fungi for which no sexual production of spores is known.

Fungicide—An agent that inhibits or kills fungi.

Fungistat—A chemical or physical agent that prevents fungi from developing but does not kill them.

Fungus—A single- or many-celled, naked or covered, irregular or filamentous organism, usually with a chitinous cell wall. Lacking chlorophyll and incapable of manufacturing its own food, it feeds on dead or living plant or animal matter.

G

Gall - An unusual enlargement on some portion of a plant.

Germinate—To begin growth of a seed or spore.

Giant Cells—Large, usually multinucleate cells formed by abnormal cell fusions or failure of proper cell wall formation following growth and nuclear division. Associated with nematode feeding.

Girdle—To circle and cut through; to destroy vascular tissue, as in a canker or knife cut that encircles the stem.

Gram-negative—A negative reaction to the standard Gram's stain for bacteria.

H

Haploid—The chromosome number of the gametophytic genera-tion or phase or having a single complete set of chromosomes.

Haustorium—A modified mycelial branch that grows into a plant cell, makes intimate contact with the protoplast, and absorbs food.

Hemibiotroph: A plant pathogenic fungus that initially requires living host cells but after killing the host cell grows on the dead and dying cells.

Hemiparasites: Parasitic plants that have chlorphyl and can make some of their own sugar but still rely on thier host for water and other nutrients.

Heteroecious—Requiring two or more unrelated hosts for completing the life cycle of a rust.

Heterothallic—Producing fusing gametes on separate and distinct mycelia.

Holoparasites: Parasitic plants that do not have chlorophyl and rely on thier host for all nutrients.

Homothalic—Producing fusing gametes on the same mycelium.

Host—The plant on or in which a parasite lives and from which it obtains its food.

Hyaline—Clear, translucent.

Hyperplasia - A symptom due to an abnormal increase in the number of individual cells.

Hypersensitive response: Plant responds to pathogen infection by quickly killing the infected cells, blocking the advance of the pathogen.

Hypertrophy - A symptom due to an abnormal increase in the size of individual cells.

Hyphae - Fungal filaments which collectively form the mycelium of a fungus.

Hypoplasia—The underdevelopment of cells, tissues, or organs.

I

Immune - Cannot be infected by a given pathogen.

Immunity—A relationship between a plant and a causal agent in which the plant does not become diseased.

Incubation period: The period of time between penetration of a pathogen to the host and the first appearance of symptoms on the plant.

Indexing—Determining presence of disease in a plant by removing buds or other parts for inoculation of a susceptible indicator plant that exhibits specific symptoms of a transmissible disease.

Indicator plants: Certain plant species or cultivars that show characteristic symptoms of infection.

Infection court - Specific area on a plant where a pathogen gains entrance to the host.

Infection: The initiation and establishment of a parasite within a host plant.

Infest - To overrun or contaminate.

Infestation—Presence in numbers (e.g., of insects, mites, or nematodes). Do not confuse with "infection," a term that applies only to living, diseased plants or animals.

Inoculation - The process of transferring inoculum to host.

Inoculum density: The number of infective units in a given volume or area

Inoculum potential: The growth or threshold of fungus available for colonization at host.

Inoculum: That portion of pathogen which is transferred to plant and cause disease.

Intercellular—Between the cells.

Intracellular—Within the cells.

Invasion: The penetration and spread of a pathogen in the host.

J

Juvenile- Immature, non-reproductive stage of nematodes.

K

Klendusity—Ability of an otherwise susceptible variety of plant to escape infection because of the way it grows (e.g., early-maturing plants escape late-season diseases).

L

Latent—Present but not manifest or visible, as a symptomless infection.

Lesion—A local injury or delimited diseased area..

Local invasion - That involving only a portion of the plant.

Local Necrosis—The death or disintegration of cells and tissues in a localized area of an organ.

M

Macrocyclic: Rusts that produce all five spore types.

Macroscopic—Visible to the naked eye, without the aid of a microscope.

Mechanical transmission: Virus transmission from plant to plant by infected plant sap.

Microcyclic; Rusts that lack one or more of the five spore types.

Micron—A millionth of a meter (or, a thousandth of a millimeter).

Microscopic—Visible only with the aid of magnification.

Migratory- Describes a life style of plant parasitic nematodes that move through the host as they feed.

Monocyclic disease: A disease where only one disease cycle is completed each year or growing season.

Monotrichous—Having only one flagellum.

Mosaic—Disease symptom characterized by nonuniform foliage coloration, with a more or less distinct intermingling of normal and light green or yellowish patches. Usually caused by a virus.

Mottle—An irregular pattern of light and dark areas.

Multiple cycle disease (Polycyclic): Some pathogens specially a fungus, can complete a number of life cycles within one crop season of the host plant and the disease caused by such pathogens is called multiple cycle disease e.g. wheat rust, rice blast, late blight of potato etc.

Mummification—The drying up and shriveling of fruits and other plant parts.

Mummy—A dried and shriveled fruit.

Mushroom—A conspicuous fleshy fungus fruiting body.

Mutualism: Symbiosis of two organisms that are mutually helpful or that mutually support one another.

Mycelium—The mass of interwoven threads (hyphae) making up the vegetative body of a fungus.

Mycoplasma—Degenerate bacteria that do not have cell walls. Mycoplasmas are smaller than bacteria but larger than viruses. They cause animal and human diseases.

Mycorrhiza—A symbiotic association of a fungus with the roots of a plant.

N

Necrosis : A symptom marked by rapid death of the host or parts of the host.

Necrotroph: A pathogenic fungus that kills the host and survives on the dying and dead cells.

Nematicide—A chemical or physical agent that kills, inhibits, or protects against nematodes.

Nematodes—Generally microscopic tubular worms, usually living free in moist soil, water, and decaying matter, or as parasites of plants and animals.

Non-persistant transmission: Vector trasmission of a virus where the vector quickly picks up virus particles on its mouthparts and is infective for a short period of time .

O

Obligate parasite - An obligate parasite is an organism that can live only on living tissue.

Oogonium—Female egg cell of oomycete fungi.

Oomycete—A group of fungi that produce oospores such as *Pythium, Phytophthora,* and *Aphanomyces.*

Oospore—Thick-walled, sexually-derived resting spore of oomycete fungi.

Overwinter—To survive over the winter period.

P

Parasite—An organism that lives within or upon another living organism from which it derives nourishment and in which it may cause various degrees of injury.

Parasitism—The phenomenon of the growth of one organism, the parasite, at the expense of another, the host.

Pathogen— An entity, usually a micro-organism that can cause the disease.

Pathogenesis: It is a process caused by an infectious agent (pathogen) when it comes in contact with a susceptible host.

Pathogenicity—An entity's capacity for producing a disease.

Pathology - The study of disease

PCR: Polymerase chain reaction – technique to amplify sequences of DNA. Can be used to detect specific sequences of pathogen DNA.

Pectinase—The enzyme that breaks down pectic substances to simple carbohydrates.

Perithecium—A round to flask-shaped, thick-walled spore case containing asci and with an ostiole (pore).

Peritricous— Having flagella all over the outside of the cell.

Pesticide—Any chemical or physical agent that destroys pests (e.g., fungicide, insecticide, miticide).

Phage: Virus that attacks bacteria.

Phycomycetes—A group of fungi that may consist of one cell or have filaments (hyphae) with few or no cross walls and that reproduce sexually by union of two sex cells.

Phyllody—Change from a normal flower to leafy structures. Characteristic of certain phytoplasma infections.

Physiogenic Disease—A disease produced by some unfavorable physical or environmental factors .

Physiologic race: One or a group of microorganisms similar in morphology but dissimilar in certain cultural, physiological or pathological characters.

Physiology - The study of metabolic processes, activities and phenomena related to life.

Phytoplasma—Microorganisms found in phloem tissue that resemble mycoplasmas in all respects except that they cannot yet be grown on artificial nutrient media. Formerly known as mycoplasma like organism (MLO).

Phytotoxic—Injurious to plants.

Plasmodium—A naked, multinucleate, vegetative (fungal) body capable of amoeboid motion.

Polymorphism—The existence of several asexual spore stages in the life cycle of an organism.

Predisposition: The effect of one or more environmental factors which makes a plant vulnerable to attack by a pathogen.

Preventative: Chemical control method aimed at preventing infection of the pathogen.

Primary infection: The first infection of a plant by the over wintering or over summering of the pathogen.

Primary Inoculum—Inoculum, usually from an overwintering source, that initiates disease in the field, as opposed to inoculum that spreads disease during the season.

Propagative transmission: Vector trasmission of a virus where virus particles are replicated in the vector. In this case the vector retention time is longer than with circulative transmission and, in some cases, the virus can be transovarially transmitted.

Propagule—The part of an organism that may be spread so as to reproduce the organism.

Prophylaxis - Methods used to preserve health and prevent spread of disease.

Protectant—A chemical applied to a plant surface in advance of the pathogen to prevent infection.

Pustule—A local elevation of the epidermis that may rupture to expose the causal agent (e.g., rust, smut).

Pycnidium—The asexual, globose or flask-shaped fruiting body of fungi-producing conidia.

Q

Quarantine—Regulation forbidding sale or shipment of plants or plant parts, usually to prevent disease, insect, nematode, or weed invasion of an area.

Quorum sensing; Dependence of bacterial behavior and pathogenicity on thier cells reaching a certain density by sensing the concentration of certain signal molecules.

R

Race—A strain of a pathogen characterized by the limitation of its host range to certain species and varieties of plants.

Resistance—The sum of the qualities of the host and causal agent that retard the activities of the causal agent.

Rhizoid—Intercellular thallus branch that absorbs food and provides anchorage.

Rhizomorph—An aggregation of hyphae into a cordlike or rootlike strand.

Rickettsia—A single-celled animal and human disease--causing organism with a partial cell wall that has not been grown in culture.

Ringspot—Symptom of a disease characterized by yellowish or dead (necrotic) rings with green tissue inside them, as in certain virus diseases.

Rogue—To remove and destroy undesired individual plants from a planting on the basis of disease infection, not being true-to-type, insect infestation, or other reason.

Rot—Softening, discoloration, and often disintegration of succulent plant tissue as a result of fungal or bacterial infection.

Rugose—Wrinkled.

Russet—Yellowish-brown or reddish-brown scar tissue on the surface of fruit.

Rust - Used to describe a particular fungus, any of its stages or the disease caused by any of the stages.

S

Sanitation—Destroying all infested and infected plant parts during the season.

Saprophyte—An organism that derives its nourishment from dead organic matter.

Scab—Crustlike disease lesion.

Sclerotium—A small, compact, hardened mass of hyphae that may bear fruiting bodies. Can help fungus survive adverse environments.

Scorch—"Burning" of plant tissue from infection, lack or excess of some nutrient, or weather conditions.

Secondary Infection—Infection resulting from the spread of infectious material produced after a primary infection.

Sedentary- Describes a life style of plant parasitic nematodes that stay in one place and set up a feeding site.

Semi-pertsistant transmission: Vector trasmission of a virus where virus particles enter the vectors foregut. In this case the vector also picks up the virus quicly but is infective for somewhat longer (days) than with non-persistant transmission.

Senesce—To decline with maturity or age, often hastened by stress from environment or disease.

Shothole—Disease symptom characterized by the dropping out of small, round fragments of leaves, making them look as if riddled by shot.

Sign - The structure of the pathogen itself.

Single cycle disease (Monocyclic): This type of disease is referred to those caused by the pathogen (fungi) that can complete only one life cycle in one crop season of the host plant. e.g. downy mildew of rapeseed, club root of crucifers, sclerotinia blight of brinjal etc.

Soilborne—Refers to many fungi able to survive in the soil as saprophytes. Also called "soil inhabitant."

Sorus—A compact aggregation of spores and/or sporophores growing out to the surface of the host.

Spiroplasma—A single-celled, wall-less, spiral, filamentous organism associated with corn stunt and citrus stubborn disease.

Sporangiophore—A sporangium-bearing hypha.

Sporangium—A fruiting body that produces asexual spores within a more or less spherical wall.

Spore - A fungal reproductive unit or seed that serves as an agent of dispersal and propagation.

Sporodochium—A cushion-shaped spore-producing body of a fungus.

Sporogenous—Capable of forming spores.

Sporulation—The process of producing spores.

Sterilant—Any agent or chemical that destroys all living organisms in a substance such as soil.

Stomata- A small pore or opening in the epidermis of leaves and stems through which gases pass.

Streak—An elongated lesion with irregular sides.

Stroma—A compacted mass of hyphae that supports sexual fruiting bodies.

Stunt—A wide range of parasitic and nonparasitic agents.

Stunted—An unthrifty plant reduced in size and vigor due to unfavorable environmental conditions.

Stylet—Slender, tubular mouthparts in plant-parasitic nematodes or aphids.

Substrate—The substance or object on which an organism lives and from which it gets nourishment.

Sun Scald—Plant tissues burned or scorched by too much sun exposure and other unfavorable conditions.

Susceptibility—The sum of the qualities of a plant and causal agent that allows the development of the causal agent.

Symbiosis: A mutually beneficial association of two or more different kinds of organisms.

Symptoms: The external and internal reaction or alterations of a plant as a result of disease.

Systemic aquired resistance: Whole plant resistance response that occurs following an earlier localized exposure to a pathogen.

Systemic—Pertaining to a disease in which an infection leads to general spread throughout the plant body. Also, a chemical that spreads internally through a plant.

T

Teliomorph—Sexual stage of a fungus.

Teliospore—Thick-walled resting spore produced by some fungi, notably rusts and smuts, that germinates to form a basidium.

Thallus—The vegetative body of the lower plant that has not differentiated into stems and leaves.

Ti-plasmid: Tumor inducing plasmid of *Agrobacterium tumefaciens* that causes gall formation and opine production by infected plants.

Tolerance—Ability of the plant to endure the development of the parasite without showing marked symptoms of disease.

Transgenic plants: Plants that have been genetically manipulated to express a gene from a different species.

Transovarial transmission: Viral transmission from an insect vector to its offspring, meaning offspring of an infected vector are also infective.

Transposons: A segment of chromosmal DNA that can move around in the genome.

Tumor—A swelling or protuberance.

Tylosis—A bladderlike intrusion of the protoplasm from a parenchymatous cell through a pit into the lumen of a xylem cell.

Type three secretion system: Protein sectretion system used by some bacteria to inject bacterial proteins into a host cell.

V

Variety—One or more races of a pathogen that are characterized by the limitation of their host range to a certain genus or genera. Also, a group of closely related plants of common origin and similar characteristics within a species.

Vector—An agent, such as an insect, nematode, or fungus, that may transmit a pathogen.

Vein-banding—Symptom of a virus disease in which regions along the veins are darker green than the tissue between the veins.

Viroid—An infectious nucleic acid without a protein coat that causes potato spindle tuber or chrysanthemum stunt.

Virulence: The degree of infectivity of a given pathogen

Viruliferous—Capable of transmitting a virus.

Virus—Submicroscopic, infectious agent, too small to be seen with a compound microscope, that multiplies only in living cells. A virus consists of nucleic acid surrounded by a protein coat.

W

Water-soaked—Describing plants or lesions that appear wet and dark and are usually sunken and translucent.

Wilt—Lack of freshness and turgor and drooping of leaves from lack of water; a vascular disease that interrupts the plant's normal uptake and distribution of water.

Witches' Broom—Abnormal, brush-like development of many weak shoots.

Y

Yellowing—The yellow color of plant parts resulting from the excessive proportion of yellow pigments, in turn produced by the underdevelopment or partial destruction of the green pigments.

Yellows—A disease characterized by yellowing and stunting of affected parts (caused by fungi, virus, bacteria, or deficiency of essential elements).

Z

Zoospore—Fungus spore with flagella, able to move in water.

Zygospore—A fungal resting spore produced by the fusion of equal gametes.

Chapter - 42

References

Abd-El-Khair, H. and Waff, M.H.(2007).Application of some Egyptian Medicinal plants Extracts against potato late and early blights. *Research Journal of Agriculture and Biological Sciences.* **3 (3):** 166-175.

Acedo, A.L. Jr., Acedo, J.Z. and Evangelio, M.F.N.(1999). Post harvest biocontrol of bacterial soft rot of cabbage using botanicals. Philippine *Journal of Crop Science.* **24 (1):** 12.

Agnihotri, N P.(2000). Pesticide consumption in agriculture in India- an update. *Pesticide Res. Jour.***112:** 150-155.

Ahmad , J.S and Baker.(1990).Implications of rhizosphere competence of Trichoderma harzianum. *Can. J. Microbiology.***34:** 229..

Ahmad, I. and Beg, A.Z. (2001). Antimicrobial and phytochemical studies on 45 Indian medicinal plants against multi-drug resistant human pathogens. *Journal of Ethnopharmacology.***74:** 113–123.

Akhtar, J. and Divedi, R.R.(2002). Effect of different oil cakes on radial growth and mycelia dry weight of Colletotrichum graminicola in vitro conditions. *Indian Phytopath.*, **55(3):** 383.

Anandalakshmi R (2013).Application of RNAi for engineering disease tolerance in crops with special reference to horticultural crops. *J. Mycol. Pl. Pathol.* **43(1):** 111.

Andrews, j.A. (1983). Future strategies for integrated control, Chapter 40, In: Challenging Problem in Plant Health, T. Kommedahl and P.H. Williams (Eds.). *American Phytopathological Society, St. Paul, Minnesota.* p.538.

Baker, K.E., and Cook, R.J. (1983).The future of biological and cultural control of plant diseases. In: Challenging Problem in Plnat Health, T Kommedahl and P.H.Williams (Eds), *Ameriacan Phytopathological Society (APS) Press, St. Paul, Minnesota.* p. 217.

Baker, R.(1990).An overview of current and future strategies and models for biological control. *In : Biological Control of Soil borne Plant Pathogens. D. hornby (Ed.), 375, CAB International Wallingford, United kingdom.*

Bambawale OM, Saradana HR, Arora S (2008) Expanding dimensions of plant protections as per current needs . *Crop Care.* **34 (2):** 15-21.

Bauer, A.W., Kirby, W. M.M. and Sherris, J.C.(1996). Antibiotic susceptibility testing by a standardized single disk method. *Am. J. Clin. Pathol.* 493-496.

Baysal, O. (1997). Determination of microorganisms decomposing essential oils of *Thymbra spicata* L. var. spicata and effect of these micro-organisms on some soil borne pathogens. M. Sc. Thesis, Akdenniz University, Antalya.

Bhojwani, S.S. and M.K. Razdan.(1996). *Plant tissue culture: Theory and Practice: Developments in crop science Vol. 5. Elsevier, Amsterdam.*

Brown DCW, Thorpe TA .(1995).Crop improvement through tissue culture. *World J. Microbiol & Biotechnol.* **11:** 409-415.

Bowers, J.H., and Locke, J. C.(2000). Effect of botanical extracts on the population density of *Fusarium oxysporum* in soil and control of Fusarium wilt in the green house. *Plant Dis.* **84:** 300-305.

Brent, K. J. and Hollomon, D. W. (1998). Fungicide resistance: the assessment of risk. FRAC, *Global Crop Protection Federation, Brussels, Monograph.* **2:** 1-48.

C., Warmington, J. R., and Wyllie, S.G. (1998). Tea tree oil causes K+ leakage and inhibits respiration in *Escherichia coli. Letters in Applied Microbiology*, **26:** 355–358.

Canillac, N. and Mourey, A.(2001). Antibacterial activity of the essential oil of *Picea excelsa* on *Listeria, Staphylococcus aureus* and coliform bacteria. *Food Microbiology*, **18:** 261–268.

Cannell R J P. Natural Products Isolation. New Jersey: Human Press Inc; 1998. pp. 165–208.

Chahal SS (2012). Indian Agriculture: Challenges and Opportunities in post Borlaug era. *Souvenir, 3rd Glo. Conference on Plant. Pathology & Food Security*, pp. 48-55

Chakarbarti A, Ganapathi TR, Mukherjee PK and Bapat VA .(2003). MSI-99, a magainin analogue, im7parts enhanced disease resistance in transgenic tobacco and banana. *Planta.* **216:** 587-596.

Chakraboty, B.N., Biswas. R.D. and Sharma, M.(2007). Induction of resistance in tea plants against Alternaria alternate by foliar application of leaf extracts. *J.Mycol. Pl. Pahtol.* **37 (1):** 60-64.

Chand, H. and Singh , S.(2005). Control of chickpea wilt using bioagents and plant extracts. *Indian J. of Agric. Sci.* **75 (2):** 115-116.

Chattopadhyay, C. (1999). Yield loss attribute to Alternaria blight of sunflower in India and some potentially effective control measures . *Int. J. Pest Manag.* **45(1):** 15-21.

Chaube, H.S. and Singh , Ramji.(2004). *Introductory Plant Pathology. Army Printing Press Lucknow* : p.444

Chaube, H.S. and Singh, U.S.(1990). *Plant Disease Management: principles and Practices. CRC Press, New York,* . 329.

Chaudhari PJ, Shrivastava P and Khadse AC (2011). Substrate evaluation for mass cultivation of trichoderma viride. *Asiatic Journal of Biotechnology Resources.* **4 :** 441-446.

Chern MS, Fitzgerald HA, Yadav RC, Canlas PE, Dong X , Ronald PC .(2001). Evidence for adisease resistance pathway in rice similar to the NPRI- mediated signaling pathway in Arabidopsis. *Plant J.* **27:** 101-103

Clark MF, Adams AN .(1977). Characteristics of the microplate method of enzyme – linked immunosorbent assay (ELASA) for the detection of plant viruses. *J. Gen. Virol.* **34 :** 475-483.

Coa, K.Q. and Ariena, H.C. Van B.(2001). Inhibitory efficacy of several plant extracts and plant products on Phytophthora infestans. *J.of Ahric. Univ. of Hebei.* **24(2):** 1-9.

Cosa P, Vlietinck A J, Berghe D V, Maes L. (2006).Anti-infective potential of natural products: How to develop a stronger *in vitro* 'proof-of-concept' *.J Ethnopharmacol.***106:** 290–302.

Cox, S. D., Gustafson, J. E., Mann, C. M., Markham, L., Liew, Y. C., Hartland, R. P., Bell, H. (2008) . *Crop care. Official magazine of Crop Care Federation of India* .**34(2):** 1-100.

Doubrara, N.S., Dean, R.A. and Kuc, J.(1998).Induction of systemic induced resistance to anthracnose caused by *Colletotrichum lagenarium* in cucumber by oxalate and extracts from spinach and rhubarb leaves. *Physiol. And Mol. Pl. Pathol.* **33:** 69-79.

Dubey, R. K., Rajesh, K.Jaya, and Dubey, N. K. (2007). Evaluation of *Eupatorium cannabinum* Linn. Oil in enhancement of shelf life of mango fruits from fungal rotting. *World Journal of Microbiology and Biotechnology.*

Dubey, S. C., Suresh, M. and Singh, B.(2007). Evaluation of *Trichoderma* species against *Fusarium oxysporum* f. sp. *ciceris* for integrated management of chickpea. *Biological Control.***40:** 118-127.

Eberhardt T L, Li X, Shupe T F, Hse C Y.(2007). Chinese Tallow Tree (Sapium Sebiferum) utilization: Characterization of extractives and cell-wall chemistry. *Wood Fiber Sci.* **39:** 319–324.

Ehteshamul Hague, Zaki, M.J., Vahidy, A.A and Abaul Graffas.(1998). Effect of organic amendments on the efficacy of Pseudomonas aeruginosa in the control of root rot diseases of sunflower. *Pakistan J.Botany.* 30 (1): 45-50.

Elgayyar, M., Draughon , F. A., Golden, D. A. and Mount, J. R. (2001). Antimicrobial activity of essential oils from plants against selected pathogenic and saprophytic microorganisms. *Journal of Food Protection*, **64:** 1019-1024.

Enikuomehin, O.A., Ikotun, T. and Ekpo, E. J.A.(1998). Evaluation of ash from some tropical plants of Nigeria for the control of Sclerotium rolfsii sacc. On wheat. *Mycopathologia.* 142(1): 81-87.

Esteshamul Hague, Zaki, M.J., Vahidy, A.A. and Abaul Graffas.(1998). Effect of organic amendments on the efficacy of *Pseudomonas aeruginosa* in the control of root rot diseases of sunflower. *Pakistan J.Botany.* **30 (1):** 45-50.

Fabricant D S, Farnsworth N R.(2001). The value of plants used in traditional medicine for drug discovery. *Environ Health Perspect.***109:** 69–75.

Fan X H, Cheng Y Y, Ye Z L, Lin R C, Qian Z Z.(2006).Multiple chromatographic fingerprinting and its application to the quality control of herbal medicines. *Anal Chim Acta.***555:**217–224.

Fry, W.E.(1977). Integrated control of potato late blight effects of polygenic resistance and techniques of timing fungicide applications. *Phytopathology.* **67:** 415-20.

Fry, W.E. (1982). Principles of plant disease management. *Academic press, New york, U.S.A.*

Ganguly, Dutta .(2012). Plant parasitic nematodes: An emerging problem under changing climate and agricultural practices. *J. Mycol. Pl. Pathol.* **43(1):** 541.

Garrett, S.D.(1970). *Pathogenic Root Infecting Fungi , Cambridge University Press, Cambridge. p.294.*

Gaur VK, Sharma LC. (1989). Variability in single spore isolates of *Fusarium udum* Butler. *Mycopathol.* **107:** 9–15.

Ghose, S.(1996). Biocontrol characterization of *Trichoderma harzianum Rifai*, isolate -3 and its protoplast fusion with *Gliocladium virens* Miller, et.al . *M.Sc., Thesis, G.B Pant University of Agric. And Tech., Pantnagar.* p.a75

Gopalakrishnan S, Sharma RK, Rajkumar KA, Joseph M, Singh MP, Singh AK, Bhat KV, Singh NK, Mohapatra T.(2007). Integrating marker assisted background analysis with foreground selection for identification of superior bacterial blight resistant recombinants in Basmati rice. *Pl. Breed.* **127:** 131-139.

Guleria S, Aggarwal R, Thind TS, Sharma TR .(2007). Morphological and pathological variability in rice isolates of *Rhizoctonia solani* and molecular analysis of their genetic variability. *J. Phytopathol.* **155:** 654-661.

Hamburger M O, Cordell G A.(1987). A direct bioautographic TLC assay for compounds possessing antibacterial activity. *J Nat Prod.* **50:**19–22.

Harmon , G.E. and Bjoorman, T.(1998).Potential and existing uses of Trichoderma and Gliocladium for plant disease control and plant growth enhancement. *In : Trichoderma and Gliocladium, vol. II. G.E. Harman and C.K. Kubicek, (Eds), 229, London: Taylor and Francis Ltd.*

Hewitt, H.G. (1998). *Fungicdes in crop protection. CAB International Wallingford, U.K.* 221 pp.

Hjeljord LG and Tronsmo A .(1998). *Trichoderma* and *Gliocladium* in biocontrol: an overview. In: *Trichoderma* and *Gliocladium*, edited by Kubicek CP, Harman GE Taylor and Francis (London, United Kingdom) .135-151.

Homans A L, Fuchs A.(1970). Direct bioautography on thin-layer chromatograms as a method for detecting fungitoxic substances. *J Chromatogr.***51**:327–329.

Hooda, K.S. and Srivastava, M.S.(1998). Impact of neem coatd urea and potash on the incidence of rice blast. *Plant Dis. Research.* 13(1):

Huie C W.(2002). A review of modern sample-preparation techniques for the extraction and analysis of medicinal plants. *Anal Bioanal Chem.***373:**23–30.

Hui-Hung, Y., Jin-Shu,C., Pin-Jui, H.and Yei- Shung , W.(2009). Effects of fungicides triadimefon and propiconzole on soil bacterial communities. *J. Environ. Sci. Health.***44:** 681-689.

Hundekar, A.R., Anahosur, K.H., Patil, M.S., Kalapannavar. I.K. and Chattannavar, S.N.(1998). *In vitro* evaluation of orgnic amendments against stalk rot of sorghum. *J.Mycol. and Plant Pathol.* **28 (1):** 26-30.

Harding K.(2010).Plant and algal cryopreservation: issues in genetic integrity, concepts in cryobionomics and current applications in cryobiology. Aspac *J. Mol. Biol.Biotechnol.***18(1):** 151-154

Isman, M. B.(2006). Botanical insecticides, deterrents, and repellents in modern agriculture and an increasingly regulated world. *Annual Review of Entomology.***51:** 45–66.

Jain, C. and Trivedi, P.C.(1997). Nematicidal activity of certain plants against root knot nematode, *Meloidogyne incognita* infecting chickpea, *Cicer arietinum. Annals of Plant Protection Sciences.* **5(2):** 171-174.

Jalali BL.(2008). Molecular plant pathology: where do we stand. *J. Mycol. Pl. Pathol.* **38(3):** 419-429.

Jha, M.M., Kumar , S. and Hasan, S.(2004). Effect of botanicals on maydis leaf blight of maize *in vitro. Annals of Biology.* **20 (2):** 173-176.

Joshi Sharda.(2000). Pathogenic Variability in Pigeonpea Wilt Pathogen *Fusarium udum* Butler in Nepal. Nepal Agric. *Re. J.* **4 & 5:** 64-65.

Katan, J.(1987). *Soil solarization , In: Innovation Approaches to Plnt Diseases Control (I. Chet, Ed.), John Wiley and Sons, New York*, p.77.

Katan, J.(1996). *Cultural practices and soil borne disease management m In: Management of soil borne diseases, R.S. Utkhde and V.K. Gupta (Eds) , kalyani Publishers, India*, p. 100.

Kohler G, Milstein C (1975)Continuous culture of fused cells secreting antibody of predefined specificity. *Nature* **.256:** 495-497

Kolte SJ .(2006) .Carrers in Plant Pathology: Plant pathologists have reasons to be proud of their profession. *J Mycol Pl Pathol* . **36(3):** 360-364.

Krishnaraj .(2013). Post transcriptional gene silencing: a tool to develop virus disease resistance *J. Mycol. Pl. Pathol.* **43(1):** 133.

Kumar A, Kumar V, Bhattacharya BK, Singh Niranjan, Chattopadhyay .(2013). Integrated disease management : need for climate resilient technologies. *J. Mycol Pl. Pathol.* **43(1):** 28-36.

Kumar A. (2013). Forewarning models for Alternaria blight in mustards (*Brassica juncea*) crops *Ind. J. Agri. Sci.* **81:** 116-119.

Kumar Prasad T and Palakshappa M.G .(2009). Evaluation of suitable substrates for on farm production of antagonist *Trichoderma harzianum Karnataka Journal of Agricultural. Science.,* **22(1):** 115-117.

Kumar Ranavay., Kumar Sanjeev and Upadhyay, J.P .(2012). Effect of different solid and liquid media on growth and sporulation of *T. viride*. *Advance Applied Research*. **4 (2):** 131-132.

Kumar S & Gupta Om .(2012). *Expanding dimensions of Plant Pathology JNKVV Res. J.* **46(3):** 286-293

Kumar Sanjeev.(2013). *Trichoderma*; a biological weapon for managing plant diseases and promoting sustainability. *International Journal of Agricultural Sciences. & Vetenary Medicine* **1(3):** 1-16.

Kumar Sanjeev, Upadhyay, JP. (2013). Cultural, morphological and pathogenic variability in isolates of *Fusarium udum* causing wilt of pigeonpea. *J. Mycol. Pl. Pathol.* **(43):**76-79.

Kumar Sudheer .(2013). Molecular diagnostics in plant pathogens: Recent advances. *J. Mycol Pl. Pathol.* **43 (1):** 135.

Kumar Vinod, Chauhan, VD, Srivastava, JP. (2007). Pathogenic and biochemical variability in *F udum*, causing pigeonpea wilt. *Indian Phytopath.* **60:** 281 288.

Kumar, R., Mishra, A. K., Dubey, N. K. and Tripathi, Y. B. (2007). Evaluation of *Chenopodium ambrosoides* oil as a potential source of antifungal, antiaflatoxigenic and antioxidant activity. *International Journal of Food Microbiology*.**115:** 159-164.

Kumar, Sanjeev, Upadhyay, JP. (2009). Variablility in isolates of *Fusarium udum* inciting pigeonpea wilt in Bihar. *Int. con. on grain legumes:quality improvement,value addition and trade, IIPR, Kanpur, India,* pp.295

Kumar,A and Gupta. J.P.(2000). Variation in the enzymatice activity of tebuconazole tolerant biotypes of Trichoderma viride, *In: proceeding of Indian Phytopathological Society, Golden Jubilee, International Conference on Integrated Plant Disease Managemnt for Sustainable Agriculture,* P. 391.

Kurucheve, V., Ezhilan, J.G. and Newaskar. V.B.(1988). Effect of different fungicides and neem products for control of leaf spot of groundnut. *J.Soils and Crops*. **8 (1):** 44-49.

Lal Sahab Yadav .(2012). Antagonistic activity of *Trichoderma* sp and evaluation of various agro wastes for mass production. *Indian Journal of Plant Sciences.* **1(1):**109-112.

Lale, N. E. S.(1992). A laboratory study of the comparative toxicity of products from three spices to the maize weevil. *Postharvest Biology and Technology*. **2:** 612- 664.

Lalithakumari D.(2000). Development of effective technology for strain improvement of Trichoderma spp. *In: Proceeding of Indian Phytopathological Society; Golden Jubilee. International Conference on Integrated Plant Disease Managemnt for Sustainable Agriculture.* P. 851.

Leadbeater A (2012). The role of FRAC in resistant management. *J. Mycol Pl. Pathol*. **42(1):** 25.

Leadbeater, A. and Staub, T. (2007). Exploitation of induced resistance: A commercial perspective. *In: Induced Resistance for Plant Defence. D. Walter, A. Newton, and G. Lyon, eds Blackwell, Oxford ,UK.*, pp.229-242.

Li H B, Jiang Y, Chen F.(2004). Separation methods used for *Scutellaria baicalensis* active components. *J Chromatogr B*.**812:** 277–290.

Lokhande, N.M., Lanjewar . R. D. and Newaskar. V.B. (1998). Effect ofdifferent fungicides and neem products for the control of leaf spot of groundnuts. J.Soils and Crops. 8(1): 44-49.

Lewin, B. 2004 Genes VIII, Oxford University Press, New York.

Mahadevan, A.(1982).Biochemical aspects of disease resistance part I. *Performed inhibitory substances prohibitions. Today and Tomorrow's Printers and Publishers, New Delhi, India*, 425 p.

Mahesh M, Saifulla, M, Prasad, P.S. and Sreenivasa, S. (2010). Studies on Cultural variability of *Fusarium udum* isolates in India. *I. J. S. N.* **2 :** 219-225.

Maji , M.D., Chattopadhyay, S., Kumar. P. and Saratchandra, B.(2005). *In vitro* screening of some plant extracts against fngal pathogens of mublberry. Archies . *Phytopathology and Plant Protection.* **38 (3):**157-164.

Mararishi, R.P.(1993). Management of chilli diseases by neem based preparations. *World neem conference. Bangalore, India*:34.

Mariappan,V.(1998). Neem for the management of crop diseases. Associated Publishing Company, New Delhi. Pp. 220.

Mauch, F., Mauch- mani, B. and BOller, T.(1998). Antifungal hydrolases in pea tissue. II. Inhibition of funga growth by combinations of chitinase and â-1,3-glucanase. Plant Physiol. 88: 936-942.

Mayee CD.(2006). Plant pathology in growth of Indian Agriculture. *J. Mycol Pl. Pathol.* **36 (3):** 355-359

Mayee CD.(2008).Molecular Pathology assisted agriculture growth in India. *J. Mycol. Pl. Pathol.* **38(2):** 151-157.

Meena , R.L., Rathore, R.S. and kusum, M.(2003). Evaluation of fungicides and plant extracts against banded leaf and sheath blight of maize. *Ind. J. Plant. Prot.* **31(1):** 94-97.

Mesapogu, Sukumar, Achala Bakshi, Babu Bandamaravuri Kishore, Reddy SS, Sangeeta Saxena, Arora K Dilip.(2012). Genetic diversity and pathogenic variability among Indian isolates of *Fusarium udum* infecting pigeonpea. *Int. Res. J. of Agri. Sci. and Soil. Sci.* **2:** 051-057.

Metcalfe, R.J. *et al.* (2000). The effect of dose and mobility on the strength of selection for DMI (sterol demethylation inhibitors) fungicide resistance in inoculated field experiments. *Plant Pathology* **49**: 546-557 .

Millardet, P.M.A and Gyan, U.(1887). Researches nouvelles sur l' action que less preparations cuiveren ses exercent sur le peronospora de la vigne. *J.Agric. Prat.* **51:** 123-129, 151-161.

Mishra, A. K. and Dubey, N. K.(1994). Evaluation of some essential oils for their toxicity against fungi causing deterioration of stored food commodities. *Applied and Environmental Microbiology*. **60:** 1101-1105.

Mojumdar, V. and Mishra, S.D.(1992). Effect of seed soaking in aqueous extracts of neem seed on germination on ungbean and penetration of second stage juveniles of *Meloidogyne incognita. Annals of Agricultural Research.* **13:** 297-299.

Mondal KK, Chatterjee SC, Viswakarma N, Bhattacharya RC, Grover A .(2003). Chitinase-mediated inhibitory activity of Brassica transgenic on growth of *Alternaria brassicae*. *Curr. Microbiol.* **47:** 171-173.

Monte E, Rubio MB, Dominguez S, Moran- Diez E, Nicolas E and Hermosa R.(2012). Molecular cross –Talk between Trichoderma and Plants . *J. Mycol Pl. Pathol.* **42(1):** 24.

Montealegre, J., Varnero, M.T. and Sepulveda, C.(1993). A method of biomass production of Trichdoerma harzianum strain V: growth evaluation , *Fitopathol.* **28:** 99.

Mukherjee, P.K.(1991).Biological control of chickpea wilt complex. *Ph.D. Thesis, G.B. Pant University of Agric. & Tech. Pantnagar*, p.188.

Mukhopadhyay AN (2012) Trichoderma for plant disease management- A gift of god to humankind. *J. Mycol Pl. Pathol.* **42(1):** PP 23.

Nagarajan .(1990). Effect of plant extracts and oils on rice yellow dwarf infection. *Madras Agric. J.* **77:** 197-201.

Nagarajan S.(2000). Plant Pathology and Indian Agriculture- past, present and future. *Indian Phytopath.***53(2):** 121-128.

Nair, R and Chanda, S.(2005). Anticonidial activity of *Punica granatum* exhibited in different solvents. *Pharm. Biol.* **43:** 21-25.

Nene, Y. L., Kannaiyan, J., Haware, M. P. and Reddy, M. V. (1979). Review of work done at ICRISAT on soil borne diseases of pigeonpea and chickpea. In : *Proceedings of the Consultant Group Discussion on the Resistance to Soil borne Diseases of Legumes*, ICRISAT, Patancheru, Andhra Pradesh, India, pp.3

Nene, Y. L., Sheeila, V. K. and Sharma, S. B. (1996). *A world list of chickpea and pigeonpea pathogens. Fifth Edition, ICRISAT, Patancheru, Andhra Pradesh, India*, pp. 19-20.

Nene, Y.L. and Thapliyal, P.N.(1987).*Fungicides in plant disease control. Oxford and IBH publishing Co. Pvt. Ltd. New Delhi*, pp 691.

Okonkwo, E. U. and Okoye, W. I. (1996). The efficacy of four seed powders and the essential oils as protectants of cowpea and maize grains against infestation by *Callosobruchus maculatus* (Fabricius) (Coleoptera: Bruchidae) and *Sitophilus zeamais* (Motschulsky) (Coleoptera: Curculionidae) in Nigeria. *International Journal of Pest Management*, **42:** 143-146.

Oxenham, S. K. (2003).Classification of an *Ocimum basilicum* germplasm collection and examination of the antifungal effects of the essential oil of basil. *Ph.D. thesis, University of Glasgow, Glasgow, UK.*

Old, R.W. and Primrose, S.B. 1990. *Principles of Gene Manipulation, An Introduction to Genetic Engineering. Blackwell Science Publishers, London.*

Palti, J.(1981). *Cultural Practices and Infection Crop Diseases, Springer- Verlag, Berlin*,p.243.

Papavizas , G.C., Dunn, Mt. Lewis, J.A., and Beagle- Ristaino, J.E.(1984). Liquid fermentation technology for experimental production of biocontrol fungi.*Phytopathology.* **74:**1171.

Patel SI, Patel RL, Desai AG, Patel DS. (2011) Morphological, Cultural and Pathogenic Variability among *Fusarium udum* and Root Dip Inoculation Technique for Screening Pigeonpea Germplasm. *J. Mycol. Pl. Pathol.*, **41**: 2011.

Pathak VN .(2000). The dividing walls are transparent.*J.Mycol. Pl. Pathol.* **30(2):** 137-142.

Patil, M.J., Ukey , S.P. and Raut, B.T.(2003). Evaluation of fungicides and botanicals for the management of early blight of tomato. *PKV Research Journal*. **25 (1):** 49-51.

Patni C.S., Kolte, S.J and Awasthi , R.P.(2005 b).Inhibitory effect of some plant extracts against Alternaria brassicae, causing Alternaria blight of mustard. *Journal of Research SKUAT-J.***4 (1):**71-79.

Patni, C.S., Kolte, S.J and Awasthi, R.P.(2005a).Efficacy of botanicals against Alternaria blight of mustard. *Indian Phtopath*. **58 (4):** 426-430.

Paul, P.K and Sharma, P.D.(2002). *Azadirachta indica* leaf extract induces resistance in barley against leaf stripe disease. *Physiol. Mol. Pl. Pathol.* **61:** 3-13.

Paul.YS .(2012). Role of Plant clinics in global food security. *Souvenir, 3rd Glo. Con. Pl. Path. & Food Security.*34p

Penna, C., Marino, S., Vivot, E., Cruanes, M. C., Munoz, J. de D., Cruanes, J., Ferraro, G., Gutkind, G. and Martino, V.(2001). Antimicrobial activity of Argentine plants used in the treatment of infectious diseases. Isolation of active compounds from *Sebastiania brasiliensis. Journal of Ethnopharmacology*, **77:** 37-40.

Perez, C., Paul, M. and Bazerque, P.(1990). An antibiotic assay for the agar well diffusion method. *Acta Biol. Med. Exp.* **15:** 113-115.

Pharmacopoeia of the People's Republic of China, author. *The Pharmacopeia Commission of PRC. English ed. Beijing*: 2000.

Ponnanna, K.M. and Adiver, S.S.(2001). Fungicidal management of grey mildew of cotton. *Plant Pathology Newsletter.* **19:** 6-8.

Pozo, C., Rodelas, B., Salmeron, V., Martinez-Toledo, M.V., Vela, G.R. and Gonzalez-Lopez, J. (1994).Effects of fungicides maneb and mancozeb on soil microbial populations. *Toxicol. Environ. Chem.* **43:** 123-132.

Prabha K, Baranwal VK .(2009). Emerging viral menace in plants : an Overview. *Indian Farming* PP 51-56.

Pramanick , T.C. and Phookan, A.K.(1998). Effect of plant extracts in the management of sheath rot of rice. *J.Agric. Sci. North East India*. **11(1):** 85-87.

Prasad , C.S.., Gupta, v., Tyagi, A. and Pathak, S.(2003). Biological control of Sclerotium rolfsii Sacc., the incitant of cauliflower collar rot. *Annals. Of Plant Protection Sciences.* **11(1):** 61-63.

Prasad , M.S., Lakshmi, B.S. and Shaik Mohiddin.(1998). Survival of sclerotia of *Rhizoctonia solani* in rice soils amended with oil cakes and green leaf manures. *Ann. Agric. Res.* **19(1):** 44-48.

Prasad ,R.D.and Rangshwaran, R.(2000). Shelf life and bioefficacy of *Trichoderma harzianum* formulated in various carrier materials. *Plant Dis. Res.* 15:38.

Prashar M .(2012). Tackling threat of Ug99 or wheat rust variants. *J. Mycol. Pl. Pathol.* **42(1):** 28.

Raghuvanshi, N.S., Dubey , K.S. and Kumar, B.(2006). Effect of soil extracts amended with some organic materials on conidial germination of *Colletotrichum falcatum. Indian J.Plant Pathology.* **24 (1&2):** 117-118.

Rahalison L, Hamburger M, Hostettmann K, Monod M, Frenk E.(1991). A bioautographic agar overlay method for the detection of antifungal compounds from higher plants.*Phytochem Anal.***2:**199–203.

Rai B, Upadhyay RS (1982). *Gibberella indica*: The perfect stage of *Fusarium udum*. *Mycologia.* **74:** 343.

Ramanujam.B., Prasad R.D., Sriram.S and Rangeswaran.R.(2010). Mass production,formulation, quality control and delivery of *Trichoderma* for plant disease management *The Journal of Plant Protection Sciences*.**2 (2) :** 1-8.

Rauha, J.P., Remes, S., Heinonen, M., Hopia, A., Kahkonen, M., Kujala, T., Pihlaja, K., Vuorela, H. and Vuorela, P. (2000). Antimicrobial effects of Finnish plant extracts containing flavonoids and other phenolic compounds. *International Journal of Food Microbiology*, **56:** 3- 12.

Razeena, B.P.M and Ahmad,R.(2007). Control of seed borne fungi of okra with Pseudomonas fluorescens and aqueous extract of Heena . *J.Mycol. Pl. Pathol.* **37 (3):** 485-487.

Reddy ENP and Basu Chaudhary KC. (1985). Variation in *Fusarium udum* . *Phytopathoogy.* **38** :72.

Reddy M V, Raju TN. (1993). Pathogenic variability in pigeonpea wilt pathogen *Fusarium udum*. *Pl. Dis. Prob. in Central India*. 32-34.

Reddy, M. V., Sharma, S. B. and Nene, Y. L. (1990). Pigeonpea : Disease management. *In : The Pigeonpea (Eds. Y. L. Nene, S. D. Hall and V. K. Sheila), CAB International, Wallingford, U.K.* 303-347 pp.

Rini and Sulochana.(2007). Substrate evaluation for multiplication of *Trichoderma* spp. *Journal of Tropical. Agriculture.* **45 (1-2):** 58–60.

Sahayaraj, K., Mamasivayam, S.K.R, and Borgio, J.A.F.(2006). Influence of three plant extracts on Fusarium oxysporum f. sp. ciceris mycelia growth. *J.Plant Ptotec. Res.* **46(4):** 235-238.

Salie, F., Eagles, P.F.K. and leng, H.M.F.(1996). Preliminary antimicrobial screening of four South African Asteraceae species. *J. Ethonopharmacol.* **52:**27-33.

Sataraddi AR. (1998). Variability in *Fusarium udum* causing wilt of pigeonpea. *Ph.D Thesis. Univ. Agri. Sci., Dharwad,* 112 pp.

Satish, S., Raveesha, K.A. and Janardhana, G.R.(1999). Antibacterial activity of plant extracts on phytopathogenic Xanthomonas campestris pathovars. *Letters in Applied Microbiology.* **28:** 145-147.

Saxena RK, Saxena KB, Kumar RV, Hoisington DA, Varshney RK. (2010). Simple sequence repeat-based diversity in elite pigeonpea genotypes for developing mapping populations to map resistance to *Fusarium* wilt and sterility mosaic disease. *Plant Breed.* **129:**135-14.

Saxena, R.C., Khan, Z.R. and Bajet, N.B.(1987). Reduction of tungro virus transmission by Nephotettix virescens in neem cake treated rice seedlings. *J.Econ. Entomol.* **80 (5):** 1079-1082.

Schillhorn van Veen, T. W. (1999). Agricultural policy and sustainable livestock development. *Int. J. Parasitol.,* **29:** 7-15, ISSN: 0020-7519.

Schnabel, G., and Jones, A. L.(2001). The 14a-demethylase (CYP51A1) gene is overexpressed in *V. inaequalis* strains resistant to myclobutanil. *Phytopathology* **91**:102-110.

Sesha Kiran, K., Ligaraju, S. and Adiver, S.S.(2006). Effect of plant extracts on Slerotium rolfsii, the incitant of stem rot of groundnut. *J. Mycol. Pl. Pathol.* **36 (1):** 77-78.

Shahverdi A R, Abdolpour F, Monsef-Esfahani H R, Farsam H A.(2007). TLC bioautographic assay for the detection of nitrofurantoin resistance reversal compound. *J Chromatogr B.***850:**528–530.

Sharma TM and Singh BM.(1995b). *In vitro* microrhizome production in *Zinger officinale. Plant Cell Rep.* **15:** 274-277.

Sharma TR and Tewari JP.(1998).RAPD analysis of three Alternaira species pathogenic to crucifers. *Mycol. Res.* **102:** 807-81.

Sharma YP (2012) Wheat stem rust Ug 99- A threat to food security. *Proceedings of the 21st training on Recent Advances in Plant Disease Management, Pantnagar.* PP 171-173

Sharma, N. and Tripathi,A.(2006). Fungitoxicity of the essential oils of *Citrus sinensis* on post harvest pathogens *.Worls J.Microbiol. Biotech.* **22 (6):** 587-593.

Sharma, S.N. and Chandel, S.S.(2003). Screening of biocontrol agents *in vitro* against *Fusarium oxysporum f. sp. gladioli* and their mass multiplication on different organic substrates. *Plant Disease Reseaarch.Ludhiana.* **18:** 135-138.

Sharma, U., Thakur, P.D., Handa, A., Bhalik, A. and Gupta, D.(2007). Effect of *Centella asiatica* and *Vitex negundo* against TUMV infectiong radish. *J.Pl.Dis. Sci.* **2(1):** 22-25.

Shekhawat GS (2000) Management of potato diseases through host resistance. *J.Mycol. Pl. Pathol.* **30(2):**143-150

Shoyama Y, Tanaka H, Fukuda N.(2003). Monoclonal antibodies against naturally occurring bioactive compounds. *Cytotechnology.***31**:9–27.

Sierotzki, Helge .(2000). Mode of resistance to respiration inhibitors at the cytochrome bc1 enzyme complex of *Mycosphaerella fijiensis* field isolates *Pest Management Science* **56**:833-841

Singh (2012) Commercialization of biocontrol agents. *J. Mycol Pl. Pathol.* **42 (1):** 25

Singh , U.P. and Prithiviraj, B.(1997). Neem Azal. A product of neem , induces resistance in pea against *Erysiphe pisi. Physiological and Molecular Plant Pathology.* **51(3):** 181-194.

Singh ,N and Singh , R.S.(1983). Inhibition of *Fusarium udum* (Pigeon pea wilt) by ether distillate of margosa cake amended soil. *Indian Journal of Mycol. & Pl.Pathol.* **13(3):** 329-330.

Singh HP, Malhotra SK.(2010).Research and development in vegetables- issues and strategies. *Indian Horticulture*. PP 3-10

Singh P.K and Dwivedi, R.S.(1987). Effect of oils on *Sclerotium rolfsii* causing root rot of barle. *Indian Phytopath*. **40:** 531-533.

Sinha P, Banik S.(2009).Plant disease forecasting and monitoring: An imoerative in precision agriculture. Indian Farming. **59 (8):** 46-50.

Sinha, R.K.P. and Sinha, B.B.P.(2004). Effect of potash , botanicals and fungicides against wilt disease complex of lentil. *Annls. Pl. Protec. Sci.* **12(20:** 454-455.

Sobita Simon.(2011).Agro-based Waste Products as a Substrate for Mass Production of *Trichoderma spp. Asian Journal of Agriculture Science.***3:** 05-10.

Somasekhar N, Praseas JS, Ganguly AK.(2010). Impact of climate change on soil nematodes-implications for sustainable agriculture. *Ind. J. Nemat.* **40:** 125-134.

Somasekhara, Y.M., Natishan, B.M and Muniyappa, V.(1998).Evaluation of neem products and insecticides against west fly (*Bemesia tabaci*) a vector of tomato leaf curl Gemini virus diseases. *Neem News letter.***15 (2):** 16.

Song J, Bradeen M, Naess SK, Raasch JA , Wielgus SM, Heberlach GT, Liu J, Kuang H, Phillips Austin S, Buell CR Helgeson JP and Jiang J .(2003). Gene RB cloned from solanum bulbocastanum confers broad spectrum resistance to potato late blight Proc. *Natl Acad Sci USA*. **100:** 9128-33.

Srinivasulu, B., Doraiswamy, S., Aruna, K., Rao, D.V.R., Rabindran, R.(2002). Efficacy of biocontrol agen, chemicals and botanicals on *Ganoderma sp*., the coconut basal stem rot pathogen. *J. Planta. Crops*. **30(3):** 57-59.

Suhr, K. I. and Nielsen, P. V.(2003). Antifungal activity of essential oils evaluated by two different application techniques against rye bread spoilage fungi. *Journal of Applied Microbiology*. **94:** 665-674.

Sundaram , R.M.(1996). Biocontrol characterization of *Trichoderma harzianum* Rifai, isolate -1 and its protoplast fusion with *Trichoderma harzianum Rifai* , isolate -3. *M.Sc.Thesis G.B.Pant University of Agric. And Tech. Pantnagar*. p.91.

Sundaram RM, Manne R, Vishnupriya R, Biradar SK, Laha GS, Reddy GA, Rani NS, Sharma NP, Sonti RV. (2008) .Marker assisted introgression of bacterial blight resistance in *Samba Mahsuri* , and *elite indica* rice variety. *Euphytica*. **160 :** 411-422.

Suryawanshi, A.P., Ladkat, G.M., Dhoke, P.K., Surayawanshi , S.D. and Pensalwar, S.N. .(2007).Evaluation of some plant extracts against *Sclerotium rolfss* on pigeonpea. *J.Pl. Sis. Sci*. **2(1):** 32-33.

Singer, M. and Berg, P. 1991. Genes and Genomes, University Science Books, Mill Valley, California and Blackwell Science Publishers.

Singh, B.D. (1998).*Biotechnology, Kalyani publishers, New Delhi*

Slater, A., Scott, N. and Fowler, M. (2003). *Plant Biotechnology: The Genetic Manipulations of Plants, Oxford University Press.*

Street, H. E. (1977).*Plant Cell and Tissue Culture, Blackwell, London.*

Thorpe T (2007). History of plant tissue culture. *J. Mol. Microbial Biotechnol.* **37:** 169-180.

Tai TH, Dahlbeck D, Eszter TC, Paresh G, Romela P, Maureen C, Whalen RE, Stall RE & Staskawicz.(1999).Expression of the Bs2 pepper gene confers resistance to bacterial spot disease in tomato. *Proc. Natl. Acad. Sci. USA*. **96:** 14153-14158.

Tewari , A.K.(1996). Biological control of chickpea wilt complex using differential formulation of Gliocladium virens through seed treatment. *Ph.D Thesis, G.B. Pant University of Agric. & Tech. Pantnagar, India.*167.

Thakur RP .(1999). Pathogen diversity and plant disease management. *Indian Phytopath*. **55 (1)**:1-9

Thind T.S(2012).Fungicides in crop health security-the road ahead *Indan Phytopath* .**65(2):** 109-115.

Thind, T.S., Singh, P.P., Sokhi and Grewal, R.K.(1991). Application timing and choice of fungicides for the control of downey mildew of muskmelon. *Pl. Dis. Res*. **6:** 49-53.

Threshs, J.M. Temporal patterns of virus spread. *Ann. Rev. Phytopathol*.**12:** 111-128.

Tiwari, A. K., Kumar, K., Razdan, V. K. and Rathor, T. R.(2004).Mass production of *Trichoderma viride* on indigenous substrates. *Annals of Plant Protection Sciences*.**12:** 71-74.

Tripathi, P., Dubey , N.K., Banerji, R, and Chansouria, J.P.N., 2004. Evaluation of some essential oils as botanical fungitoxicvants in management of post harvest rotting of citrus fruits. *World J. Microbiol. Biotech*.**20 (3):** 317-21.

Tripathi, R.K.R. and Tripathi, R.N.(1982). Reduction in bean common mosaic virus (BCMV) infectivity vis-a vis crude leaf extracts of some higher plants. *Experimentia* .**38 (3):** 349.

Tsao R, Deng Z.(2004). Separation procedures for naturally occurring antioxidant phytochemicals. *J Chromatogr B*. **812:** 85–99.

Tygi, S.A. and Alam M.M.(1995). Efficacy of oil seed cakes against plant parasitic nematodes and soil inhabiting fungi on mungbean and chickpea. *Bioresource Technology*. **51:** 233-239.

Upadhyay,J. P ., Lal, H.C.and Roy, S.(2004). Effect of fungicides , cakes and plant byproducts on the development of *Trichoderma viride* . *Journal of Mycology and Plant Pathology* **34:** 313.

Upadhyay., J. P. and Mukhopadhyay, A. N.(1986). Biological control of *Sclerotium rolfsii* by *Trichoderma harzianum* in sugarbeet.*Tropical pest Management*. **32:** 215-220.

Ushamalini, C., Rajappan,K. and Gangadhran , K., 1997. Suppression of charcoal rot and wilt pathogens of cowpea by botanicals. *Plant Disease Research*. **12(2):** 113-117.

Varma, J. and Dubey, N. K. 1999. Perspective of botanical and microbial products as pesticides of tomorrow. *Current Science*. **76:** 172-179.

Verma S. and Dohroo, N.P.(2003). Evaluation of botanicals *in vitro* against *Fusarium oxysporum f. sp. pisi* causing wilt of pea. *Plant Dis. Res*. **18(2):** 131-134.

Vidhyasekaran, P.(1992). *Principles of Plant Pathology. CBS Printers and Publishers, New Delhi.*

Vishunavat K .(2012). Advancement of seed health testing techniques for better disease management. *Proceedings of the 21st training on Recent Advances in Plant Disease Management, Pantnagar*. PP. 87-91.

Wani SH, Sanghera GS, Singh NB (2013). Biotechnology and plant disease control-Role of RNA interference. *Amer. J.Pl.Sci*.**1:**55-68.

Waugh MM, Kim DH, Ferrin DM and Stanghellini ME.(2003). Reproductive potential of *Monosporascus cannonballus*. *Plant Dis*. **87:** 45-50.

Yadav, V.K. and Thirmurty, V.S.(2006). Fungitoxicity of some medicinal plant extracts against Sarocladium sryze causing sheath rot of rice. *Indin J.Plant pathology*. **24 (1&2) :** 93-96.

Yamada, T., Hiramotoa, T., Tobimatsu, T., Shiraishi, T. and Oku. H.(1990). Elicitor like substances present in barley and wheat seeds. *J.Phytopathology*. **128:** 89-98.

Yokoyama, K., Aist, J.R. and Bayles, C.J., 1991:Plant growth regulating extract that induced resistance to barley powdery mildew. *Physiol. And Mol. Pl. Pathol*. **35:** 166-175.

Young, H.C., Prescott, J.M. and Saari, E.E.(1978). Role of disease monitoring in pre epidemics. *Ann. Rev. Phytopathol.* **16:** 263-285.

Zwiers, L. H. *et al.* (2003). ABC transporters of the wheat pathogen *Mycosphaerella graminicola* function as protectants against biotic and xenobiotic toxic compounds *Molecular Genetics and Genomics.* **269**: 499-507.

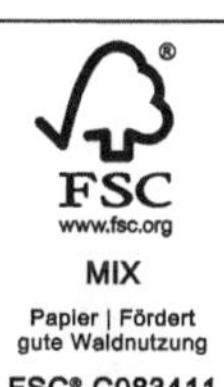

Zeitfracht Medien GmbH
Ferdinand-Jühlke-Straße 7
99095 Erfurt, Deutschland
produktsicherheit@kolibri360.de